Assessment Scales in Old Age Psychiatry

Second Edition

Alistair Burns MD FRCP FRCPsych

Head, School of Psychiatry & Behavioural Sciences
Professor of Old Age Psychiatry
University of Manchester, Wythenshawe Hospital
Manchester, UK

Brian Lawlor MD FRCPI FRCPsych

Consultant Psychiatrist
Department of Psychiatry of the Elderly
Jonathan Swift Clinic, St James's Hospital
Dublin, Ireland

Sarah Craig MB MSc MRCPsych

Consultant in Old Age Psychiatry
The Royal Bolton Hospitals NHS Trust
Bolton, UK

With a contribution by

Robert Coen PhD

Mercer's Institute for Research on Aging
St James's Hospital
Dublin, Ireland

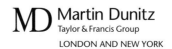 **Martin Dunitz**
Taylor & Francis Group
LONDON AND NEW YORK

© 1999, 2004 Martin Dunitz, an imprint of the Taylor & Francis Group plc

First published in the United Kingdom in 1999
by Martin Dunitz, an imprint of the Taylor & Francis Group plc,
11 New Fetter Lane, London EC4P 4EE

Tel.: +44 (0) 20 7583 9855
Fax.: +44 (0) 20 7842 2298
E-mail: info@dunitz.co.uk
Website:, http://www.dunitz.co.uk

Second edition 2004

A CIP record for this book is available from the British Library.

ISBN 1 84184 168 4

Distributed in the USA by
Fulfilment Center
Taylor & Francis
10650 Toebben Drive
Independence, KY 41051, USA
Toll Free Tel. +1 800 634 7064
E-mail: taylorandfrancis@thomsonlearning.com

Distributed in Canada by
Taylor & Francis
74 Rolark Drive
Scarborough, Ontario M1R 4G2, Canada
Toll Free Tel.: +1 877 226 2237
E-mail: tal_fran@istar.ca

Distributed in the rest of the world by
Thomson Publishing Services
Cheriton House
North Way
Andover, Hampshire SP10 5BE, UK
Tel.: +44 (0)1264 332424
E-mail: salesorder.tandf@thomsonpublishingservices.co.uk

Composition by Scribe Design, Gillingham, Kent, UK
Printed and bound in Italy

Contents

Foreword by *Idris Williams*   xi

Preface   xiii

Introduction   xv

1 DEPRESSION   1
Geriatric Depression Scale (GDS)   2
Geriatric Depression Scale (Residential)   4
A Collateral Source Version of the Geriatric Depression Rating Scale   5
Hamilton Depression Rating Scale   6
Beck Depression Inventory (BDI)   7
Montgomery and Åsberg Depression Rating Scale (MADRS)   8
Cornell Scale for Depression in Dementia   9
Brief Assessment Schedule Depression Cards (BASDEC)   10
SELFCARE (D)   11
Center for Epidemiological Studies - Depression Scale (CES-D)   13
OARS Depressive Scale (ODS)   14
Depressive Signs Scale (DSS)   15
Carroll Rating Scale (CRS)   16
Mood Scales – Elderly (MS–E)   18
Mania Rating Scale   19
Checklist Differentiating pseudodementia from dementia   21
NIMH Dementia Mood Assessment Scale (DMAS)   23
Emotionalism and Mood Disorders after Stroke   26
EURO-D scale   28
Brief Assessment Scale for Depression   29
The Even Briefer Assessment Scale for Depression (EBAS-DEP)   31
Short Anxiety Screening Test   32

2 DEMENTIA   33

2a COGNITIVE ASSESSMENT   35
Mini-Mental State Examination (MMSE)   36
The Severe MMSE   38
Standardized Mini-Mental State Examination (SMMSE)   40
The Modified MMSE (3MS) Examination   42
Mental Test Score (MTS)/Abbreviated Mental Test Score (AMTS)   44
Blessed Dementia Scale   46
ADAS/ADAS-Cog, ADAS-Non-Cog   48
Mattis Dementia Rating Scale (DRS)   50
Clock Drawing Test   51

The Ten-Point Clock Test   55
Clifton Assessment Procedures for the Elderly (CAPE)   56
The Mini-Cog   60
Brief Cognitive Rating Scale (BCRS)   61
Cambridge Neuropsychological Test Automated Battery (CANTAB)   63
Short Portable Mental Status Questionnaire (SPMSQ)   64
SET Test   66
Short Mental Status Questionnaire   67
Short Orientation–Memory–Concentration Test   68
Syndrom Kurztest (SKT)   69
Cognitive Abilities Screening Instrument (CASI)   70
Cognitive Drug Research Assessment System (COGDRAS)   71
Kew Cognitive Test   73
Severe Impairment Battery (SIB)   74
Mental Status Questionnaire (MSQ)/Face–Hand Test (FHT)   75
Cognitive Capacity Screening Examination   76
7-Minute Neurocognitive Screening Battery   77
Revised Hasegawa's Dementia Scale (HDS-R)   78
The Time and Change Test   79
Memory Impairment Screen   80
Structured Telephone Interview for Dementia (STIDA)   81
Détérioration de Cognition Observée (DECO)   83
Objective Assessment of Praxis   84
Lay Person-Based Screening for Early Detection of AD   85
The Telephone Interview for Cognitive Status   86
Observation List for Early Signs of Dementia (OLD)   88
Early Signs of Dementia Checklist   89
A Cognitive Screening Battery for Dementia in the Elderly   90
Test Battery for the Diagnosis of Dementia in Individuals with Intellectual Disability   91
The Test for Severe Impairment (TSI)   92
The Frontal Behavioral Inventory   93
The General Practitioner Assessment of Cognition (GPCOG)   95
Computerized Cognitive Examination of the Elderly (ECO)   97
The Neuropsychological Impairment Scale – Senior (NIS–S)   98
Short and Sweet Screening Instrument (SAS-SI)   100
Middlesex Elderly Assessment of Mental State (MEAMS)   101
The Executive Interview   102
Short Cognitive/Neuropsychologic Test Battery for First-Tier Fitness-to-Drive
    Assessment of Older Adults   103

Neuropsychological Tests   **104**
Buschke Selective Reminding Test   106
Rey Auditory Verbal Learning Test   107
Rey Osterrieth Complex Figure   108
Trail Making Test   109
Wechsler Adult Intelligence Scale (WAIS-III)   110
Wechsler Memory Scale (WMS-III)   111
Wisconsin Card Sorting Test (WCST)   112
National Adult Reading Test (NART)   113
Verbal Fluency: FAS Test/Category Fluency   114

Stroop Colour–Word Test   115
Boston Naming Test   116
Stepwise Comparative Status Analysis (STEP)   117

2b NEUROPSYCHIATRIC ASSESSMENTS   **123**
Personality Inventory   124
BEHAVE-AD   125
Neuropsychiatric Inventory (NPI)   128
Neuropsychiatric Inventory with Caregiver Distress Scale   129
Columbia University Scale for Psychopathology in AD (CUSPAD)   130
Manchester and Oxford Universities Scale for the Psychopathological Assessment
   of Dementia (MOUSEPAD)   133
Present Behavioural Examination (PBE)   137
CERAD Behavioural Rating Scale   138
Rating Scale for Aggressive Behaviour in the Elderly (RAGE)   142
Overt Aggression Scale (OAS)   144
Neurobehavioural Rating Scale (NRS)   146
Caretaker Obstreperous Behaviour Rating Assessment (COBRA) scale   148
Nurses' Observation Scale for Inpatient Evaluation (NOSIE)   150
Disruptive Behavior Rating Scales (DBRS)   152
Ryden Aggression Scale   154
Agitated Behavior Mapping Instrument (ABMI)   157
Brief Agitation Rating Scale (BARS)   158
Cohen-Mansfield Agitation Inventory (CMAI) – Long Form   159
Observed Agitation in Patients with DAT (SOAPD)   160
Dementia Behavior Disturbance Scale   162
Pittsburgh Agitation Scale (PAS)   163
Dysfunctional Behaviour Rating Instrument (DBRI)   165
Irritability, Aggression and Apathy Scale   166
Apathy Scale for Parkinson's Disease   168
BEAM-D   169
Clinical Rating Scale for Symptoms of Psychosis in AD (SPAD)   171
Georagsobber Vatieschaal voor de Intramurale Psychogeriatrie (GIP)   173
Nursing Home Behavior Problem Scale (NHBPS)   174
The California Dementia Behavior Questionnaire Caregiver and Clinical Assessment
   of Behavioral Disturbance   175
Harmful Behaviours Scale   176
The Challenging Behaviour Scale (CBS)   177
Behavioural Activities in Demented Geriatric Patients   178
Behavior Rating Scale for Dementia (BRSD)   179
Resistiveness to Care Scale (RTC-DAT)   181
The Agitated Behavior in Dementia Scale   182
Rating Anxiety in Dementia (RAID)   183

2c ACTIVITIES OF DAILY LIVING   **185**
Instrumental Activities of Daily Living Scale (IADL)   186
Interview for Deterioration in Daily Living Activities in Dementia (IDDD)   188
Barthel Index   190
Progressive Deterioration Scale (PDS)   191

Functional Activities Questionnaire (FAQ)   192
Daily Activities Questionnaire (DAQ)   194
Bristol Activities of Daily Living Scale   195
Direct Assessment of Functional Status (DAFS)   197
Activities of Daily Living (ADL) Index   199
Cleveland Scale for ADL (CSADL)   200
Cognitive Performance Test   201
Present Functioning Questionnaire (PFQ) and Functional Rating Scale (FRS)   202
Dressing Performance Scale   205
Rapid Disability Rating Scale – 2 (RDRS–2)   207
Functional Dementia Scale (FDS)   209
Performance Test of Activities of Daily Living (PADL)   210
Structured Assessment of Independent Living Skills (SALES)   212
Direct Assessment of ADL in AD   215
Refined ADL Assessment Scale (RADL)   216
Bayer Activities of Daily Living Scale (B-ADL)   218
The Disability Assessment for Dementia (DAD)   219
The Alzheimer's Disease Functional Assessment and Change Scale (ADFACS)   220
Physical Self-Maintenance Scale and Instrumental Activities of Daily Living (IADL)   221
Dependence Scale   222
The Alzheimer's Disease ADL International Scale (ADL-IS)   223

2d GLOBAL ASSESSMENTS/QUALITY OF LIFE   **225**
The Texas Functional Living Scale   227
EuroQol   228
Quality of Life in Dementia   229
Lancashire QoL Profile (Residential)   230
QoL in AD: Patient and Caregiver Report (QOL-AD)   232
Functional Assessment Staging (FAST)   235
Global Deterioration Scale (GDS)   236
Clinical Dementia Rating (CDR)   238
Clinicians' Global Impression of Change   240
Crichton Royal Behavioural Rating Scale (CRBRS)   241
Psychogeriatric Dependency Rating Scales (PGDRS)   243
Dementia Rating Scale   245
GBS Scale   246
Geriatric Rating Scale (GRS)   247
PAMIE Scale   248
Stockton Geriatric Rating Scale   250
Hierarchic Dementia Scale   251
Sandoz Clinical Assessment – Geriatric (SCAG)   253
Comprehensive Psychopathological Rating Scale (CPRS)   255
Validity and Reliability of the Alzheimer's Disease Co-operative Study – Clinical, Global
   Impression of Changes (ADCS-CGIC)   256
Echelle Comportement et Adaptation (ECA) Scale   257
CarenapD   258
The FSAB Battery   259
Milan Overall Dementia Assessment   260
Cognitively Impaired Life Quality Scale (CILQ)   262
Quality of Life Assessment Schedule (QOLAS)   263

The Dementia Quality of Life Instrument 264
An Instrument for Assessing Health-Related QoL in Persons with AD (ADRQL) 265
Cornell–Brown Scale for QoL in Dementia 266
The Bedford Alzheimer Nursing Severity Scale for the Severely Demented 267
Quality of Well-Being Scale 268
Community Screening Instrument for Dementia (CSI-D) 269

3 GLOBAL MENTAL HEALTH ASSESSMENTS 271
Brief Psychiatric Rating Scale (BPRS) 272
Relative's Assessment of Global Symptomatology (RAGS) 274
Structured Interview for the Diagnosis of the Alzheimer's Type and Multi-infarct
    Dementia and Dementias of other Aetiology (SIDAM) 275
Global Assessment of Psychiatric Symptoms (GAPS) 276
The Core Assessment and Outcomes Package for Older People 277
Psychogeriatric Assessment Scales (PAS) 278
Geriatric Mental State Schedule (GMSS) 279
Canberra Interview for the Elderly (CIE) 280
Survey Psychiatric Assessment Schedule (SPAS) 281
Multidimensional Observation Scale for Elderly Subjects (MOSES) 284
Cambridge Mental Disorders of the Elderly Examination (CAMDEX) 286
Nurses' Observation Scale for Geriatric Patients (NOSGER) 288
Comprehensive Assessment and Referral Evaluation (CARE) 290
The Philadelphia Geriatric Center Multilevel Assessment Instrument 292
PRIME-MD 293
Camberwell Assessment of Need for the Elderly (CANE) 294
Easycare: Elderly Assessment System 295
The MOS 36-Item Short-Form Health Survey (SF-36) 296
Health of the Nation Outcome Scales for Older People (HoNOS 65+) 297

4 PHYSICAL EXAMINATION 299
Cambridge Neurological Inventory 301
Webster Scale 302
Tardive Dyskinesia Rating Scale (TDRS) 304
Neurological Evaluation Scale (NES) 305
Quantification of Physical Illness in Psychiatric Research in the Elderly 306
London Handicap Scale 307
General Medical Health Rating (GMHR) 309
Simpson–Angus Scale (SAS) 310
Barnes Akathisia Rating Scale (BAS, BARS) 311

5 DELIRIUM 313
Delirium Symptom Interview (DSI) 314
Confusion Assessment Method (CAM) 315
Delirium Rating Scale (DRS) 317
The Delirium Index (DI) 319

6 CAREGIVER ASSESSMENTS 321
Problem Checklist and Strain Scale 322
Ways of Coping Checklist: Revision and Psychometric Properties 324
Screen for Caregiver Burden (SCB) 326

Burden Interview   327
Caregiving Hassles Scale   328
Marital Intimacy Scale   330
Revised Memory and Behavior Problems Checklist   332
Caregiver Activity Survey (CAS)   333
General Health Questionnaire (GHQ)   334
TRIMS Behavioral Problem Checklist (BPC)   336
Geriatric Evaluation by Relative's Rating Instrument (GERRI)   337
Zung Self-Rating Depression Scale   339
Behavioural and Mood Disturbance Scale (BMDS)   340
The Pleasant Events Schedule – AD   341
Caregiver Time Use   343
Multidimensional Caregiver Burden Inventory   344

7 MEMORY FUNCTIONING   **345**
Cognitive Failures Questionnaire (CFQ)   346
Informant Questionnaire on Cognitive Decline in the Elderly (IQCODE)   348
Metamemory in Adulthood (MIA) Questionnaire   350
Memory Functioning Questionnaire (MFQ)   351
The Knowledge of Memory Aging Questionnaire   352

8 OTHER SCALES   **355**
Multiphasic Environmental Assessment Procedure (MEAP)   356
Philadelphia Geriatric Center Morale Scale   357
Cumulative Illness Rating Scale (CIRS)   359
Measurement of Morale in the Elderly   360
Retrospective Postmortem Dementia Assessment (RCD-1)   364
Quality of Interactions Schedule (QUIS)   365
INSIGHT   366
Ischaemic Score   367
The CAGE Questionnaire   368
MAST-G   369
AUDIT   370
Mini Nutritional Assessment   371
The Resource Utilization in Dementia (RUD) Instrument   372
The Alzheimer's Disease Knowledge Test   373

APPENDIX
What to use and when   377

ALPHABETIC LIST OF SCALES   **381**

Foreword

It is a pleasure to write the Foreword to the second edition of this book. I am told that the first edition has been very successful and this does not surprise me. In the piece I wrote five years ago I described many of the reasons why I thought success would be achieved; most, indeed I would say all of these, still stand.

It is in the nature of a compilation that it will expand. All the scales that were in the first edition are included in this one. A sizable number of new ones have been added, including a new section covering neuropsychological tests. This subject is complex, and I thought the authors' introduction was very helpful in clarifying the purpose of such assessments.

The added 'new' scales are not necessarily new chronologically but their inclusion adds to the range of choice. The result again enhances the comprehensiveness of the publication and also its international scope. There is a skill in relating scales to local culture and also to their employment in a general or specialist way. The commentaries included in each scale are very helpful in gaining an understanding of their usage.

Practice continues to change. In the UK over the past five years care of older people has become more focused; this has been facilitated by a series of National Service Frameworks. A result is to widen the range of professional workers who are involved in the assessment process. The introduction of a single assessment programme has meant health and social workers collaborating closely together in the care of older people with mental health problems. The scales included in the sections on Activities of Daily Living and Care Givers are relevant to this.

Finally what I said in the Foreword to the first edition about the importance of accurate diagnosis, proper treatment/ management and monitoring of outcomes still applies. This is the purpose of the scales in this book and because of this it is very welcome. I must congratulate the authors for maintaining the high standards of presentation and sensible comment.

Idris Williams OBE
Chairman
Morecambe Bay Hospitals NHS Trust
Emeritus Professor of General Practice
University of Nottingham

Preface

We were as surprised as anyone about the success of the first edition of *Assessment Scales in Old Age Psychiatry*. Sales have been strong but, more importantly for us, we know through personal contacts and through reviews that the book is widely used and, in some ways, widely appreciated. We hope that there is sufficient information attached to each scale to allow its use, at least at a superficial level, without recourse to the original article. However, we must emphasise again the issue of copyright, and this is particularly well illustrated with the Mini Mental State Examination where we are now unable to reproduce it in full.

The stimulus for a second edition arose out of what usually happens. We felt that the book needed to retain a freshness, although as most of the material we present is retrospective, the issue of keeping up to date is not as important as with other publications. We hope that we have included some more of the scales which have been written, or at least information on scales which have matured since the first edition. However, a critical reviewer will spot that probably the majority of the additional scales could well have been included in the first edition.

Apart from an increase in the bulk of the text, we hope we have made some improvements. We are indebted to Robert Coen, who has contributed an excellent section on more detailed neuropsychological tests. While these remain the perview of an experienced neuropsychologist, and have to be interpreted in the light of a skilled clinical assessment, we felt that their inclusion for the general reader might be of some interest and help. We hope the referencing section makes the scales easier to find. The layout has been altered slightly.

We would like to thank those authors who have provided additional information about their scales and to those who have reminded us that theirs were not included in the first edition. We are grateful for the continuing support of our publishers, Martin Dunitz, in the guise of Clive Lawson and Pete Stevenson. We are grateful again to Idris Williams for writing a generous preface. Most of all, we are indebted to Barbara Dignan, who has done all the hard work and without whom this book would not have appeared at all.

AB, BL, SC

Introduction

There were several aims behind producing this compendium of scales. The first was simply to bring together in one volume as many scales as was practical for ease of reference. Other publications have expertly summarized smaller numbers of scales, but not since the book by Israel et al of 1984,[1] and the *Psychopharmacology Bulletin* supplement of 1988 (Vol. 24, no. 4), has there been an attempt to synthesize the whole field. Also, a great number of scales have been published in the last decade and a half, and an update seemed appropriate. Presenting them in an ordered form with information about the completion of the instrument would be convenient and allow the reader to see at a glance the scope of the scale and its application. The compendium may also act as a reference guide and allow readers to interpret the use of scales they may read about in journal articles. We have concentrated on scales available in the English language literature and on those which can be completed relatively easily. We have not, therefore, attempted to include detailed neuropsychological tests, which are the remit of specialist neuropsychology. The scales are approximately in the order of their annualized citation index.

The second aim was to provide the reader with a document allowing them to pick whichever scale was appropriate to the question being asked. Care protocols and clinical guidelines with an emphasis on outcomes are now commonly adopted in clinical practice, and it is important for clinicians to be aware of ways in which performance can be measured. Formal documentation of clinical variables allows individual patients (and thereby a service) to be evaluated. This must obviously be carried out carefully using valid and appropriate instruments, and should be led by clinicians of any discipline (ideally the process should be multidisciplinary). Awareness of the range of measures available is essential to this process. We have therefore included in each chapter a short summary of the main scales which, from reading the literature and from knowledge of the field, we feel would be the most appropriate for the researcher, hospital specialist or general practitioner. A caveat is that the best scale depends on the question being asked and not the clinical discipline of the inquirer. The characteristics of an ideal scale can easily be summarized in terms of reliability (test retest, inter-rater) and validity (content, face and construct validity). However, in practice, this can seldom be interpreted with clarity – it is comparatively easy to document reliability in any clinically based scale, and validity can usually be demonstrated by comparison with an existing instrument, especially if the two are similar. Clever statistical manipulation can prove most things (or at least cannot disprove them). Information enabling one to recommend the ideal scale (in terms of psychometric characteristics, ease of administration and predictive in terms of outcomes) is simply not available. We would have liked to present a standardized account of each scale, with reliability, validity, cut-off points, sensitivity and specificity measurements, drawbacks, advantages and disadvantages, but this information is simply not available. To have confined ourselves to scales which provide that level of detail would have resulted in a very different book. We have preferred to be inclusive (we will be accused of being overinclusive) and allow the reader to make up his or her own mind. There are now more scales than there are measurable facets of illness, and so duplication is inevitable. For instance, there are only a limited number of ways in which to test for disorientation in time by direct questioning (i.e. what time, date, year, day and season is it?). Variations occur in terms of the individual characteristics of a scale such as adaptation to a particular environment (e.g. a scale specifically for nursing homes) or brevity (reductionism facilitates ease of administration).

The third aim was to inform anyone considering constructing a scale of the large number available and that referring back to a previous scale, perhaps with modification, would be more cost-effective than starting from scratch.

The fourth, and most indulgent, aim was to put together a collection of scales, many of which have been used only occasionally but which form a body of work supporting the concept of accurate, reliable and valid measurement of signs and symptoms of disease in older people. Some of these are only of historical interest and have not stood the test of time, but many have been adapted to inform the development of later, more commonly used scales.

---

[1]Israel L, Kozarevic D, Sartorius N (1984) *Source book of geriatric assessment* Vols I & II. Basel: S Karger AG.

Chapter 1

Depression

Depression can mean either a mild feeling of lowered mood which is transient and may reflect an individual response to life circumstances or a major illness with biological features (e.g. weight loss, diurnal variation in mood, sleep disturbance). It also covers anything in between. Scales which measure depressed mood do so at a symptomatic level with the general assumption that there is a linear relationship between the score and the severity of the illness. Particular difficulties with the measurement of depression unique to older people include the tendency of older people to deny feelings of depression, the atypical presentation of depression (more somatic complaints) and the coexistence of depression and cognitive impairment. The symptoms of depression, however, are sufficiently commonly recognized that there is general agreement about what should be asked. Some questions have to be addressed carefully – many a centenarian has roared with laughter when asked by a nervous interviewer what they feel about the future. In practice, this demonstrates a valuable point of amending what is said to the situation: asking that question to a younger person conjures up thoughts of months and perhaps years in the future; in a centenarian, the time scale should be adapted, at least when trying to elucidate depression, to the next day or so. DSM IV criteria for major depressive illness include five or more of the following symptoms, present during the same two-week period and representing a change from previous function:

- Depressed mood most of the day, nearly every day;
- Markedly diminished interest or pleasure in all, or almost all activities;
- Significant weight loss, or decrease or increase in appetite nearly every day;
- Insomnia or hypersomnia;
- Psychomotor agitation or retardation;
- Fatigue or loss of energy;
- Feelings of worthlessness or excessive or inappropriate guilt;
- Diminished ability to think or concentrate, or indecisiveness;
- Recurrent thoughts of death, suicidal ideation with or without a plan.

Scales can be self reports, interviews by trained or non-trained staff and informant-based measures. The Hamilton Depression Rating Scale (page 6) is probably the gold standard of depression scales and in general psychiatry probably has yet to be beaten. It is often used in studies of older people to act as an anchor by which to measure new instruments, although it was not designated for use with elderly people. This is because the psychometric properties have not been well established for that age group and some of the questions are not really appropriate for older people. For example, it has a number of questions relating to somatic symptoms and therefore depression in the elderly may be overdiagnosed. Another disadvantage is that it is based on a skilled interview procedure by a competent clinician. The Montgomery and Åsberg Depression Rating Scale (MADRS; page 8) taps ten domains of depression and has been used in a number of drug studies, having been shown to be sensitive to change. It can be used by any trained interviewer. The Geriatric Depression Scale (GDS; page 2) is essentially a self-reported inventory with a simple yes/no format which lends itself to ease

of administration by the older person or by an interviewer. It is the most widely used in old age psychiatry and has several versions, going from a 30-item to a 15-item (the most commonly used) to a 4-item test. Self-report questionnaires like the Beck Depression Inventory (BDI; page 7) have been used with older people, and contain a severity rating and a suicide item. The SELFCARE (D) (page 11) is adapted from a larger rating scale and has been used in general practice, as has the Center for Epidemiological Studies – Depression Scale (CES-D; page 13), which has been validated in epidemiological samples. The Mood Scales – Elderly (MS-E; page 18) and the Carroll Rating Scale (CRS; page 16) are more lengthy interviews and could not be used for screening (the latter has not been used specifically in elderly people but is validated against the dexamethasone depression test). The OARS Depressive Scale (ODS; page 14) can be used by trained interviewers where a diagnosis of depression against DSM criteria is required.

Depression in special settings

In medical inpatients, the necessity of interviewing in a noisy atmosphere makes a sensitive and private interview problematic. This led to the development of the Brief Assessment Schedule Depression Cards (BASDEC; page 10), adapted by using a set of cards which the patient simply puts into piles (true/false or don't know). The CRS is essentially a self-rated version of the Hamilton Depression Rating Scale with many of the advantages. It has been used in neuroendocrine studies with the dexamethasone test, but data relating to its use in the elderly are lacking.

The assessment of depression in dementia is an important clinical issue, and a number of scales reflect this. The special circumstances of interviewing a patient with cognitive impairment have been addressed in scale design, particularly emphasizing the need for direct observation of the patient and the difficulties of an informant answering on behalf of the patient. The elucidation of depressive symptomatology in patients with severe cognitive impairment is problematic. There is some evidence that there are two situations where depression occurs in dementia. In the early stages there is a reactive, almost understandable, reaction to loss of cognitive powers and fears for the future, whereas in the later stages the depression is more related to biological changes in the disease. The level of cognitive loss below which the communication of complex depressive ideation cannot be expressed by the patient (or captured by the interviewer) is not known (although guessed at by many), but there is general agreement that as the severity of dementia increases, determination of depressive symptoms direct from the patient becomes less reliable and proxy measures become necessary. The Cornell Scale for Depression in Dementia (page 9) set the standard for assessment in this area. Other scales (e.g. the Hamilton Depression Rating Scale) can be used if adapted appropriately for the clinical situation. Care must be taken in these circumstances to ensure that phenomena are assessed accurately, perhaps by checking with an informant after the examination rather than having them interrupt during an interview (Schneider, personal communication). The Depressive Signs Scale (DSS; page 15) has been less used in the rating of depressive symptoms, but has been validated against the dexamethasone suppression test.

Geriatric Depression Scale (GDS)

Reference: **Yesavage JA, Brink TL, Rose TL, Lum O, Huang V, Adey M, Leirer O (1983)
Development and validation of a geriatric depression screening scale: a preliminary report.**
Journal of Psychiatric Research 17: 37–49

Time taken 5–10 minutes (reviewer's estimate)

Rating self-administered

Main indications

To rate depression in elderly people, the emphasis being on a scale that was simple to administer and did not require the skills of a trained interviewer.

Commentary

The Geriatric Depression Scale (GDS) was devised by gathering 100 questions relating to depression in older people, then selecting the 30 which correlated best with the total score. Each question has a yes/no answer, with the scoring dependent on the answer given. Some 100 subjects took part in the validation study, using the Hamilton Depression Rating Scale (page 6) and the Zung Self-Rating Depression Scale (page 339). Internal consistency was assessed in four ways and found to be higher for the GDS than for the other two scales. Test/retest reliability was assessed by 20 subjects completing the questionnaire twice, one week apart, with a correlation of 0.85. The GDS correlated well with the number of research diagnostic criteria symptoms for depression. Sensitivity and specificity of the GDS had been shown in a previous study (Brink et al, 1982), and a cut-off of 11 had an 84% sensitivity and 95% specificity rate whereas a cut-off of 14 decreased the sensitivity rate to 80% but increased the specificity rate to 100%.

A 15-item version of the GDS has been described by Shiekh and Yesavage (1986). This has a cut-off of between 6 and 7 and correlates significantly with the parent scale. Logistic regression analysis has been used to derive a four-point item of the GDS with specificity of up to 88% with a cut-off of 1/2 and sensitivity of 93% with a cut-off of 0/1 (Katona, 1994). Shah et al (1997) have reported that both the 4- and 10-item versions can be used for screening successfully. The GDS has also been used to assess depression in dementia of the Alzheimer type, the results suggesting it does not maintain validity in that population (Burke et al, 1989).

Additional references

Brink T, Yesavage J, Lum O et al (1982) Screening tests for geriatric depression. *Clinical Gerontologist* 1: 37–43.

Burke WJ, Houston MJ, Boust SJ et al (1989) Use of the Geriatric Depression Scale in dementia of the Alzheimer type. *Journal of the American Geriatrics Society* 37: 856–60.

Katona C (1994) *Depression in old age.* Chichester: John Wiley & Sons.

Shah A, Herbert R, Lewis S et al (1997) Screening for depression among acutely ill geriatric inpatients with a short geriatric depression scale. *Age and Ageing* 26: 217–21.

Shiekh J, Yesavage J (1986) Geriatric Depression Scale; recent findings and development of a short version. In Brink T, ed. *Clinical gerontology: a guide to assessment and intervention.* New York: Howarth Press.

Address for correspondence

JA Yesavage
Department of Psychiatry and Behavioral Sciences
Stanford University Medical Center
Stanford
CA 94395
USA
www.stanford.edu/~yesavage/GDS.html

Geriatric Depression Scale (GDS)

Choose the best answer for how you felt the past week

1. Are you basically satisfied with your life?
2. Have you dropped many of your activities and interests?
3. Do you feel that your life is empty?
4. Do you often get bored?
5. Are you hopeful about the future?
6. Are you bothered by thoughts you can't get out of your head?
7. Are you in good spirits most of the time?
8. Are you afraid that something bad is going to happen to you?
9. Do you feel happy most of the time?
10. Do you often feel helpless?
11. Do you often get restless and fidgety?
12. Do you prefer to stay at home, rather than going out and doing new things?
13. Do you frequently worry about the future?
14. Do you feel you have more problems with memory than most?
15. Do you think it is wonderful to be alive now?
16. Do you often feel downhearted and blue?
17. Do you feel pretty worthless the way you are now?
18. Do you worry a lot about the past?
19. Do you find life very exciting?
20. Is it hard for you to get started on new projects?
21. Do you feel full of energy?
22. Do you feel that your situation is hopeless?
23. Do you think that most people are better off than you are?
24. Do you frequently get upset over little things?
25. Do you frequently feel like crying?
26. Do you have trouble concentrating?
27. Do you enjoy getting up in the morning?
28. Do you prefer to avoid social gatherings?
29. Is it easy for you to make decisions?
30. Is your mind as clear as it used to be?

Code answers as Yes or No

Score 1 for Yes on: 2–4,6,8,10–14,16–18,20,22–26,28
Score 1 for No on: 1,5,7,9,15,19,21,27,29,30

0–10 = Not depressed
11–20 = Mild depression
21–30 = Severe depression
GDS 15: 1,2,3,4,7,8,9,10,12,14,15,17,21,22,23 (cut-off of 5/6 indicates depression)
GDS 10: 1,2,3,8,9,10,14,21,22,23
GDS 4: 1,3,8,9 (cut-off of 1/2 indicates depression)

Reprinted from *Journal of Psychiatric Research*, Vol. 17, Yesavage JA, Brink TL, Rose TL, Lum O, Huang V, Adey M, Leirer O, Development and validation of a geriatric depression scale: a preliminary report, 1983, with permission from Elsevier Science.

Geriatric Depression Scale (Residential)

Reference: **Sutcliffe C, Cordingley L, Burns A, Godlove-Mozley C, Bagley C, Huxley P, Challis D (2000) A new version of the Geriatric Depression Scale for Nursing and Residential Home Populations: The Geriatric Depression Scale (Residential) (GDS-12R).** *International Psychogeriatrics* 12: 173–81

Time taken 5–10 minutes

Main indications

To measure depression in nursing home residents.

Commentary

A study in nursing in residential homes has suggested that a 12-item Geriatric Depression Scale was more suitable for people living in such places. The three items excluded from the original scale were 'Do you prefer staying in rather than going out and doing new things?', 'Do you feel you have more problems with memory than most?' and 'Do you think that most people are better off than you?' Deleting these three items increased the Cronbach's alpha from 0.76 to 0.81.

Address for correspondence

Professor Alistair Burns
University of Manchester
School of Psychiatry & Behavioural Sciences
Education & Research Centre
Wythenshawe Hospital
Manchester M23 9LT
e-mail: a_burns@man.ac.uk

A Collateral Source Version of the Geriatric Depression Rating Scale

Reference: Nitcher RL, Burke WJ, Roccaforte WH, Wengel SP (1993) A collateral source version of the Geriatric Depression Rating Scale. *American Journal of Geriatric Psychiatry* 1: 143–152

Time taken approximately 15–20 minutes

Rating by trained rater

Main indications

The scale is used to detect symptoms of depression in patients with mild to moderate cognitive impairment. It is designed to include information supplied by an informed collateral source.

Commentary

The Geriatric Depression Scale correlates well with the clinical diagnosis of depression in cognitively intact patients, but as the questions are based on how individuals have felt in the past week, the scale performs no better than chance in mildly demented subjects with dementia of the Alzheimer's type. The Collateral Source Version of the Geriatric Depression Rating Scale (CSGDS) consists of the same 30 items as the original GDS, is in the same 'yes/no' format, and the reference time frame is still 1 week. The CSGDS, however, has been developed simply by changing the pronoun 'you' on the GDS to 'they'. In the original study, all patients were evaluated by one of three geriatric psychiatrists who were blinded to the GDS and CSGDS results. During the year's study period 194 patients were evaluated. Major depression was diagnosed in 37 (22%).

They found a high prevalence of symptoms reported by the collateral source. This could be explained by the caregiver's mood, the quantity of contact with the patient, and the amount of sympathy or empathy for the patient. The collateral sources tend to endorse more depressive symptoms than patients. Therefore, if the scales are used a higher cut-off point should be used on the CSGDS than on the GDS.

Additional references

MacKenzie TB, Robiner WN, Knopman DS (1989) Differences between patient and family assessments of depression in Alzheimer's disease. *American Journal of Psychiatry* **146**: 1174–8.

Burke WJ, Rubin EH, Morris J et al (1988) Symptoms of depression in senile dementia of the Alzheimer type. *Alzheimer Disease and Associated Disorders* **2**: 356–62.

Address for correspondence

Dr WJ Burke
Department of Psychiatry
University of Nebraska Medical Center
600 S 42nd St
Omaha
NE 68198-5575
USA

Hamilton Depression Rating Scale

Reference: Hamilton M (1960) A rating scale for depression. *Journal of Neurology, Neurosurgery and Psychiatry* 23: 56–62

Time taken 20–30 minutes

Rating by semi-structured interview with trained interviewer

Main indications

To assess the severity of depression for clinical research purposes, in patients of any age.

Commentary

This is a widely used and reliable scale. Although not specific to the elderly, it is the most commonly used depression scale. Nine items are scored 0–4, and a further eight items are scored 0–2 as they represent variables which cannot be expressed quantitatively. The last four items do not measure intensity of depression, and are commonly omitted to give the 17-item version. The scale has been devised primarily for use on patients already diagnosed as suffering from affective disorders, and is used for quantifying results of interviews. Its value depends on the skill of the interviewer in eliciting the necessary information. A cut-off of 10/11 is generally regarded as appropriate for the diagnosis of depression.

Additional reference

Hamilton M (1967) Development of a rating scale for primary depressive illness. *British Journal of Social and Clinical Psychology* **6**: 278–96.

www.members.optusnet.com.au/bill54/depresstest.htm

Hamilton Depression Rating Scale

1.	DEPRESSION (MOOD)	0–4	12.	SOMATIC SYMPTOMS (GASTRO INTESTINAL)	0–2
2.	DEPRESSION (GUILT)	0–4	13.	GENERAL SOMATIC SYMPTOMS	0–2
3.	DEPRESSION (SUICIDE)	0–4	14.	SOMATIC SYMPTOMS (GENITAL SYMPTOMS)	0–2
4.	INSOMNIA (INITIAL)	0–2	15.	HYPOCHONDRIASIS	0–4
5.	INSOMNIA (MIDDLE)	0–2	16.	LOSS OF INSIGHT	0–2
6.	INSOMNIA (DELAYED)	0–2	17.	LOSS OF WEIGHT	0–2
7.	WORK AND INTERESTS	0–4	18.	DIURNAL VARIATION	0–2
8.	RETARDATION	0–4	19.	DEPERSONALISATION ETC.	0–4
9.	AGITATION	0–4	20.	PARANOID SYMPTOMS	0–4
10.	ANXIETY (PSYCHIC SYMPTOMS)	0–4	21.	OBSESSIONAL SYMPTOMS	0–2
11.	ANXIETY (SOMATIC SYMPTOMS)	0–4			

(0–4):
0 = Absent
1 = Doubtful or slight (trivial)
2 = Mild
3 = Moderate
4 = Severe

(0–2):
0 = Absent
1 = Doubtful or slight (trivial)
2 = Clearly present

Reproduced with permission of the BMJ Publishing Group, BMA House, Tavistock Square, London WC1H 9JR.

Beck Depression Inventory (BDI)

Reference: **Beck AT, Ward CH, Mendelson M, Mock J, Erbaugh J (1961) An inventory for measuring depression.** *Archives of General Psychiatry* 4: 53–63

Time taken 20 minutes (reviewer's estimate)

Rating self-rating

Main indications

Self-rating scale for depression.

Commentary

The Beck Depression Inventory (BDI) like the Zung Self-Rating Depression Scale (page 339) is not used specifically for older people but, along with the Zung Scale, is included here because of its widespead use. It represents the gold standard for self-rating depression scales and is often used in assessing depression in carers of patients with dementia, many of whom are younger. The original paper described the administration of the scale to two groups of subjects (409 in total) showing excellent external consistency and validation as scored by independent ratings by psychiatrists. A cut-off of 12/13 is taken to indicate the presence of depression.

Address for correspondence

Center for Cognitive Therapy
Room 602
133 South 36th Street
Philadelphia
PA 19104
USA

www.criminology.unimelb.edu.au/victims/resources/assessment/affect/bdi.html

---

Beck Depression Inventory (BDI) – summary

The BDI is a 21-item scale with a series of statements rated 0, 1, 2 and 3 denoting increasing severity of symptoms. The person completing the questionnaire is asked to read each group of symptoms and then pick the one that best describes the way that they have felt in the past week. Examples of questions include feelings of sadness, concerns about the future, suicidal ideation, tearfulnesss, sleep, fatigue, interests, worries about health, sexual interest, appetite, weight loss and general enjoyment.

Montgomery and Åsberg Depression Rating Scale (MADRS)

Reference: **Montgomery SA, Åsberg M (1979) A new depression scale designed to be sensitive to change.** *British Journal of Psychiatry* 134: 382–9

Time taken 20 minutes

Rating by trained interviewer

Main indications

The scale is designed as a sensitive measure of change in the treatment of depression. The scale may be used for any time interval between ratings, be it weekly or otherwise, but this must be recorded.

Commentary

The Montgomery and Åsberg Depression Rating Scale (MADRS) was developed from 65 original items from the Comprehensive Psychopathological Rating Scale (CPRS; page 255) (Åsberg et al, 1978). The 17 most common items were reduced to 10. These 10 variables specifically deal with the treatment of depression, apparent sadness, reported sadness, inner tension, reduced sleep, reduced appetite, concentration difficulties, lassitude, an ability to feel pessimistic thoughts and suicidal thoughts. Inter-rater reliability was >0.90. Validation studies were carried out on inpatients and outpatients in England and Sweden with concurrent validity tested by the Hamilton Depression

Scale (page 6) and shown to be satisfactory. The scale is now probably the most widely used in drug treatment trials, in young and older patients.

Additional references

Åsberg M, Montgomery S, Perris C et al (1978) A comprehensive psychopathological rating scale. *Acta Psychiatrica Scandinavica, Supplement* **271**: 5–27.

Montgomery S, Åsberg M, Jörnestedt L et al (1978) Reliability of the CPRS between the disciplines of psychiatry, general practice, nursing and psychology in depressed patients. *Acta Psychiatrica Scandinavica, Supplement* **271**: 29–32.

Address for correspondence

Stuart A Montgomery
Emeritus Professor of Psychiatry
Faculty of Medicine
Imperial College
Paterson Centre
20 South Wharf Road
London W2 1PD

Montgomery and Åsberg Depression Rating Scale (MADRS)

1. Apparent sadness	6. Concentration difficulties
2. Reported sadness	7. Lassitude
3. Inner tension	8. Inability to feel
4. Reduced sleep	9. Pessimistic thoughts
5. Reduced appetite	10. Suicidal thoughts

Score:
0 = No difficulties/normal
2 = Fluctuating/fleeting difficulties or feelings
4 = Continuous/pervasive feelings or thoughts
6 = Unrelenting/overwhelming feelings or thoughts

Cornell Scale for Depression in Dementia

Reference: Alexopoulos GS, Abrams RC, Young RC, Shamoian CA (1988) Cornell Scale for Depression in Dementia. *Biological Psychiatry* 23: 271–84

Time taken 20 minutes with the carer, 10 with the patient

Rating by clinician interview

Main indications

The diagnosis of depression in patients with a dementia syndrome.

Commentary

The importance of diagnosing depression in the setting of dementia is self-evident in terms of improved diagnosis and recognition of a potentially treatable condition. The authors state that most other depression scales are completed with information provided by the patient – something not always possible in dementia – hence the combination of observed and informant-based questions. The difference from other scales is therefore mainly in the method of administration rather than based on an analysis of the different phenomenology of depression in the setting of dementia. The 19-item scale is rated on a three-point score of absent, mild or intermittent and severe, with a note when the score was unevaluable. Twenty-six subjects were examined, with an inter-rater reliability kappa of 0.67, satisfactory internal consistency (0.84) and validity when measured against research diagnostic criteria and the Hamilton Depression Rating Scale (page 6). A score of 8 or more suggests significant depressive symptoms.

Address for correspondence

GS Alexopoulos
Department of Psychiatry
Cornell University Medical College
New York Hospital – Westchester Division
21 Bloomingdale Road
White Plains
NY 10605
USA

Cornell Scale for Depression in Dementia

A. Mood-Related Signs
1. Anxiety
   anxious expression, ruminations, worrying
2. Sadness
   sad expression, sad voice, tearfulness
3. Lack of reactivity to pleasant events
4. Irritability
   easily annoyed, short tempered

B. Behavioral Disturbance
5. Agitation
   restlessness, handwringing, hairpulling
6. Retardation
   slow movements, slow speech, slow reactions
7. Multiple physical complaints
   (score 0 if GI symptoms only)
8. Loss of interest
   less involved in usual activities (score only if change occurred acutely, i.e. in less than 1 month)

C. Physical Signs
9. Appetite loss
   eating less than usual
10. Weight loss
   (score 2 if greater than 5 lb in 1 month)

11. Lack of energy
   fatigues easily, unable to sustain activities
   (score only if change occurred acutely, i.e. in less than 1 month)

D. Cyclic Functions
12. Diurnal variation of mood
   symptoms worse in the morning
13. Difficulty falling asleep
   later than usual for this individual
14. Multiple awakenings during sleep
15. Early morning awakening
   earlier than usual for this individual

E. Ideational Disturbance
16. Suicide
   feels life is not worth living, has suicidal wishes, or makes suicide attempt
17. Poor self-esteem
   self-blame, self-depreciation, feelings of failure
18. Pessimism
   anticipation of the worst
19. Mood-congruent delusions
   delusions of poverty, illness, or loss

Rating:
a = Unable to evaluate; 0 = Absent; 1 = Mild or intermittent; 2 = Severe
All based on week prior to interview

Brief Assessment Schedule Depression Cards (BASDEC)

Reference: **Adshead F, Day Cody D, Pitt B (1992) BASDEC: a novel screening instrument for depression in elderly medical inpatients.** *British Medical Journal* **305: 397**

Time taken 3½ minutes (range 2–8 minutes)

Rating the patient chooses the response prompted by an interviewer

Main indications

Screening for depression in geriatric inpatients.

Commentary

The Brief Assessment Schedule Depression Cards (BASDEC) is based on the Brief Assessment Schedule (Macdonald et al, 1982), with the novel development that, because of the difficulties of questions being overheard on geriatric wards, the patients themselves would choose from a deck of cards the answers to particular questions. The BASDEC comprises 19 cards with enlarged black print on a white background. The cards are presented one at a time. Every response of 'true' gains 1 point except 'I have given up hope' and 'I seriously considered suicide', which score 2. The maximum score available is 21 and answers of 'Don't know' score half a point. A validation study was carried out on 79 subjects comparing the responses with the 30-item Geriatric Depression Scale (GDS; page 2) and the BASDEC (using a cut-off score of less than 7 as a non-case and 7 or greater as a case of depression). The GDS and the BASDEC performed identically well with a sensitivity of 71%, specificity of 78%, positive predictive value of 74% and negative predictive value of 86% against a psychiatric diagnosis.

Additional reference

Macdonald A, Mann A, Jenkins R et al (1982) An attempt to determine the impact of 4 types of care upon the elderly in London by the study of matched groups. *Psychological Medicine* 12: 193–200.

www.webenet.com/geriatricscales.htm

Brief Assessment Schedule Depression Cards (BASDEC)

BASDEC (BRIEF ASSESSMENT SCHEDULE DEPRESSION CARDS)

Each item in this scale is reproduced on a separate large-print card. The instructions for its administration are as follows

1 Remove TRUE and FALSE cards from pack
2 Shuffle pack of cards
3 Hand the cards, one by one, to the patient
4 Ask the patient to place the cards in one of two piles 'TRUE' or 'FALSE'
5 Any cards which cause confusion or doubt should be placed in a 'don't know' pile (these may form a useful focal point for discussion)

The cards

I've been depressed for weeks at a time in the past
I am a nuisance to others being ill
I'm not happy at all
I seem to have lost my appetite
I have regrets about my past life
I'm kept awake by worry and unhappy thoughts
I've felt very low lately
I've seriously considered suicide
I feel anxious all the time
I feel life is hardly worth living
I feel worst at the beginning of the day
I'm too miserable to enjoy anything
I'm so lonely
I can't recall feeling happy in the past month
I suffer headaches
I'm not sleeping well
I've lost interest in things
I've cried in the past month
I've given up hope
True
False

Scoring

Each 'TRUE' card has a value of ONE POINT. Each 'DON'T KNOW' card has a value of HALF A POINT. The cards in the 'FALSE' pile do not score. The exceptions to this are the cards

I've given up hope
I've seriously considered suicide

which have value of TWO POINTS if 'TRUE' and ONE POINT if 'DON'T KNOW'.

A patient scoring a total of SEVEN or more points may well be suffering from a depressive disorder

---

This table was first published in the *BMJ* [Adshead F, Day Cody D, Pitt B, BASDEC: a novel screening instrument for depression in elderly medical inpatients, 1992, Vol. 305, p. 397] and is reproduced with kind permission of the *BMJ*.

SELFCARE (D)

Reference: **Bird AS, MacDonald AJD, Mann AH, Philpot MP (1987) Preliminary experience with the SELFCARE (D): a self-rating depression questionnaire for use in elderly, non-institutionalized subjects.** *International Journal of Geriatric Psychiatry* **2: 31–8**

Time taken 15 minutes (reviewer's estimate)

Rating self-rating

Main indications

A self-rating depression scale for use with elderly subjects in general practice.

Commentary

The SELFCARE (D) was devised from the larger Comprehensive Assessment and referral Evaluation (CARE) schedule (Gurland et al, 1977). The items were chosen as the ones previously known to discriminate subjects with and without depression. The results were compared with an independent assessment in 75 patients, using a cut-off of 5/6, attending their general practitioners in London. The sensitivity of the scale at detecting depression was 77% and specificity 98% with a positive predictive value of 96%. Kappa reliability scores were 0.77.

Additional references

Beck AT, Ward CH, Mendelson M et al (1961) An inventory for measuring depression. *Archives of General Psychiatry* **4**: 53–63.

Gurland B, Kuriansky J, Sharpe L et al (1977) The Comprehensive Assessment and Referral Evaluation (CARE) – rationale, development and reliability. *International Journal of Ageing in Human Development* **8**: 9–42.

Address for correspondence

MP Philpot
Section of Old Age Psychiatry
Institute of Psychiatry
Denmark Hill
London SE5 8AF
UK

SELFCARE (D)

(1) In general, how is your health compared with others of your age?
- Excellent ☐
- Good ☐
- * Fair ☐
- Don't know what is meant by question ☐

(2) How quick are you in your physical movements compared with a year ago?
- Quicker than usual ☐
- About as quick as usual ☐
- * Less quick than usual ☐
- * Considerably slower than usual ☐
- Don't know what is meant by question ☐

(3) How much energy do you have, compared to a year ago?
- More than usual ☐
- About the same as usual ☐
- * Less than usual ☐
- * Hardly any at all ☐
- Don't know what is meant by question ☐

(4) In the last month, have you had any headaches?
- Not at all ☐
- About the same as usual ☐
- * Some of the time ☐
- * A lot of the time ☐
- * All of the time ☐
- Don't know what is meant by question ☐

(5) Have you worried about things this past month?
- Not at all ☐
- Only now and then ☐
- * Some of the time ☐
- * A lot of the time ☐
- * All of the time ☐
- Don't know what is meant by question ☐

(6) Have you been sad, unhappy (depressed) or weepy this past month?
- Not at all ☐
- Only now and then ☐
- * Some of the time ☐
- * A lot of the time ☐
- * All of the time ☐
- Don't know what is meant by question ☐

(7) In the past month, have you been lying awake at night feeling uneasy or unhappy?
- Not at all ☐
- Once or twice ☐
- * Quite often ☐
- * Very often ☐
- Don't know what is meant by question ☐

(8) Do you blame yourself for unpleasant things that have happened to you in the past?
- Not at all ☐
- About one thing ☐
- * About a few things ☐
- * About everything ☐
- Don't know what is meant by question ☐

(9) How do you feel about your future?
- Very happy ☐
- Quite happy ☐
- All right ☐
- * Unsure ☐
- * Don't care ☐
- * Worried ☐
- * Frightened ☐
- * Hopeless ☐
- Don't know what is meant by question ☐

(10) What have you enjoyed doing lately?
- Everything ☐
- Most things ☐
- Some things ☐
- * One or two things ☐
- * Nothing ☐
- Don't know what is meant by question ☐

(11) In the past month, have there been times when you've felt quite happy?
- Often ☐
- Sometimes ☐
- * Now and then ☐
- * Never ☐
- Don't know what is meant by question ☐

(12) In general, how happy are you?
- Very happy ☐
- Fairly happy ☐
- * Not very happy ☐
- * Not happy at all ☐
- Don't know what is meant by question ☐

Score 1 for each asterixed item ticked; scoring is made with reference to symptoms experienced over the past month.
Non-case/case cut point = 5–6
Don't know >4 = unreliable

Reproduced from Bird AS, MacDonald AJD, Mann AH, Philpot MP (1987) Preliminary experience with the SELFCARE (D): a self-rating depression questionnaire for use in elderly, non-institutionalized subjects. *International Journal of Geriatric Psychiatry* **2**: 31–8. Copyright John Wiley & Sons Limited. Reproduced with permission.

Center for Epidemiological Studies – Depression Scale (CES-D)

Reference: Radloff LS, Teri L (1986) Use of the Center for Epidemiological Studies – depression scale with older adults. *Clinical Gerontologist* 5: 119–37

Time taken 5 minutes

Rating self-administered

Main indications

To detect depressive symptoms, particularly to be used for research purposes or screening.

Commentary

The sensitivity and specificity of the Center for Epidemiological Studies – Depression Scale (CES-D) compare favourably with scales such as the Beck Depression Inventory (BDI; page 7) and Zung Self-Rating Depression Scale (page 339). Although originally developed for a large general population study of depressive symptoms the instrument has been found to be particularly useful in

older adults. The scale should be used cautiously in visually or cognitively impaired elderly individuals.

The CES-D was developed from a large community study reporting depression symptoms (Radloff, 1977) and consists of 20 items. Scores range from 0 to 60.

Test/retest reliability over weeks averaged 0.57 and interval consistency was high (0.92). Validity was satisfactorily assessed by correlation with other depression rating studies. A cut-off of 16 has been suggested to differentiate patients with mild depression from normal controls and 23 and over to indicate significant depression.

Additional reference

Radloff L (1977) The Center for Epidemiological Studies Depression Scale. A self-report depression scale for research in the general population. *Applied Psychological Measurements* 3: 385–401.

Center for Epidemiological Studies – Depression Scale (CES-D)

During the past week:

1. I was bothered by things that usually don't bother me. (S)
2. I did not feel like eating; my appetite was poor. (S)
3. I felt that I could not shake off the blues even with help from my family or friends. (D)
4. I felt that I was just as good as other people. (P)
5. I had trouble keeping my mind on what I was doing. (S)
6. I felt depressed. (D)
7. I felt that everything I did was an effort. (S)
8. I felt hopeful about the future. (P)
9. I thought my life had been a failure.
10. I felt fearful.
11. My sleep was restless. (S)
12. I was happy. (P)
13. I talked less than usual.
14. I felt lonely. (D)
15. People were unfriendly. (I)
16. I enjoyed life. (P)
17. I had crying spells. (D)
18. I felt sad. (D)
19. I felt that people disliked me. (I)
20. I could not get 'going'. (S)

Rating:
Rarely/None of the time (< 1 day)
Some/Little of the time (1–2 days)
Occasionally/Moderate amount of time (3–4 days)
Most/All of the time (5–7 days)
D = Depressed affect
P = Positive affect
S = Somatic/vegetative signs
I = Interpersonal distress

OARS Depressive Scale (ODS)

Reference: **Blazer D (1980) The diagnosis of depression in the elderly.** *Journal of the American Geriatrics Society* 28: 52–8

Time taken 20 minutes (reviewer's estimate)

Rating by trained interviewer

Main indications

Indentification of elderly people with depressive symptomatology, based on DSM-III.

Commentary

For the OARS Depressive Scale (ODS), Blazer described 18 items derived from DSM-III indicators of depressive symptomatology and assessed internal reliability and construct validity, and compared this scale with the Zung Self-Rating Depression Scale (page 339). The ODS was assessed on a random sample of 997 people over the age of 65. Split half reliability was 0.74 and the coefficient alpha was 0.801, confirming the reliability of the instrument. Factor analysis revealed three factors – factor 1 relating to the symptoms of dysphoria, factor 2 items assessing the criteria for assessing diagnosis of depressive disorder and factor 3 around items assessing general pessimism for the future. When compared with clinical diagnosis, it was found that the ODS was specific but not quite as sensitive as other assessment instruments. People scoring at least four of the DSM-III symptoms for depression (poor appetite, weight loss, sleep disturbance, fatigue, agitation/retardation, loss of interest, guilt, poor concentration and suicidal ideas) were rated as positive on the ODS scale.

Factors: feelings of uselessness, can't get going, mind works slower, feelings of guilt, decreased self-confidence, decreased life satisfaction, loss of interest, weakness, poor appetite, difficulty concentrating, sadness, frequent worry, restlessness, pessimism about the future.

Additional references

Micro D (1978) Revision in the diagnostic criteria of DSM-III 1/15/78 draft. Prepared by the Task Force on Nomenclature and Statistics of the American Psychiatric Association. Washington DC.

Zung WWK (1965) A Self-Rating Depression Scale. *Archives of General Psychiatry* 12: 63–70.

Address for correspondence

Dan Blazer
Duke University Medical Center
Box 3173
Duke Medical Center
Durham
NC 27710
USA

OARS Depressive Scale (ODS)

Do you have a good appetite?
Is your daily life full of things that keep you interested?
Do you find it hard to keep your mind on a task or job?
Have you had periods of days, weeks or months when you couldn't take care of things because you couldn't get going?
Much of the time, do you feel you have done something wrong or evil?
Are you happy most of the time?
Do you feel useless at times?
Do you feel weak all over much of the time?
Do you feel your sins are unpardonable?
Do you frequently find yourself worrying about something?

Do you have periods of such great restlessness that you cannot sit long in a chair?
Does your mind seem to work more slowly than usual at times?
Do you usually expect things will turn out well for you?
Do you sometimes feel unhappy because you think you are not useful?
In general, how happy would you say you are – very happy, fairly happy or not happy?
Taking everything into consideration, how would you describe your satisfaction with life in general at the present time – good, fair or poor?

The above items are all rated yes or no, except the last two, where a three-point choice is given.

Reproduced from Blazer D (1980) The diagnosis of depression in the elderly. *Journal of the American Geriatrics Society*, Vol. 28, no. 2, pp. 52–8.

Depressive Signs Scale (DSS)

Reference: Katona CLE, Aldridge CR (1985) The Dexamethasone Suppression Test and depressive signs in dementia. *Journal of Affective Disorders* 8: 83–9

Time taken 10 minutes (reviewer's estimate)

Rating by interview with subject followed by interview with informant

Main indications

Depressive symptoms in patients with dementia.

Commentary

The authors were initially looking at the characteristics of patients with dementia who were non-suppressors on the Dexamethasone Depression Test (DST) (Carroll, 1982). The Depressive Signs Scale (DSS) aims to detect depressive signs in people with severe dementia. Failure of suppression was found in 10 out of 20 patients with dementia, who scored higher on the DSS. Inter-rater reliability was 0.98.

Additional reference

Carroll BJ (1982) The Dexamethasone Suppression Test for melancholia. *British Journal of Psychiatry* 140: 292–304.

Address for correspondence

Professor Cornelius Katona
Dean
Kent Institute of Medicine and Health Sciences
University of Kent at Canterbury
Kent CT2 7PD
UK

Depressive Signs Scale (DSS)

1.   Sad appearance
1.1   Reactivity of sad appearance
2.   Agitation by day
3.   Slowness of movement
4.   Slowness of speech

5.   Early waking
6.   Loss of appetite
7.   Diurnal variation in mood (mornings worst)
8.   Interest in surroundings

Score:
2 = Marked/consistent or persistent
1 = Intermediate/mild or intermittent
0 = Absent

Except:
8–2 = Never, 1 = Occasional, 0 = Equally
and
1.1–1 = Absent, 0 = Present

Carroll Rating Scale (CRS)

Reference: **Carroll BJ, Feinberg M, Smouse PE, Rawson SG, Greden JF (1981) The Carroll Rating Scale for Depression. I. Development, reliability and validation.** *British Journal of Psychiatry* **138: 194–200**

Time taken 15 minutes (reviewer's estimate)

Rating self-rating

Main indications

Screening for depressive illness.

Commentary

The Carroll Rating Scale (CRS) was developed from the 17-item Hamilton Depression Rating Scale (page 6). Concurrent validity was measured against other scales of depression, e.g. the Hamilton Depression Rating Scale and the Beck Depression Inventory (BDI; page 7). External validity was measured using a clinical rating of the severity of depression. A cut-off score of 10 or above indicates the presence of at least mild depression. Reliability was assessed using a test/retest and split half reliability, and sensitivity was measured in its ability to discriminate depressed and non-depressed subjects. All were satisfactory. The same authors in companion papers assessed the factor structure of the CRS and compared it to other available scales.

The CRS has not been used specifically in elderly people, but it is included here as a very well validated and reliable instrument.

Additional references

Feinberg M, Carroll B, Smouse P et al (1981) The Carroll Rating Scale for Depression. III. Comparison with other rating instruments. *British Journal of Psychiatry* **138**: 205–9.

Smouse P, Feinberg M, Carroll B et al (1981) The Carroll Rating Scale for Depression. II. Factor analyses of the feature profiles. *British Journal of Psychiatry* **138**: 201–4.

Carroll Rating Scale (CRS)

1. I feel just as energetic as always
2. I am losing weight
3. I have dropped many of my interests and activities
4. Since my illness I have completely lost interest in sex
5. I am especially concerned about how my body is functioning
6. It must be obvious that I am disturbed and agitated
7. It am still able to carry on doing the work I am supposed to do
8. I can concentrate easily when reading the papers
9. Getting to sleep takes me more than half an hour
10. I am restless and fidgety
11. I wake up much earlier than I need to in the morning
12. Dying is the best solution for me
13. I have a lot of trouble with dizzy and faint feelings
14. I am being punished for something bad in my past
15. My sexual interest is the same as before I got sick
16. I am miserable or often feel like crying
17. I often wish I were dead
18. I am having trouble with indigestion
19. I wake up often in the middle of the night
20. I feel worthless and ashamed about myself
21. I am so slowed down that I need help with bathing and dressing
22. I take longer than usual to fall asleep at night
23. Much of the time I am very afraid but don't know the reason
24. Things which I regret about my life are bothering me
25. I get pleasure and satisfaction from what I do
26. All I need is a good rest to be perfectly well again
27. My sleep is restless and disturbed
28. My mind is as fast and alert as always
29. I feel that life is still worth living
30. My voice is dull and lifeless
31. I feel irritable or jittery
32. I feel in good spirits
33. My heart sometimes beats faster than usual
34. I think my case is hopeless
35. I wake up before my usual time in the morning
36. I still enjoy my meals as much as usual
37. I have to keep pacing around most of the time
38. I am terrified and near panic
39. My body is bad and rotten inside
40. I got sick because of the bad weather we have been having
41. My hands shake so much that people can easily notice
42. I still like to go out and meet people
43. I think I appear calm on the outside
44. I think I am as good a person as anybody else
45. My trouble is the result of some serious internal disease
46. I have been thinking about trying to kill myself
47. I get hardly anything done lately
48. There is only misery in the future for me
49. I worry a lot about my bodily symptoms
50. I have to force myself to eat even a little
51. I am exhausted much of the time
52. I can tell that I have lost a lot of weight

Code: Yes or No on all

In addition, Visual Analogue Scale of how patient feels on day of test from worst ever to best ever

Depression – 32,16,34,48
Guilt – 14,20,24,44
Suicide – 12,17,29,46
Initial insom – 9,22
Middle insom – 19,27
Delayed insom – 11,35
Work and interests – 3,7,25,42
Retardation – 21,28,30,47
Agitation – 6,10,37,43
Psychological anxiety – 8,23,31,38
Somatic anxiety – 13,18,33,41
Gastrointestinal – 36,50
General somatic – 1,51
Libido – 4,15
Hypochondriasis – 5,39,45,49
Loss of insight – 26,40
Loss of weight – 2,52

Reproduced from the *British Journal of Psychiatry*, Carroll BJ, Feinberg M, Smouse PE, Rawson SG, Greden JF (1981), The Carroll Rating Scale for Depression. I. Development, reliability and validation. Vol. 138, pp. 194–200. © 1981 Royal College of Psychiatrists. Reproduced with permission.

Mood Scales – Elderly (MS–E)

Reference: **Raskin A, Crook T (1988) Mood Scales – Elderly (MS-E).** *Psychopharmacology Bulletin* **24: 727–32**

Time taken 25 minutes (reviewer's estimate)

Rating self-rating

Main indications

Assessment of depression in elderly people.

Commentary

The Mood Scales – Elderly (MS-E) consists of 50 adjectives taken from a number of sources. The individual is asked to complete the scale on a five-point choice from 'not at all' through to 'extremely'. The validity of the scale was assessed using a factor analysis – seven factors were described: tense/irritable; considerate; cognitive disturbances; inept/helpless; depressed; fatigued and energetic/capable. Internal consistency was good, with a Cronbach's alpha of 0.8 or higher for the factors. Validity was asssessed by the scale's ability to differentiate between diagnostic groups and a high correlation was found

between the MS-E and that of other ratings of psychopathology. Good sensitivity is reported with regard to the ability of the MS-E to detect change with treatment.

Additional references

Raskin A, Crook T (1976) Sensitivity rating scales completed by psychiatrists, nurses and patients to antidepressant drug effect. *Journal of Psychiatric Research* **13**: 31–41.

Zuckerman M (1960) The development of an affect adjective checklist for the measurement of anxiety. *Journal of Consulting Psychology* **24**: 457–62.

Address for correspondence

Allen Raskin
7658 Water Oak Point Road
Pasedena
MD 21122
USA

Mood Scales – Elderly (MS-E)

1. Sad	14. Relaxed	27. Lively	40. Jittery
2. Tense	15. Good natured	28. Efficient	41. Sarcastic
3. Angry	16. Worthless	29. Depressed	42. Kind
4. Happy	17. Sleepy	30. Restless	43. Absent-minded
5. Warmhearted	18. Active	31. Annoyed	44. Lonely
6. Tired	19. Forgetful	32. Considerate	45. Able to work
7. Full of pep	20. Able to concentrate	33. Weary	46. Clumsy
8. Confused	21. Unhappy	34. Alert	47. Bewildered
9. Able to think clearly	22. Friendly	35. Blue	48. Energetic
10. Downhearted	23. Cheerful	36. Nervous	49. Helpless
11. On edge	24. Capable	37. Rude	50. Carefree
12. Irritable	25. Useless	38. Awkward	
13. Sluggish	26. Worn out	39. Troubled	

Score: 1 = Not at all
2 = A little
3 = Moderately
4 = Quite a bit
5 = Extremely

Reproduced from Raskin A, Crook T (1988) Mood Scales – Elderly (MS-E). *Psychopharmacology Bulletin* **24**: 727–32.

Mania Rating Scale

Reference: **Bech P, Rafaelsen OJ, Kramp P, Bolwig TG (1978) The Mania Rating Scale: scale construction and inter-observer agreement.** *Neuropharmacology* 17: 430–1

Time taken 15–30 minutes

Rating by clinician

Main indications

To quantify the severity of manic states, and said to be useful in clinical trials in patients of all ages.

Commentary

The Mania Rating Scale was developed to measure manic symptomatology based on a previous attempt to devise a scale (Petterson et al, 1973). Eleven variables were described: activity (motor and verbal), flight of ideas, voices/noise level, hostility/destructiveness, mood (feeling of well-being), self esteem, contacts, sleep, sexual interest and activity, work activity. Each item scores 0–4, giving a maximum score of 44. Inter-rater reliability was over 0.85. The suggested inclusion criterion for clinical trials of mania is 15 or above out of 44. Scores of 6–14 indicate partial response to treatment, scores less than 5 indicate full remission.

Additional references

Petterson V, Fyrö B, Sedvall G (1973) A new scale for longitudinal rating of manic status. *Acta Psychiatrica Scandinavica* **49**: 248–56.

Mania Rating Scale

1. ACTIVITY (motor)
   0. Normal motor activity, adequate facial expressions
   1. Slightly increased motor activity, lively facial expression
   2. Somewhat excessive motor activity, lively gestures
   3. Outright excessive motor activity, on the move most of the time
      Rises one or several times during interview
   4. Constantly active, restlessly energetic, even if urged, patient cannot sit still

2. ACTIVITY (verbal)
   0. Normal, verbal activity
   1. Somewhat talkative
   2. Very talkative, no spontaneous intervals in the conversation
   3. Difficult to interrupt
   4. Impossible to interrupt, dominates completely the conversation

3. FLIGHT OF THOUGHTS
   0. Cohesive speech, no flight of thoughts
   1. Vivid associations, maintaining cohesive speech
   2. Sporadic clang associations
   3. Several clang associations
   4. Difficult to impossible to follow the patient's clang association

4. VOICE–NOISE LEVEL
   0. Natural volume of voice
   1. Speaks loudly without being noisy
   2. Voice discernible at a distance, and somewhat noisy
   3. Vociferous, voice discernible at a long distance, is noisy
   4. Shouting, screaming, singing or using other sources of noise due to hoarseness

5. HOSTILITY–DESTRUCTIVENESS
   0. No signs of impatience or hostility
   1. Touchy, but irritation easily controlled
   2. Markedly impatient, or irritable. Provocation badly tolerated
   3. Provocative, makes threats, but can be calmed down
   4. Overt physical violence. Physically destructive

6. MOOD (feelings of well-being)
   0. Neutral mood
   1. Slightly elevated mood, optimistic, but still adapted to situation
   2. Moderately elevated mood, joking, laughing
   3. Markedly elevated mood, exuberant both in manner and speech
   4. Extremely elevated mood, quite irrelevant to situation

7. SELF ESTEEM
   0. Normal self esteem, slightly boasting
   1. Slightly increased self esteem, slightly boasting
   2. Moderately increased self esteem, boasting. Frequent use of superlatives
   3. Bragging, unrealistic ideas
   4. Grandiose ideas which cannot be correct

8. CONTACT
   0. Normal contact
   1. Slightly meddling, putting his oar in
   2. Moderately meddling and arguing
   3. Dominating, arranging, directing, but still in context with the setting
   4. Extremely dominating and manipulating without context with the setting

9. SLEEP (average of last 3 nights)
   0. Habitual duration of sleep
   1. Duration of sleep reduced by 25%
   2. Duration of sleep reduced by 50%
   3. Duration of sleep reduced by 75%
   4. No sleep

10. ACTIVITY (sexual)
    0. Habitual sexual interest and activity
    1. Slight increase in sexual interest and activity. Slightly flirtatious
    2. Moderate increase in sexual interest and activity
    3. Clearly flirtatious. Dress provocative
    4. Completely and inadequately occupied by sexuality

11. ACTIVITY (work and interests)
    0. Habitual work activities
    1. Work slightly up and/or quality slightly down
    2. Work somewhat up, but quality clearly down. Attention easily distracted
    3. Unable to work, tries to do several things at the same time, but nothing is brought to an end
       In hospital, rate 3 if patient does not spend at least 3 hr per day in activities (hospital, job or hobbies)
    4. Unable to work, purposelessly occupied all the time. In hospital, rate 4 if patient often has to be helped with personal needs

Reprinted from *Neuropharmacology,* Vol. 17, Bech P, Rafaelsen OJ, Kramp P, Bolwig TG, The Mania Rating Scale: scale construction and inter-observer agreement, pp. 430–1, copyright © 1978, with kind permission from Elsevier Science Ltd, The Boulevard, Langford Lane, Kidlington OX5 1GB, UK.

Checklist Differentiating Pseudodementia from Dementia

Reference: **Wells CE (1979) Pseudodementia.** *American Journal of Psychiatry* **136: 895–900**

Time taken 15 minutes

Rating by a semi-structured interview with an experienced rater

Main indications

To differentiate pseudodementia from dementia.

Commentary

The Checklist Differentiating Pseudodementia from Dementia is a 22-item instrument focusing on clinical history, behaviour and an assessment of mental capacities. It was validated with a psychometric test battery, computerized tomography and electroencephalogram (EEG). The instrument is for clinical use only.

Checklist Differentiating Pseudodementia from Dementia

Clinical course and history	Pseudodementia	Dementia
1. Family awareness of dysfunction and its severity:		
aware	☐	
unaware		☐
2. Onset dated with:		
some precision	☐	
only within broad limits		☐
3. Duration of symptoms before medical help sought:		
short	☐	
long		☐
4. Progression of symptoms after onset:		
rapid	☐	
slow		☐
5. History of previous psychiatric dysfunction:		
present	☐	
absent		☐
Complaints and clinical behavior		
6. Patient complains of cognitive loss:		
much	☐	
little		☐
7. Patient's complaint of cognitive dysfunction:		
detailed	☐	
vague		☐
8. Attitude towards disability:		
emphasizes disability	☐	
conceals disability		☐
9. Response to achievements:		
highlights failures	☐	
delights in accomplishments, even if trivial		☐
10. In performing even simple tasks:		
patient makes little effort	☐	
patient struggles		☐
11. In order to keep up with things:		
patient does not try	☐	
patient relies on notes, calendars etc.		☐
12. In emotional situations:		
patient communicates strong sense of distress	☐	
patient often appears unconcerned		☐

cont.

		Pseudodementia	Dementia
13.	Affective change:		
	pervasive	☐	
	labile and shallow		☐
14.	Social skills:		
	prominent and early loss	☐	
	retained		☐
15.	Congruence between performance and apparent cognitive dysfunction:		
	behavior incompatible	☐	
	behavior compatible		☐
16.	Nocturnal accentuation of dysfunction:		
	not present	☐	
	occurs		☐

Clinical assessment of mental capacities

		Pseudodementia	Dementia
17.	Attention and concentration:		
	well preserved	☐	
	faulty		☐
18.	Typical answers to questions:		
	'don't know'	☐	
	'near-miss'		☐
19.	Answers in tests of orientation:		
	'don't know'	☐	
	inappropriate, replaces usual with 'unusual', e.g. 'home' when patient in hospital		☐
20.	Memory loss for recent and remote events:		
	equally severe	☐	
	more severe for recent than for remote		☐
21.	Memory gaps for specific periods or events:		
	present	☐	
	memory loss not patchy		☐
22.	Performance on tasks similar in difficulty:		
	marked variability	☐	
	consistently poor		☐

NIMH Dementia Mood Assessment Scale (DMAS)

Reference: **Sunderland T, Alterman IS, Yount D, Hill JL, Tariot PN, Newhouse PA, Mueller EA, Mellow AM, Cohen RM (1988) A new scale for the assessment of depressed mood in dementia patients.** *American Journal of Psychiatry* **145: 955–9**

Time taken 20–30 minutes

Rating by direct observation and a semi-structured interview of the patient by trained raters

Main indications

A measure of mood in cognitively impaired subjects.

Commentary

The NIMH Dementia Mood Assessment Scale (DMAS) was validated on 21 patients with primary degenerative dementia to the 24-item scale. It is not a diagnostic instrument for depression in dementia but a measure of mood in people with mild to moderate dementia. The first 17 items of the 24-item scale assess depression, the last 7 severity of dementia. There were high inter-rater reliability and intra-class correlations, and validation was against other instruments – the Geriatric Depression Scale (GDS; page 2) and Montgomery and Åsberg Depression Rating Scale (MADRS; page 8) – to focus on observable mood and functional capacities of dementia patients. The DMAS is in part derived from the Hamilton Depression Rating Scale (page 6).

Additional reference

Sunderland T, Hill J, Lawlor B et al (1988) NIMH Dementia Mood Assessment Scale (DMAS). *Psychopharmacology Bulletin* **24**: 747–53.

Address for correspondence

Trey Sunderland
Unit of Geriatric Psychopharmacology
Laboratory of Clinical Science, NIMH
Building 10
Room 3D41
Bethesda
MD 20892
USA

NIMH Dementia Mood Assessment Scale (DMAS)

1. Self-Directed Motor Activity
0 = Remains active in day-to-day pursuits.
2 = Participates in planned activities but may need some guidance structuring free time.
4 = Needs much direction with unstructured time but still participates in planned activities.
6 = Little or no spontaneous activity initiated. Does not willingly participate in activities even with much direction.

2. Sleep (Rate A and B)
A. Insomnia
0 = No insomnia/restlessness.
2 = Restlessness at night or occasional insomnia (greater than one hour). May complain of poor sleep.
4 = Intermittent early morning awakening or frequent difficulty falling asleep (greater than one hour).
6 = Almost nightly sleep difficulties, insomnia, frequent awakening, and/or agitation, which is profoundly disturbing the patient's sleep–wake cycle.
B. Daytime Drowsiness
0 = No apparent drowsiness.
2 = May appear drowsy during the day with occasional napping.
4 = May frequently nod off during the day.
6 = Continuously attempts to sleep during the day.

3. Appetite (Rate either A or B)
A. Decreased Appetite
0 = No decreased appetite.
2 = Shows less interest in meals.
4 = Reports loss of appetite or shows greater than 1 pound/week weight loss.
6 = Requires urging or assistance in eating or shows greater than 2 pounds/week weight loss.

B. Increased Appetite
0 = No increased appetite.
2 = Shows increased interest in meals and meal planning.
4 = Snacking frequently in addition to regular meal schedule or weight gain of greater than 1 pound/week.
6 = Excessive eating through the day or weight gain of greater than 2 pounds/week.

4. Psychosomatic Complaints
0 = Not present or appropriate for physical condition.
2 = Overconcern with health issues (i.e. real or imaginery medical problems).
4 = Frequent physical complaints or repeated requests for medical attention out of proportion to existing conditions.
6 = Preoccupied with physical complaints. May focus on specific complaints to the exclusion of other problems.

5. Energy
0 = Normal energy level.
2 = Slight decrease in general energy level.
4 = Appears tired often. Occasionally misses planned activities because of 'fatigue'.
6 = Attempts to sit alone in a chair or lie in bed much of the day. Appears exhausted despite low activity level.

6. Irritability
0 = No more irritable than normal.
2 = Overly sensitive, showing low tolerance to normal frustrations; sarcastic.
4 = Impatient, demanding, frequent angry reactions.
6 = Global irritability that cannot be relieved by diversion or explanation.

7. Physical Agitation
0 = No physical restlessness or agitation noted.
2 = Fidgetiness (i.e. plays with hands or taps feet) or bodily tension.
4 = Has trouble sitting still. May move from place to place without obvious purpose.
6 = Hand wringing or frequent pacing. Unable to sit in one place for structured activity.

8. Anxiety
0 = No apparent anxiety.
2 = Apprehension or mild worry noted but able to respond to reassurance.
4 = Frequent worries about minor matters or overconcern about specific issues. Tension usually obvious in facial countenance or manner. May require frequent reassurances.
6 = Constantly worried and tense. Requires almost constant attention and reassurance to maintain control of anxiety.

9. Depressed Appearance
0 = Does not appear depressed and denies such when questioned directly.
2 = Occasionally seems sad or downcast. May admit to 'spirits' being low from time to time.
4 = Frequently appears depressed, irrespective of ability to express or explain underlying thoughts.
6 = Shows mostly depressed appearance, even to casual observer. May be associated with frequent crying.

10. Awareness of Emotional State
0 = Fully acknowledges emotional condition. Expressed emotions are congruent with current situation.
2 = Occasionally denies feelings appropriate to situation.
4 = Frequently denies emotional reactions. May display some appropriate feelings with focused discussion of individual issues.
6 = Persistently denies emotional state, even with direct confrontation.

11. Emotional Responsiveness
0 = Smiles and cries in appropriate situations. Establishes eye contact regularly. Speaks and jokes spontaneously in groups.
2 = Occasionally avoids eye contact but able to respond appropriately when addressed by others. Sometimes may appear distant when sitting in social situations, as if not paying attention.
4 = Often sitting with blank stare while with others. Responses usually show limited variation of facial expression.
6 = Does not seek social interaction. Shows little emotion, even when in the presence of loved ones. Seems unable to react to emotional situations, either positively or negatively (i.e. calm or 'bland').

12. Sense of Enjoyment
0 = Appears to enjoy activities, friends, and family normally.
2 = Reduced animation. May display less pleasure.
4 = Infrequent display of pleasure. May show less enjoyment of family or friends.
6 = Rarely expresses pleasure or enjoyment, even when taking part in formerly consuming interests.

13. Self-Esteem
0 = No obvious loss of self-esteem or sense of inferiority.
2 = Mild decrease in self-esteem noted ocasionally. May be unable to identify strengths and accomplishments.
4 = Spontaneously self-deprecating. May display feeling of worthlessness out of proportion to objective observations.
6 = Persistent feelings of worthlessness that cannot be dispelled with reassurance.

cont.

14. Guilt Feelings

0 = Absent.

2 = Self-reproach.

4 = Spontaneously talks of being a burden to the family or caretakers. May be overly concerned with ideas of guilt or past errors but can be reassured by others.

6 = Preoccupied with guilty thoughts or feelings of shame.

15. Hopelessness/Helplessness

0 = No evidence of hopelessness or helplessness.

2 = Questions ability to cope with life and future. May ask for assistance with simple tasks or decisions that are within his/her capacity.

4 = Pessimistic about the future but can be reassured. Frequently seeks assistance regardless of need.

6 = Feels hopeless about the future. Expresses belief of having little or no control over life.

16. Suicidal Ideation

0 = Absent. Denies any thoughts of suicide.

2 = Feels life is not worth living or states that others would be better off without him/her. Not consciously pursuing any plans for self-harm.

4 = Thoughts of possible death to self; may wish to die in his/her sleep or pray for 'God to take me now'.

6 = Any attempt, gesture, or specific plan of suicide.

17. Speech

0 = Normal rate and rhythm with usual tonal variability. Speech is audible, clear, and fluent.

2 = Noticeable pauses during conversation. Voice may be low, soft, or monotonous.

4 = Reduced spontaneous speech. Responses to direct questions are less fluent or mumbled. Initiates little conversation; difficult to hear.

6 = Rarely speaks spontaneously. Speech is difficult to understand.

18. Diurnal Mood Variation

A. Note whether mood appears worse in morning or evening. If no diurnal variation, mark 'none'.

0 = None.

1 = Worse in morning.

2 = Worse in evening.

B. When present, mark the severity of the variation. Mark 'none' if no variation is present.

0 = None.

2 = Mild.

4 = Moderate.

6 = Severe.

19. Diurnal Cognitive Variation

A. Note whether general cognitive abilities appear worse in morning or evening. If no diurnal variation, mark 'none'.

0 = None.

1 = Worse in morning.

2 = Worse in evening.

B. When present, mark the severity of the variation. Mark 'none' if no variation is present.

0 = None

2 = Mild.

4 = Moderate.

6 = Severe.

20. Paranoid Symptoms

0 = None

2 = Occasionally suspicious of harm or watching others closely. Guarded with personal questions.

4 = Shows intermittent ideas of reference or frequent suspiciousness.

6 = Paranoid delusions or overt thoughts of persecution.

21. Other Psychotic Symptoms

0 = None.

2 = Occasionally misinterprets sensory input or experiences illusions.

4 = Frequently misinterprets sensory input.

6 = Overt hallucinations or nonparanoid delusions.

22. Expressive Communication Skills

0 = Able to make self understood, even to strangers.

2 = Sometimes has difficulty communicating with others, but is able to make self understood with additional effort (e.g. visual cues).

4 = Frequently has trouble expressing ideas to others.

6 = Marked difficulty communicating ideas to others, even family members and significant others.

23. Receptive Cognitive Capacity

0 = Appears to grasp ideas normally.

2 = Experiences occasional difficulty understanding complex statements expressed by others.

4 = Frequently misunderstands or fails to comprehend issues when addressed directly, despite repeated attempts.

6 = Needs multiple modalities of communication (e.g. verbal, visual, and/or physical prompts) to comprehend basic task.

24. Cognitive Insight

0 = Normal cognitively or shows insight into deficits.

2 = Admits to some, but not all of his/her cognitive difficulties.

4 = Intermittently denies cognitive deficits even when pointed out by others.

6 = Denies cognitive difficulties even when they are obvious to casual observers.

Scoring for DMAS 17 (1–17) = max 102

DMAS 18–24 (last 7 items) = max 42

DMAS 17 corresponds to mood scale

DMAS 18–24 – dementia severity

Emotionalism and Mood Disorders after Stroke

References: House A, Dennis M, Molyneux A, Warlow C, Hawton K (1989a) Emotionalism after stroke. *British Medical Journal* 298: 991–4

House A, Dennis M, Hawton K et al (1989b) Methods of identifying mood disorders in stroke patients: experience in the Oxfordshire Community Stroke Project. *Age and Ageing* 18: 371–9

Time taken 15 minutes (reviewer's estimate)

Rating by clinician, nurse or carer

Main indications

For the assessment of emotional lability post-stroke.

Commentary

The original paper described the prevalence using the emotionalism scale in 128 patients post-stroke. Emotionalism was associated with higher measures of mood disorder and psychiatric illness, more cognitive impairment and larger lesions on CT scan, particularly in the left frontal and temporal regions. The scale asked the following questions:

(1) Have you been more tearful since the stroke than you were beforehand? Have you actually cried more in the past month (not just felt like it)?
(2) Does the weepiness come suddenly, at times when you aren't expecting it? (Suddenly means with only a few moments or no warning, not after several minutes trying to control yourself)
(3) If you feel the tears coming on, or if they have started, can you control yourself to stop them? Have you been unable to stop yourself crying in front of other people? Is that a new experience for you?

Emotionalism was present if the reply was positive to the above questions.

In a companion paper, House et al (1989b) presented a nurses' and carers' depression scale for the assessment of stroke patients, using the House Scales, the Beck Depression Inventory (BDI; page 7) and a visual analogue self-report scale. Validity measures against a standardized psychiatric interview were made. None of the measures was satisfactory – at 12 months post-stroke, a cut-off on the BDI of 6/7 gave a true-positive rate of 0.90 and a false-positive rate of 0.32 in the detection of depression.

Address for correspondence

Allan House
Professor of Liaison Psychiatry
Academic Unit of Psychiatry and Behavioural Science
School of Medicine
University of Leeds
Level 5, Clinical Sciences Building
St James' University Hospital
Leeds LS9 7TF
UK
e-mail: a.o.house@leeds.ac.uk

Carers' and Nurses' Depression Scale

In addition to the questions given in the commentary, patients were asked to complete the Beck Inventory and the MMSE. Language function was also assessed (Frenchay aphasia screening test).

Nurses' depression rating

Would you consider .... has shown evidence of the following features of depression over the past week?

Behaviour	(1)	Slowness of thought
	(2)	Social withdrawal/uncommunicativeness
	(3)	Self-neglect
Mood	(1)	Sadness or tearfulness (regardless of circumstances)
	(2)	Anxiety/lack of self-confidence
	(3)	Irritability
Thinking	(1)	Apathy – lack of motivation, interest or concentration
	(2)	Negativity – refusal to co-operate or participate
	(3)	Pessimism – hopelessness or suicidal ideas
Somatic symptoms	(1)	Disturbed sleep pattern
	(2)	Anorexia (with or without weight loss)
	(3)	Loss of libido (where appropriate)

Taking all these features into consideration, would you consider that this person is significantly depressed or otherwise emotionally disordered?

1	2	3	4
Yes definitely	Yes probably	Probably not	Definitely not

Any other comments:

_____

_____

Carer's depression rating

Would you say any of the following descriptions applied to .... as far as you have noticed over the past week?

(1)	Slowed up in thinking or movement	YES/NO
(2)	Wanting to keep away from other people or avoid conversation	YES/NO
(3)	Not looking after him/herself properly	YES/NO
(4)	Sad or tearful	YES/NO
(5)	Anxious or lacking in self-confidence	YES/NO
(6)	Irritable	YES/NO
(7)	Lacking in interest	YES/NO
(8)	Refusing to co-operate or join in things	YES/NO
(9)	Pessimistic or hopeless	YES/NO
(10)	Feeling suicidal	YES/NO
(11)	Sleeping poorly	YES/NO
(12)	Not eating properly	YES/NO

Do you think that he/she is depressed or suffering from any other emotional problems? YES/NO

Any other comments:

_____

Reprinted from House A, Dennis M, Hawton K et al (1989) Methods of identifying mood disorders in stroke patients: experience in the Oxfordshire Community Stroke Project. *Age and Ageing* 18: 371–9. By kind permission of Oxford University Press.

EURO-D Scale

Reference: Prince MJ, Beekman ATF, Deeg DJH, Fuhrer R, Kivela S-L, Lawlor BA, Lobo A, Magnusson H, Meller I, van Oyen H, Reischies F, Roelands M, Skoog I, Turrina C, Copeland JRM (1999) Depression symptoms in late life assessed using the EURO-D scale. *British Journal of Psychiatry* 174: 339–45

Time taken approximately 10 minutes

Rating a trained rater

Main indications

For measuring the level of depression in comparative epidemiological studies.

Commentary

The Euro-D allows comparison of risk factor profiles for later life depression between European centres. When different European centres use different tools to measure depression it can be difficult to compare. Euro-D was developed to achieve consistency by collecting data derived from a variety of depression measures for the purpose of multicentre collaborative analysis of putative risk factors for late life depression. Euro-D was derived from a variety of depressive scales. The scale has 12 items originally from the Geriatric Mental State Schedule (Copeland et al 1976). The Euro-D is able to identify cases of depression with adequate sensitivity and specificity. Its validity has not, however, been checked against truly independent criteria, only other established scales.

Additional references

Copeland JR, Kelleher MJ, Kellett JM et al (1976) A semi-structured interview for the assessment of diagnosis and mental state in the elderly: the Geriatric Mental State Schedule. I. Development and reliability. *Psychological Medicine* 6: 439–49.

Prince MJ, Reischies F, Beekman ATF, Fuhrer R, Jonker C, Kivela S-L, Lawlor BA, Lobo A, Magnusson H, Fichter M, van Oyen H, Roelands M, Skoog I, Turrina C, Copeland JRM (1999) Development of the EURO-D scale – a European Union initiative to compare symptoms of depresson in 14 European countries. *British Journal of Psychiatry* 174: 330–8.

Address for correspondence

Professor Martin Prince
Section of Epidemiology & General Practice
Institute of Psychiatry
De Crespigny Park
Denmark Hill
London SE5 8AF
UK

Brief Assessment Scale for Depression

Reference: **Allen N, Amers D, Ashby D, Bennetts K, Tuckwell V, West C (1994) A Brief Sensitive Screening Instrument for Depression in Late Life.** *Age and Ageing* **23: 213–18**

Time taken 5–10 minutes (author's estimate)

Rating by experienced interviewer

Main indications

To measure depression.

Commentary

The Brief Assessment Scale consists of two scales that form part of the DEP scale and the Organic Brain Syndrome Scale (OBS) of the Comprehensive Assessment and Referral Evaluation (CARE). The DEP Scale of the BAS (BAS-DEP) consists of 21 items which are rated as the symptoms either being present or absent, with one rated on a three-point scale and another rated on a four-point scale, giving a total range of 0–24, with a cut-off point of 6/7 being suggested to indicate the presence or not of a significantly depressed state.

In this study the BAS-DEP was administered to a large population of people in local authority homes in London and Melbourne.

The need for a shorter scale of fewer than 10 items, with a higher level of internal consistency and having some form of internal logic, was deemed to be appropriate, and so the EBAS-DEP, i.e. the Even Briefer Assessment Scale for Depression, was derived consisting of 8 items with a total score of 8 (each being simply marked as either present or absent) with a score of 3 indicating the probable presence of depression. Comparison of the short and long scales and validation of the shorter scale was satisfactory, with acceptable sensitivity and specificity being achieved compared to the gold standard of the GMSS-Agecat programme (see page 279). Cronbach's alpha score was above 8 and sensitivity and specificity against a diagnosis of DSM-III-R mood disorder were 0.91 and 0.72, respectively.

A German version of the EBAS-DEP is also being developed.

Additional reference

Weyerer S, Killmann T, Ames D, Allen N (1999) The Even Briefer Assessment Scale for Depression (EBAS DEP): its suitability for the elderly in geriatric care in English- and German-speaking countries. *International Journal of Geriatric Psychiatry* 14: 473–80.

Address for correspondence

Professor David Ames
Department of Psychiatry
7th Floor
Charles Connibere Building
Royal Melbourne Hospital
Victoria 3050
Australia

Item no.	Description	Score if present
1	Admits to worrying in last month	1
*2	Worries about almost everything	1
3	Sad or depressed mood in last month	1
*4	Depression lasts longer than a few hours	1
*5	Depression worst at beginning of day	1
6	Has felt life not worth living in last month	1
7	Has not felt happy in last month	1
*8	Bothered and depressed by current loneliness	1
9	Almost nothing enjoyed lately	
10	Less enjoyment than 1 year ago	1
*11	Less enjoyment because depressed/nervous	1
*12	Has had episodes of depression longer than 1 week in duration prior to past year	1
13	Reports headaches in past month	1
*14	Poor appetite in the absence of medical cause	1
15	Slowed in physical movement compared to 1 year ago	1
*16	Difficulty sleeping due to altered moods, thoughts or tension	1
17	Has cried or felt like crying in past month	1
18i	Pessimistic or empty expectations of future	1†
ii	Thinks future bleak or unbearable	2
19i	Has wished to be dead in past month	1†
ii	Suicidal thoughts	2†
iii	Serious consideration of methods of suicide or actual attempts in past month	3
*20	Obvious self-blame present	1
21	Describes self as not very happy/not at all happy (opposed to fairly or very happy)	1

*Lead-in questions required.
†Items 18 and 19 can score >1 point.

Items of the depression scale of the BAS (maximum score)

1 *Admits to worrying (1)*
2 *Worries about almost everything (1)*
3 *Sad or depressed mood during past month (1)*
4 Depression lasts longer than a few hours (1)
5 Depression worst in the morning (1)
6 *Felt life wasn't worth living (1)*
7 Has cried or felt like crying (1)
8 Pessimistic or bleak future (2)
9 Suicidal thoughts or attempts (3)
10 *Wasn't happy in the past month (1)*
11 *Bothered and depressed by current loneliness (1)*

12 Enjoyed almost nothing (1)
13 Less enjoyment in activities than previously (1)
14 Loss of interest/enjoyment because of depression/nervousness (1)
15 Regrets about life or self-blame (1)
16 Episodes of depression lasting over a week prior to past year (1)
17 Reports headaches (1)
18 *Poor appetite in the absence of obvious medical cause (1)*
19 *Has become slowed down in movements (1)*
20 Sleep disorders due to moods (1)
21 *Not very happy at all (1)*

Notes:
1. Range: 0 (no depression)–24 (severe depression).
2. Italic type: items selected for EBAS DEP (Allen et al, 1994).

Source: Reproduced with permission from Allen N et al. Age and Ageing 1994; **23**: 213–18.

The Even Briefer Assessment Scale for Depression (EBAS-DEP)

Reference: **Weyerer S, Killmann T, Ames D, Allen N (1999) The Even Briefer Assessment Scale for Depression (EBAS DEP): its suitability for the elderly in geriatric care in English- and German-speaking countries.** *International Journal of Geriatric Psychiatry* 14: 473–80

Time taken 3–5 minutes

Rating by experienced interviewer

Main indications

To measure depression.

Commentary

A screening test for depression in later life.

Summary

The Even Briefer Assessment Scale for Depression (EBAS-DEP) was derived from the Brief Assessment Scale for Depression (see opposite). Eight of the original 21 items from the BAS-DEP were selected based on internal consistency. It has been validated against the psychiatric diagnosis of depression according to DSM-III-R mood disorder. It can be used to screen for depression in the elderly in both hospital and primary care settings.

EBAS-DEP (Even Briefer Assessment Scale for Depression)

The 8 items of this schedule require raters to make a judgement as to whether the proposition in the middle column is satisfied or not. If a proposition is satisfied then a depressive symptom is present and raters should ring '1' in the right-hand column, otherwise '0' should be ringed. Each question in the left-hand column must be asked exactly as printed but follow-up or subsidiary questions may be used to clarify the initial answer until the rater can make a clear judgement as to whether the proposition is satisfied or not. For items which enquire about symptoms over the past month, note that the symptom need not have been present for the entire month nor at the moment of interview, but it should have been a problem for the patient or troubled him/her for some of the past month.

	Question	Assessment	Rating	
1.	Do you worry? In the past month?	Admits to worrying in past month	1	0
2.	Have you beed sad or depressed in the past month?	Has had sad or depressed mood during the past month	1	0
3.	During the past month have you *ever* felt that life was not worth living?	Has felt that life was not worth living at some time during the past month	1	0
4.	How do you feel about your future? What are your hopes for the future?	Pessimistic about the future or has empty expectations (i.e. nothing to look forward to)	1	0
5.	During the past month have you at any time felt you would rather be dead?	Has wished to be dead at any time during past month	1	0
6.	Do you enjoy things as much as you used to – say like you did a year ago?	Less enjoyment in activities than a year previously	1	0
	If question 6 rated 0, then rate 0 for question 7 and skip to question 8. If question 6 rated 1, ask question 7.			
7.	Is it because you are depressed or nervous that you don't enjoy things as much?	Loss of enjoyment because of depression/nervousness	1	0
8.	In general how happy are you? (*Read out*) Are you – very happy – fairly happy – not very happy *or* not happy at all?	Not very happy or not happy at all	1	0

Total score /8

A score of 3 or greater indicates the probable presence of a depressive disorder which may need treatment and the patient should be assessed in more detail or referred for psychiatric evaluation.

Source: Weyerer S et al. *Int J Geriatr Psychiatry* 1999; **14**: 473–80. Reproduced by permission of John Wiley & Sons, Inc. © 1999.

Short Anxiety Screening Test

Reference: **Sinoff G, Ore L, Zlotogorsky D, Tamir A (1999) Short Anxiety Screening Test – a brief instrument for detecting anxiety in the elderly.** *International Journal of Geriatric Psychiatry* 14: 1062–71

Time taken 10–15 minutes

Rating by experienced interviewer

Main indications

To screen for the presence of anxiety in people over 70.

Commentary

The SAST has 10 questions graded from 1 to 4, with the suggestion that a score of 24 or over will indicate the presence of significant anxiety (based on a previous pilot study). As well as including questions found to lead to anxiety in DSM-IV, those relating to somatic symptoms were incorporated to reflect the author's belief in the importance of somatic complaints in the manifestation of anxiety in older people. The Zung Rating Scale and modified Anxiety Disorders Interview Schedule for DSM-IV were included and 312 people were assessed as part of the study. The SAST was rated at having 75.4% sensitivity, 78.7% specificity, 70.8% positive predictive value and 82.4% negative predictive value. Inter-rater test–retest reliability was very high. The SAST was effective at diagnosing anxiety even in the presence of comorbid depression.

Address for correspondence

Dr G Sinoff
Department of Geriatrics
Carmel Medical Center
7 Michal Street
Haifa 34 362
Israel
sinoff@netvision.net.il

Chapter 2

Dementia

Chapter 2a

Cognitive Assessment

The syndrome of dementia comprises three core features: a neuropsychological deficit which is progressive over time, neuropsychiatric features (sometimes called non-cognitive features and consisting of behavioural disturbances and psychiatric symptoms) and disabilities in activities of daily living (ADL).

The quantification of neuropsychological testing began in recognizable terms, in Newcastle, in the 1950s with work by Roth and Hopkins describing questions about orientation, memory and attention/concentration. These early ideas were later incorporated into the Blessed Dementia Scale (page 46) (which comprised the Information/Memory and Concentration (IMC) test, the ADL and personality change score). It was these studies that confirmed that the dementia occurring in elderly people shared the same pathology as Alzheimer's disease (until then considered a disease of younger people). They also related the severity of disease in life to the plaque count in the cerebral cortex, leading to the recognition that the pathology was related to the clinical signs of the disease, suggesting a connection between the two. The Mental Test Score (page 44) was developed from the Blessed IMC test, shortened to the Abbreviated Mental Test Score (AMTS; page 44) in a ten- or nine-item version (depending on whether another person was available for the purpose of recognition). A seven-item score was developed, and a six-item test (in the USA), the latter validated against neuropathological findings.

In the USA, Marshal Folstein published the Mini-Mental State Examination (MMSE; page 36), which has probably become the most widely used test, with a standardized version published recently which has gained wide acceptance. Jacobs produced another screening test around the same time, but it did not catch on. The Kew Cognitive Test (page 73) attempted to measure parietal lobe signs in addition to memory loss. Several other tests have also been published which measure cognition. These include the Face–Hand Test (FHT; page 75), the SET Test (page 66) and the Brief Cognitive Rating Scale (BCRS; page 61). Cognitive sections appear in a host of other instruments, such as the Structured Interview for the Diagnosis of the Alzheimer's Type and Multi-infarct Dementia and Dementias of other Aetiology (SIDAM; page 275) and the Geriatric Mental State Schedule (GMSS; page 279). The Alzheimer's Disease Assessment Scale (ADAS; page 48) contains cognitive and non-cognitive items, and the cogni-

tive section has become the gold standard of cognitive scales used in pharmaceutical trials (and is available in parallel forms). The cognitive section of the CAMDEX (page 286) (the CAMCOG) has also been widely used and validated against other measures in both clinical and community samples. The Clifton Assessment Procedures for the Elderly (CAPE; page 56) combines a cognitive and a behavioural score, the former being popular in general practice. Other cognitive tests include the Syndrom Kurztest (SKT; page 69) (which takes 15 minutes to administer), the Mattis Dementia Rating Scale (page 50) and the Severe Impairment Battery (SIB; page 74) (which can be used in the later stages of dementia to assess cognitive function). Computerized tests are also available for specialist use (the Cambridge Neuropsychological Test Automated Battery (CANTAB; page 63) and the Cognitive Drug Research Assessment System (COG-DRAS; page 71)), but with the more widespread use of computers, screening tests may become available.

Time constraints for primary care mean that one of the shorter versions is best for the assessment of cognitive function. To obtain a formal score, the Mini-Mental State Examination (MMSE; page 36) (probably the standardized version) or the much shorter AMTS (page 44) is preferred, with more detailed investigation required if the patient scores below the cut-off point. The ADAS and the CAMCOG are too lengthy for anything other than specialist use. The Clock Drawing Test (page 51) has become very popular because of its ease of use and non-threatening method of administration. This is an important aspect because traditional cognitive testing is often perceived as inappropriate, with questions being asked in a didactic manner and given little or no introduction. Testing cognitive function can be as skilled an interview technique as enquiring about delusions and hallucinations, and introducing the test with an explanation (and sometimes apologetically, if necessary) can usually secure co-operation. The use of autobiographical questions found in some early scales (e.g. asking the name of the person's school) has been used as a way around this, but the inability of the interviewer to verify the answers is a great drawback and the practicalities of obtaining an informant make this unworkable. The recently published 7 Minute Neurocognitive Screening Battery (page 77) promises much, but the lack of easily identifiable cut-offs means more work needs to be done before it is widely accepted.

Mini-Mental State Examination (MMSE)

Reference: **Folstein MF, Folstein SE, McHugh PR (1975) 'Mini-Mental State': a practical method for grading the cognitive state of patients for the clinician.** *Journal of Psychiatric Research* **12: 189–98**

Time taken 10 minutes

Rating by interview (some training desirable)

Main indications

Rating of cognitive function.

Commentary

The Mini-Mental State Examination (MMSE) is probably the most widely used measure of cognitive function. Much has been written about the MMSE and amendments have been suggested such as the Standardized Mini-Mental State Examination (SMMSE; page 40) (Molloy et al, 1991) and the Modified Mini-Mental State Examination (MMMSE) (Teng et al, 1987). A recent review of the MMSE detailed the particular measures of test/retest reliability, internal consistency and assessment of recognized cut-off points (Tombaugh and McIntyre, 1992). The MMSE has been suggested as being helpful in the early diagnosis of Alzheimer's disease with the addition of a verbal fluency test (Galasko et al, 1990), and the limits of the MMSE as a screening test have also been discussed (Anthony et al, 1982). Population norms have been reproduced (Crum et al, 1993). An analysis of the scale with a commentary by the original author has been published (Burns et al, 1998). The original paper showed that the MMSE was created to differentiate organic from functional organic disorders, and could be used as a quantitative measure of cognitive impairment in an attempt to measure change but was not intended to be used in any diagnostic sense. The authors noted originally that one of the uses of the MMSE was in teaching psychiatric trainees to become skilled in the evaluation of cognitive aspects of the mental state. The 'Mini' qualification was added because no aspects of mood, abnormal mental experiences or disordered forms of thinking were measured. The MMSE has a maximum score of 30 points, with different domains assessed: orientation to time and place (10 points), registration of three words (3 points), attention and calculation (5 points) recall of three words (3 points), language (8 points) and visual construction (1 point). Variations have included different words, e.g. *shirt,* *tree, rose, elephant* and *dog,* and great debate has surrounded whether serial 7 or spelling the word *world* backwards should be used. The original validity and reliability of the MMSE were based on 206 patients with a variety of psychiatric disorders, the scale successfully separating those with dementia, depression, and those with depression and cognitive impairment. A correlation of 0.78 was found with the Weschler adult intelligence scale for verbal IQ and 0.66 for performance IQ. Test/retest reliability was 0.89 and a combination of test/retest and inter-rater reliability was 0.83. Details of extensive subsequent validity and reliabililty studies are described by Tombaugh and McIntyre (1992).

Lowenstein et al (2000) tested the utility of an additional delayed recall of the 3 items a screening test for mild cognitive impairment. Extended delayed recall of the 3 items was at 5 minute intervals. Sensitivity of 83.3% and specificity of 90% was achieved in differentiating cases with mild cognitive impairment from individuals with normal cognition.

Additional references

Anthony J, LeResche L, Niaz U et al (1982) Limits of the 'Mini-Mental State' as a screening test for dementia and delirium among hospital patients. *Psychological Medicine* 12: 397–408.

Burns A, Brayne C, Folstein M (1998) Mini-Mental State: a practical method for grading the cognitive state of patients for the clinician. *International Journal of Psychiatry in Geriatric Practice* 134: 285–94.

Crum R et al (1993) Population-based norms for the Mini-Mental State Examination by age and educational level. *Journal of the American Medical Association* 18: 2386–91.

Galasko D, Klauber MR, Hofstetter CR et al (1990) The Mini-Mental State Examination in the early diagnosis of Alzheimer's disease. *Archives of Neurology* 47: 49–52.

Lowenstein DA, Barker WW, Harwood DG et al (2000) Utility of a modified MMSE with extended delayed recall in screening for mild cognitive impairment among community dwelling elders. *International Journal of Geriatric Psychiatry* 15: 434–40.

Molloy DW, Alemanelin E, Robert R (1991) Reliability of a standardized Mini-Mental State Examination compared with the traditional Mini-Mental State Examination. *American Journal of Psychiatry* **148**: 102–5.

Teng EL, Chang Chui H, Schneider LS et al (1987) Alzheimer's dementia: performance on the Mini-Mental State Examination. *Journal of Consulting and Clinical Psychology* **55**: 96–100.

Tombaugh TN, McIntyre NJ (1992) The Mini-Mental State Examination: a comprehensive review. *Journal of the American Geriatrics Society* **40**: 922–35.

Address for correspondence

Marshal Folstein
Department of Psychiatry
Tufts University School of Medicine
NEMC #1007
750 Washington Street
Boston
MA 02111
USA

www.nemc.org/psych/mmse.asp

The Severe MMSE

Reference: Harrell LE, Marson D, Chatterjee A, Parrish JA (2000) The Severe Mini-Mental State Examination: a new neuropsychological instrument for the bedside assessment of severely impaired patients with Alzheimer's disease. *Alzheimer Disease and Associated Disorders* 14: 168–75

Time taken 5–10 minutes

Rating by experienced interviewer

Main indications

The Severe Mini-Mental State Examination (SMMSE) (not to be confused with the Standardized Mini-Mental State Examination) was devised in an attempt to have a readily usable assessment of cognitive abilities in moderately to severely impaired patients with Alzheimer's disease.

Commentary

The SMMSE and the MMSE were administered to 182 patients with Alzheimer's disease. Performance on the two was found to be significantly correlated when the MMSE score fell below 9 points, but even as performance on the MMSE reached floor levels, patients still had a score on the SMMSE. Test–retest performance was shown to be stable over 5 months and inter-rater reliability was excellent. Construct and criterion validity was good, and scores on the scale correlated well with global ratings of dementia.

Address for correspondence

Lindy E Harrell
Professor of Neurology
Director, Alzheimer's Disease Center
The University of Alabama at Birmingham
454 Sparks Center
1720 Seventh Avenue South
Birmingham
AL 35294-0017
USA

The Severe Mini-Mental State Examination with Associated Scores for Each Item

Name: (1 point if close; 3 if completely accurate)
    First _____
    Last _____
Birthday: (1 point if any elements correct; 2 points if completely accurate)

    _____

Repeat three words (1 point for each word)
    Bird _____
    House _____
    Umbrella _____
Follow simple directions: (1 point for following command; 2 points for continuing to hold command (i.e. 5 seconds) until told to stop)
    Raise your hand _____
    Close your eyes _____
Name simple objects: (1 point for each object)
    Pen _____
    Watch _____
    Shoe _____

Draw circle from command: (1 point)
    Circle _____
Copy square: (1 point)
    Square _____
Write name: (1 point if close; 2 points if completely accurate)
    First _____
    Last _____
Animal generation: (number of animals in 1 minute)
    1–2 Animals: 1 point
    3–4 Animals: 2 points
    >4 Animals: 3 points
Spell 'CAT' forward: (1 point for each letter given in correct order)
    C _____
    A _____
    T _____

Scoring Rules for the Severe Mini-Mental State Examination

Question 1: The patient is asked to state his or her first and last names. Three points are given for each correct answer. Women, if married, must give married name.

Question 2: The patient is asked to state the month, day, and year of birth. Any order is acceptable. Two points if completely correct. One point for any of the three items.

Question 3: The examiner tells the patient that he/she is going to say three words and then ask the patient to repeat them. The examiner then says, 'bird, house, umbrella', and asks the patient to repeat them. One point is given for each correctly named item.

Question 4: The examiner shows the patient three items, one at a time, and asks the patient to name it. A pen, watch, and shoe are then shown to the patient. One point is given for each correctly named item.

Question 5: The patient is asked to follow a direction (for 5 seconds). The first direction is 'shut your eyes'; the second is 'raise your hand' (either or both hands acceptable). Two points are given for each direction if the patient follows and continues the command until told to stop by the examiner. One point is given for each command if the patient follows the command but does not maintain it until told to stop by the examiner.

Question 6: The patient is given a clean sheet of paper and a pen and is asked to write (printing or cursive acceptable) his or her first and last name. Two points are awarded for each item if totally correct and legible, one point if poorly legible or if letters are left out. Women must write their married last name.

Question 7: The patient is verbally asked to draw a circle. One point if the item drawn resembles a circle, i.e. it must be closed, may be somewhat elliptical, any size acceptable.

Question 8: A copy of a square is presented to the patient, and he/she is asked to copy it. The examiner should not identify the square orally. One point is given if the copy has four sides that touch: rectangular-appearing squares are acceptable.

Question 9: The patient is asked to generate as many animals as he/she can think of in 1 minute. One point is given for up to two animals, two points for up to four animals, three points for more than four animals.

Question 10: The patient is asked to spell the word 'CAT'. Letters must be in correct order. One point is given for each correct letter.

Source: Harrell LE et al. Alzheimer's Dis Assoc Disor 2000; 14: 168–75. Reproduced by permission.

Standardized Mini-Mental State Examination (SMMSE)

Reference: **Molloy DW, Alemayehu E, Roberts R (1991) Reliability of a Standardized Mini-Mental State Examination compared with the traditional Mini-Mental State Examination.** *American Journal of Psychiatry* **148: 102–5**

Time taken 5–10 minutes

Rating by interviewer, preferably with some training

Main indications

As per MMSE.

Commentary

The Standardized Mini-Mental State Examination (SMMSE) was developed in an attempt to improve the objectivity of the original MMSE (page 36), which, in the authors' experience, varied greatly. Up to six raters assessed eight elderly patients on three different occasions 1 week apart and, using a one-way analysis of variance, estimated inter-rater variance and intrarater variance. Inter- and intrarater variance were reduced by 86% and 76% respectively when the SMMSE was used and the intraclass correlation rose from 0.69 to 0.90. The SMMSE took slightly less time to administer than the MMSE (10.5 minutes compared with 13.4 minutes; Molloy and Standish, 1997).

Essentially, the SMMSE comes with more specific instructions as to how the scale will be measured, with specific examples of the scoring of the figures and spelling *world* backwards. Ball, car and man are three objects used, with alternatives provided for repeated testing.

A slightly expanded, modified Mini-Mental State (3MS) is also available (page 42) (Teng and Chiu, 1987).

Additional references

Molloy DW, Standish TIM (1997) A guide to the Standardized Mini-Mental State Examination. *International Psychogeriatrics* 9(Suppl 1): 37–43.

Teng E, Chiu C (1987) The modified mini-mental state. *Journal of Clinical Psychiatry* **48**: 314–18.

Address for correspondence

DW Molloy
Geriatric Research Group
McMaster University
Hamilton Civic Hospitals
Henderson General Division
711 Concession Street
Hamilton
Ontario L8V 1C3
Canada

Standardized Mini-Mental State Examination (SMMSE)

I am going to ask you some questions and give you some problems to solve. Please try to answer as best as you can.

Max Score

1. **(Allow 10 seconds for each reply)**
a) What year is this?   1
(accept exact answer only)
b) What season is this?   1
(during last week of the old season or first week of a new season, accept either season)
c) What month of the year is this?   1
(on the first day of new month, or last day of the previous month, accept either)
d) What is today's date?   1
(accept previous or next date, e.g. on the 7th accept the 6th or 8th)
e) What day of the week is this?   1
(accept exact answer only)

2. **(Allow 10 seconds for each reply)**
a) What country are we in?   1
(accept exact answer only)
b) What province/state/county are we in?   1
(accept exact answer only)
c) What city/town are we in?   1
(accept exact answer only)
d) **(In clinic)** What is the name of this hospital/building?   1
(accept exact name of hospital or institution only)
(In home) What is the street address of this house?   1
(accept street name and house number or equivalent in rural areas)
e) **(In clinic)** What floor of the building are we on?   1
(accept exact answer only)
(In home) What room are we in?   1
(accept exact answer only)

3. I am going to name 3 objects. After I have said all three objects, I want you to repeat them. Remember what they are because I am going to ask you to name them again in a few minutes.   3
(say them slowly at approximately 1 second intervals)

Ball   **Car**   **Man**

For repeated use:

Bell	**Jar**	**Fan**
Bill	**Tar**	**Can**
Bull	**War**	**Pan**

Please repeat the 3 items for me.
(score 1 point for each correct reply on the first attempt)
Allow 20 seconds for reply, if subject did not repeat all 3, repeat until they are learned or up to a maximum of 5 times.

4. Spell the word WORLD.   5
(you may help subject to spell world correctly)
Say **now spell it backwards please**. *Allow 30 seconds to spell backwards. (If the subject cannot spell world even with assistance – score 0.)*

5. Now what were the 3 objects that I asked you to remember? **3**

Ball   **Car**   **Man**

Score 1 point for each correct response regardless of order, allow 10 seconds.

6. Show wristwatch. Ask: what is this called?   1
Score 1 point for correct response. Accept 'wristwatch' or 'watch'. Do not accept 'clock', 'time', etc. (allow 10 seconds).

7. Show pencil. Ask: what is this called?   1
Score 1 point for correct response, accept pencil only – score 0 for pen.

8. I'd like you to repeat a phrase after me: "no if's, and's or but's".   1
(allow 10 seconds for response. Score 1 point for a correct repetition. Must be **exact**, e.g. no if's or but's – score 0)

9. Read the words on this page and then do what it says: Hand subject the laminated sheet with CLOSE YOUR EYES on it.   1

CLOSE YOUR EYES

If subject just reads and does not then close eyes – you may repeat: read the words on this page and then do what it says to a maximum of 3 times. Allow 10 seconds, score 1 point **only** if subject closes eyes. Subject does not have to read aloud.

10. Ask if the subject is right or left handed. Alternate right/left hand in statement, e.g. if the subject is right-handed say **Take this paper in your left hand** . . . Take a piece of paper – hold it up in front of subject and say the following: 3

'Try this paper in your right/left hand, fold the paper in half once with both hands and put the paper down on the floor'.

Takes paper in correct hand	1
Folds it in half	1
Puts it on the floor	1

Allow 30 seconds. Score 1 point for each instruction correctly executed.

11. Hand subject a pencil and paper.   1
Write any complete sentence on that piece of paper.
Allow 30 seconds. Score 1 point. The sentence should make sense. Ignore spelling errors.

12. Place design, pencil, eraser and paper in front of the subject.   1
Say: copy this design please.
Allow multiple tries until patient is finished and hands it back. Score 1 point for correctly copied diagram. The subject must have drawn a 4-sided figure between two 5-sided figures. Maximum time – 1 minute.

Total Test Score   **30**

Reproduced (with the permission of the Geriatric Research Group) from Molloy DW, Alemayehu E, Roberts R (1991) Reliability of a Standardized Mini-Mental State Examination compared with the traditional Mini-Mental State Examination. *American Journal of Psychiatry,* Vol. 140, pp. 102–5.

The Modified MMSE (3MS) Examination

Reference **Teng EI, Chui HC (1987) The Modified Mini Mental State (3MS) Examination.** *Journal of Clinical Psychiatry* **48: 314–18**

Time taken around 10 minutes

Rating by experienced interviewer

Main indications

The Modified MMSE was designed to sample a broader range of cognitive function than the traditional MMSE.

Commentary

The 3MS was designed to broaden the usefulness of the MMSE across a range of cognitive function. Four test items were added, some change in the item content and order of administration with more standardized testing procedures were adopted. The main objectives of the modifications were to extend the ceiling and floor effect of the test, to sample a wider range of cognitive abilities and to enhance the reliability and validity of the scores. The range is broadened from 0–30 to 0–100.

Details on the exact administration and scoring are relatively complex and are contained in the original paper.

Additional reference

Lowenstein DA, Barker WW, Harwood DG (2000) Utility of a modified MMSE with extended delayed recall in screening for mild cognitive impairment among community dwelling elders. *International Journal of Geriatric Psychiatry* 15: 434–40.

Subject _____ , _____ / _____ / _____ Examiner _____
                                                     yr   mo   d

Normal or DX _____ Age _____ Edu _____ M F 3MS _____ MMS _____
                                          yrs   yrs   100   30

3MS MMS

5̄

DATE and PLACE OF BIRTH   1̄0

Date: year _____, month _____, day _____
Place: town _____, state _____   6̄

3̄ 3̄

REGISTRATION (No. of presentations: _____)

SHIRT, BROWN, HONESTY
(or: SHOES, BLACK, MODESTY)
(or: SOCKS, BLUE, CHARITY)

7̄ 5̄

MENTAL REVERSAL

5 to 1
Accurate   2
1 or 2 errors/misses   0 1
DLROW   5̄ 1̄
            0 1 2 3 4 5

9̄ 3̄

FIRST RECALL

Spontaneous recall   3
After 'Something to wear'   2
'SHOES, SHIRT, SOCKS'   0 1   3̄ 1̄
Spontaneous recall   3
After 'A colour'   2
'BLUE, BLACK, BROWN'   0 1
Spontaneous recall   3
After 'A good personal quality' 2
'HONESTY, CHARITY, MODESTY' 0 1   5̄ 1̄

1̄5 5̄

TEMPORAL ORIENTATION

Year
Accurate   8   1̄0 1̄
Missed by 1 year   4
Missed by 2–5 years   0 2
Season
Accurate or within 1 month   0 1
Month
Accurate or within 5 days   2
Missed by 1 month   0 1
Day of month
Accurate   3
Missed by 1 or 2 days   2
Missed by 3–5 days   0 1   3̄ 3̄
Day of week
Accurate   0 1

5̄ 5̄

SPATIAL ORIENTATION

State   0 2
County   0 1   9̄
City (town)   0 1
HOSPITAL/OFFICE BUILDING/HOME? 0 1
NAMING (MMS: Pencil ___, Watch ___)

5̄ 2̄

Forehead ___, Chin ___, Shoulder ___
Elbow ___, Knuckle ___

FOUR-LEGGED ANIMALS (30 seconds) 1 point each

SIMILARITIES

Arm-Leg
Body part; limb; etc.   2
Less correct answer   0 1
Laughing-Crying
Feeling; emotion   2
Other correct answer   0 1
Eating-Sleeping
Essential for life   2
Other correct answer   0 1

REPETITION

'I WOULD LIKE TO GO HOME/OUT.'   2
1 or 2 missed/wrong words   0 1
'NO IFS ___ ANDS ___ OR BUTS ___'

READ AND OBEY 'CLOSE YOUR EYES'

Obeys without prompting   3
Obeys after prompting   2
Reads aloud only   0 1
(spontaneously or by request)

WRITING (1 minute)

(I) WOULD LIKE TO GOME HOME/OUT.
(MMS: Spontaneous sentence: 0 1)

COPYING TWO PENTAGONS (1 minute)

                                    Each Pentagon
5 approximately equal sides   4   4
5 unequal (.>2:1) sides   3   3
Other enclosed figure   2   2
2 or more lines   01 01
                                    Intersection
4 corners   2
Not-4-corner enclosure   0 1

THREE-STAGE COMMAND

___ TAKE THIS PAPER WITH YOUR
     LEFT/RIGHT HAND
___ FOLD IT IN HALF, AND
___ HAND IT BACK TO ME

SECOND RECALL

(Something to wear)   0 1 2 3
(Color)   0 1 2 3
(Good personal quality)   0 1 2 3

Source: Reproduced with permission from Teng EI, Chui HC. *J Clin Psychiatry* 1987; **48**: 314–18.

Mental Test Score (MTS)/Abbreviated Mental Test Score (AMTS)

References: **Hodkinson M (1972) Evaluation of a mental test score for assessment of mental impairment in the elderly.** *Age and Ageing* **1: 233–8**

Time taken MTS, 10 minutes; AMTS, 3 minutes

Rating by clinician

Main indications

A brief test to screen for cognitive impairment in the elderly.

Commentary

The Mental Test Score (MTS) was developed from the Blessed Dementia Scale (page 46), and was used in a study of over 700 patients carried out under the auspices of the Royal College of Physicians. A previous study had shown that a score of 25 and above (out of 34) was within the normal range; and the important point was made (but is often forgotten) that tests such as these do not discriminate between dementia and delirium – although longitudinal follow-up will provide quantitative changes in mental test performance. Graphic displays in the paper demonstrated questions of high and low discriminating ability. On this basis, the Abbreviated Mental Test Score (AMTS) was developed, showing that the results corresponded closely with that of the full score. The AMTS

is scored out of 10 or, if there is not the facility to carry out the recognition question, out of 9. A cut-off score of 7 or 8 out of 10 (6 or 7 out of 9) is suggested to discriminate between a cognitive impairment and normality. Qureshi and Hodkinson (1974) further validated the questionnaire in patients over the age of 60 with comparisons against the Roth and Hopkins (1953) and Denham and Jeffries (1972) questionnaires.

Additional references

Qureshi K, Hodkinson M (1974) Evaluation of a 10 question mental test of the institutionalized elderly. *Age and Ageing* **3**: 152–7

Roth M, Hopkins B (1953) Psychological test performance in patients over 60. Senile psychosis and affective disorders of old age. *Journal of Mental Science* **99**: 439–50.

Denham MJ, Jeffries PM (1972) Routine mental assessment in elderly patients. *Modern Geriatrics* **2**: 275–9.

Mental Test Score (MTS)/Abbreviated Mental Test Score

ORIGINAL TEST ITEMS

	Score
Name	0/1
Age	0/1
Time (to nearest hour)	0/1
Time of day	0/1
Name and address for five minutes recall; this should be repeated by the patient to ensure it has been heard correctly.	
Mr John Brown	0/1/2
42 West Street	0/1/2
Gateshead	0/1
Day of week	0/1
Date (correct day of month)	0/1
Month	0/1
Year	0/1
Place: Type of place (i.e. Hospital)	0/1
Name of Hospital	0/1
Name of ward	0/1
Name of town	0/1
Recognition of two persons (doctor, nurse, etc.)	0/1/2
Date of birth (day and month sufficient)	0/1
Place of birth (town)	0/1
School attended	0/1
Former occupation	0/1

Name of wife, sib or next of kin	0/1
Date of First World War (year sufficient)	0/1
Date of Second World War (date sufficient)	0/1
Name of present Monarch	0/1
Name of present Prime Minister	0/1
Months of year backwards	0/1/2
Count 1–20	0/1/2
Count 20–1	0/1/2
Total	(34)

ABBREVIATED MENTAL TEST SCORE

1. Age
2. Time (to nearest hour)
3. Address for recall at end of test – this should be repeated by the patient to ensure it has been heard correctly: 42 West Street
4. Year
5. Name of hospital
6. Recognition of two persons (doctor, nurse, ...)
7. Date of birth
8. Year of First World War
9. Name of present Monarch
10. Count backwards 20–1

(each question scores one mark)

Source: Hodkinson M (1972) Evaluation of a mental test score for assessment of mental impairment in the elderly. *Age and Ageing* 1: 233–8. By kind permission of Oxford University Press.

Blessed Dementia Scale (incorporating the Information–Memory–Concentration (IMC) Test and the Dementia Scale)

Reference: **Blessed G, Tomlinson BE, Roth M (1968) The association between quantitative measures of dementia and of senile change in the cerebral grey matter of elderly subjects.** *British Journal of Psychiatry* 114: 797–811

Time taken 30 minutes (reviewer's estimate)

Rating structured questions by observer

Main indications

Assessment of cognition and behaviour in people with dementia.

Commentary

The Blessed Dementia Scale was designed to assess quantitatively the signs of dementia to enable comparisons to be made with pathological changes. The scale is divided into two: the information–memory–concentration test (IMC) and the dementia scale. The latter incorporates changes in everyday performance habits and personality. The test has been shown to differentiate groups of demented and non-demented older persons (Roth and Hopkins, 1953; Shapiro et al, 1956). Correlation of senile plaque count and the dementia score was 0.77 and against the test score 0.59, both highly significant (on 60 patients, the direction of correlation was in keeping with the hypothesis that more pathological changes were associated with worse clinical signs). The Blessed study is one of the key papers of old age psychiatry, showing for the first time that clinical functions of dementia are related to neuropathological changes.

Additional references

Roth M, Hopkins B (1953) Psychological test performance in patients over 60. 1. Senile psychosis and the affective disorders of old age. *Journal of Mental Science* **99**: 439.

Shapiro MB, Post F, Löfving B et al (1956) 'Memory function' in psychiatric patients over sixty; some methodological and diagnostic implications. *Journal of Mental Science* **102**: 233.

www.strokecenter.org/trials/blessed_dementia.html

Blessed Dementia Scale

Changes in performance of everyday activities

1.	Inability to perform household tasks	I	½	0
2.	Inability to cope with small sums of money	I	½	0
3.	Inability to remember short list of items, e.g. in shopping	I	½	0
4.	Inability to find way about indoors	I	½	0
5.	Inability to find way about familiar streets	I	½	0
6.	Inability to interpret surroundings (e.g. to recognize whether in hospital, or at home, to discriminate between patients, doctors and nurses, relatives and hospital staff, etc)	I	½	0
7.	Inability to recall recent events (e.g. recent outings, visits of relatives or friends to hospital, etc.)	I	½	0
8.	Tendency to dwell in the past	I	½	0

Changes in habits

9.	Eating:	
	Cleanly with proper utensils	0
	Messily with spoon only	2
	Simple solids, e.g. biscuits	2
	Has to be fed	3
10.	Dressing:	
	Unaided	0
	Occasionally misplaced buttons, etc.	I
	Wrong sequence, commonly forgetting items	2
	Unable to dress	3
11.	Complete sphincter control	0
	Occasional wet beds	I
	Frequent wet beds	2
	Doubly incontinent	3

Changes in personality, interests, drive

	No change	0
12.	Increased rigidity	I
13.	Increased egocentricity	I
14.	Impairment of regard for feelings of others	I
15.	Coarsening of affect	I
16.	Impairment of emotional control, e.g. increased petulance and irritability	I
17.	Hilarity in inappropriate situations	I
18.	Diminished emotional responsiveness	I
19.	Sexual misdemeanour (appearing de novo in old age)	I
	Interests retained	0
20.	Hobbies relinquished	I
21.	Diminished initiative or growing apathy	I
22.	Purposeless hyperactivity	I
	Total	

Information–Memory–Concentration Test
Information test

Name	I
Age	I
Time (hour)	I
Time of day	I
Day of week	I
Date	I
Month	I
Season	I
Year	I
Place–	
Name	I
Street	I
Town	I
Type of place (e.g. home, hospital, etc.)	I
Recognition of persons (cleaner, doctor, nurse, patient, relative; any two available)	2
Total	

Scores lie between 0 (complete failure) and +37 (full marks)

Memory:

(1) Personal

Date of birth	I
Place of birth	I
School attended	I
Occupation	I
Name of sibs } or Name of wife }	I
Name of any town where patient had worked	I
Name of employers	I

(2) Non-personal

*Date of World War I	I
*Date of World War II	I
Monarch	I
Prime Minister	I

(3) Name and address (5-minute recall)

Mr John Brown	
42 West Street	
Gateshead	5

Total
Concentration

Months of year backwards	2	I	0
Counting I–20	2	I	0
Counting 20–I	2	I	0

*½ for approximation within 3 years.
Ascertain from relative/friend. Applies to last 6 months. Score lies between 0 (fully preserved capacity) and +28 (extreme incapacity)

Reproduced from the *British Journal of Psychiatry*, Blessed G, Tomlinson BE, Roth M (1968) The association between quantitative measures of dementia and of senile change in the cerebral grey matter of elderly subjects, Vol. 114, pp. 797–811. © 1968 Royal College of Psychiatrists. Reproduced with permission.

Alzheimer's Disease Assessment Scale (ADAS) – Cognitive and Non-Cognitive Sections (ADAS-Cog, ADAS-Non-Cog)

Reference: **Rosen WG, Mohs RC, Davis KL (1984) A new rating scale for Alzheimer's disease.** *American Journal of Psychiatry* 141: 1356–64

Time taken 45 minutes

Rating by trained observer

Main indications

Standardized assessment of cognitive function and non-cognitive features. Standard measure to assess change in cognitive function in drug trials.

Commentary

The Alzheimer's Disease Assessment Scale – Cognitive and Non-Cognitive Sections (ADAS-Cog and ADAS-Non-Cog) were designed specifically to evaluate all aspects of Alzheimer's disease. The primary cognitive function included components of memory, language and praxis, while the non-cognitive features included mood state and behavioural changes. There are 11 main sections testing cognitive function and 10 assessing non-cognitive features. ADAS-Cog tests for vascular dementia and mild cognitive impairment are being developed.

Additional references

Mohs R, Knopman D, Petersen R et al (1997) Development of cognitive instruments for use in clinical trails of antidementia drugs: additions to the Alzheimer's Disease Assessment Scale that broaden its scope. *Alzheimer Disease and Associated Disorders* 11 (suppl 2): S13–S21.

Schwarb S, Koberle S, Spiegel R (1988) The Alzheimer's Disease Assessment Scale (ADAS): an instrument for early diagnosis of dementia? *International Journal of Geriatric Psychiatry* 3: 45–53.

Standish T, Molloy DW, Bédard M et al (1996) Improved reliability of the standardized Alzheimer's Disease Assessment Scale (SADAS) compared with the Alzheimer's Disease Assessment Scale (ADAS). *Journal of the American Geriatrics Society* 44: 712–16.

Zec R, Landreth E, Vicari S et al (1992) Alzheimer Disease Assessment Scale: useful for both early detection and staging of dementia of the Alzheimer type. *Alzheimer Disease and Associated Disorders* 6: 89–102.

Address for correspondence

Dr KL Davis
Mount Sinai School of Medicine
One Gustave L Levy Place
Box 1230
New York
NY 10029-6574
USA
e-mail: Kenneth.davis@mssm.edu

Alzheimer's Disease Assessment Scale (ADAS) – Cognitive and Non-Cognitive Sections (ADAS-Cog, ADAS-Non-Cog)

Cognitive Items

1.   Spoken language ability _____
2.   Comprehension of spoken language _____
3.   Recall of test instructions _____
4.   Word-finding difficulty _____
5.   Following commands _____
6.   Naming: objects, fingers _____

High:	1	2	3	4	Fingers: Thumb
Medium:	1	2	3	4	Pinky Index
Low:	1	2	3	4	Middle Ring

7.   Constructions: drawing _____
  Figures correct: 1   2   3   4
  Closing in: Yes _____ No _____
8.   Ideational praxis _____
  Step correct:
  1   2   3   4   5
9.   Orientation _____
  Day _____ Year _____ Person _____ Time of day _____
  Date _____ Month _____ Season _____ Place _____
10.   Word recall: mean error score _____
11.   Word recognition: mean error score _____
  Cognition total _____

Noncognitive Items (all rated by examiner)

12.   Tearful _____
13.   Appears/reports depressed mood _____
14.   Concentration, distractibility _____
15.   Uncooperative to testing _____
16.   Delusions _____
17.   Hallucinations _____
18.   Pacing _____
19.   Increased motor activity _____
20.   Tremors _____
21.   Increase/decrease appetite _____
  Noncognition total _____

Total Scores

Cognitive behavior _____
Noncognitive behavior _____
Word recall _____
Word recognition _____
  Total _____

Rating: x = not assessed
  0 = not present
  1 = very mild
  2 = mild
  3 = moderate
  4 = moderately severe
  5 = severe

Spoken language – quality of speech **not** quantity.
Comprehension – do **not** include responses to commands.
Do not include finger or object naming.
Score 0–5 steps correct
  1–4 steps correct
  2–3 steps correct
  3–2 steps correct
  4–1 steps correct
  5 – cannot do one step correct

Name fingers of dominant hand and high/medium/low frequency objects.

0 = all correct; one finger incorrect and/or one object incorrect
1 = two-three fingers and/or two objects incorrect
2 = two or more fingers and three–five objects incorrect
3 = three or more fingers and six–seven objects incorrect
4 = three or more fingers and eight–nine objects incorrect

Ability to copy circle, two overlapping rectangles, rhombus and cube.

5 components in sending self a letter
1 = difficulty or failure to perform one component
2 = difficulty and/or failure to perform two components
3 = difficulty and/or failure to perform three components
4 = difficulty and/or failure to perform four components
5 = difficulty and/or failure to perform five components

Date, month, year, day of week, season, time of day, place and person.

Noncognitive behavior is evaluated over preceding week to interview.

American Journal of Psychiatry, Vol. 141, pp. 1356–64, 1984. Copyright 1984, the American Psychiatric Association. Reprinted by permission.

Mattis Dementia Rating Scale (DRS)

Reference: **Mattis S (1976) Mental status examination for organic mental syndrome in the elderly patient. In: Bellak L, Karasu T, eds.** *Geriatric psychiatry: a handbook for psychiatrists and primary care physicians.* **New York: Grune & Stratton, 77–101**

Time taken 30–45 minutes

Rating by structured interview

Main indications

For the neuropsychological assessment of patients with dementia.

Commentary

The Mattis Dementia Rating Scale is a standardized neuropsychological test battery that provides a global measure of dementia on five subscales. Its advantage is that it assesses a range of cognitive abilities and is able to monitor change in dementia. Cognitive deficits which are affected early in Alzheimer's disease are assessed, as are tests likely to be affected in other dementias (e.g. attention and initiation in subcortical dementia). This makes the scale particularly well-suited for comparisons of neuropsychological differences between different types of dementia. Rosser and Hodges (1994) found that patients with Alzheimer's disease were more impaired on memory subtests whereas patients with subcortical disease (Huntington's disease and progressive supranuclear palsy) were more impaired on the initiation/perseveration subtest. A score of less than 100 out of the total of 144 indicates moderate dementia.

Additional reference

Rosser A, Hodges J (1994) The Dementia Rating Scale in Alzheimer's disease, Huntington's disease and progressive supranuclear palsy. *Journal of Neurology* **241**: 531–6.

Address for correspondence

NFER-Nelson
Darville House
2 Oxford Road East
Windsor
Berks SL4 1DF
UK

Mattis Dementia Rating Scale: constitution and scores of the five subtests

Attention subtest		Construction subtest	
Digit span (forwards and backwards)	8	Copy geometric designs	6
Two-step commands	2		
One-step commands	2	Conceptualization subtests	
Imitation of commands	4	Similarities	8
Counting As	6	Inductive reasoning	3
Counting randomly arranged As	5	Detection of different item	3
Read a word list	4	Multiple choice similarities	8
Match figures	4	Identities and oddities	16
	(37)	Create a sentence	1
			(39)
Initiation subtest			
Fluency for supermarket items	20	Memory subtest	
Fluency for clothing items	8	Recall a sentence (I)	4
Verbal repetition (e.g. bee, key, gee)	2	Recall a self-generated sentence (II)	3
Double alternating movements	3	Orientation (e.g. date, place)	9
Graphomotor (copy alternating figures)	4	Verbal recognition	5
	(37)	Figure recognition	4
			(25)
		Total score	144

This scale is available from NFER Nelson (*see above*).

Clock Drawing Test

References: **Brodaty H, Moore CM (1997) The Clock Drawing Test for dementia of the Alzheimer's type: a comparison of three scoring methods in a memory disorders clinic.** *International Journal of Geriatric Psychiatry* **12: 619–27**

Shulman K, Shedletsky R, Silver I (1986) The challenge of time. Clock drawing and cognitive function in the elderly. *International Journal of Geriatric Psychiatry* **1: 135–40**

Sunderland T, Hill JL, Mellow AM, Lawlor BA, Gundersheimer J, Newhouse PA, Grafman JH (1989) Clock drawing in Alzheimer's disease. *Journal of the American Geriatrics Society* **37: 725–9**

Wolf-Klein GP, Silverstone FA, Levy AP, Brod MS, Breuer J (1989) Screening for Alzheimer's disease by clock drawing. *Journal of the American Geriatrics Society* **37: 730–4**

Time taken 2 minutes

Rating standardized interpretation of drawing by clinican

Main indications

As a screening measure or measure of severity in dementia.

Commentary

The Clock Drawing Test reflects frontal and temporo-parietal functioning and is an easy test to carry out. A standard assessment is that the patient is asked to draw a clock face marking the hours and then draw the hands to indicate a particular time (e.g. 10 minutes to 2). The test tends to be non-threatening but there is obviously a wide variation in the way the results can be interpreted. Three methods have been described by Brodaty and Moore (1997). Shulman et al (1986) describe a six-point hierarchical error producing a global rating assessed on 75 patients, with inter-rater reliability of 0.75, a sensitivity of 86% and specificity of 72% against the Mini-Mental State Examination (MMSE; page 36). Sunderland et al (1989) described a 10-point anchored scale tested on 150 patients and controls, with inter-rater reliability of 0.86 and sensitivity of 78% with a specificity of 96% according to diagnostic criteria for Alzheimer's disease. Wolf-Klein et al (1989) described a 10-point categorical scale assessed on 312 consecutive admissions, with a sensitivity of 0.68 in the total population and a specificity of over 0.9. Brodaty and Moore (1997), on a sample of 56 patients and controls, assessed the methods of clock drawing analysis comparing them with other measures of cognitive function. The Shulman scale, when combined with the MMSE, was felt to be a valuable screening test for mild to moderate dementia of the Alzheimer's type.

Clock Drawing Test

A priori criteria for evaluating clock drawings (10 = best and 1 = worst)

10–6. Drawing of Clock Face with Circle and Numbers is Generally Intact

10. Hands are in correct position (i.e. hour hand approaching 3 o'clock)
9. Slight errors in placement of the hands
8. More noticeable errors in the placement of hour and minute hands
7. Placement of hands is significantly off course
6. Inappropriate use of clock hands (i.e. use of digital display or circling of numbers despite repeated instructions)

5–1. Drawing of Clock Face with Circle and Numbers is Not Intact

5. Crowding of numbers at one end of the clock or reversal of numbers. Hands may still be present in some fashion.
4. Further distortion of number sequence. Integrity of clock face is now gone (i.e. numbers missing or placed at outside of the boundaries of the clock face).
3. Numbers and clock face no longer obviously connected in the drawing. Hands are not present.
2. Drawing reveals some evidence of instructions being received but only a vague representation of a clock.
1. Either no attempt or an uninterpretable effort is made.

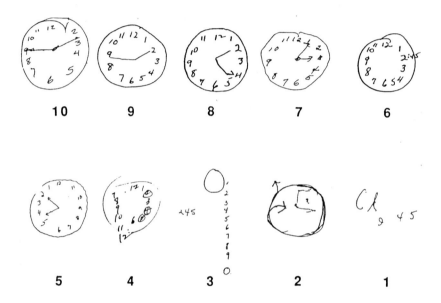

Samples of clock drawings from Alzheimer patients with evaluations of best (10) to worst (1)

Scale continued opposite

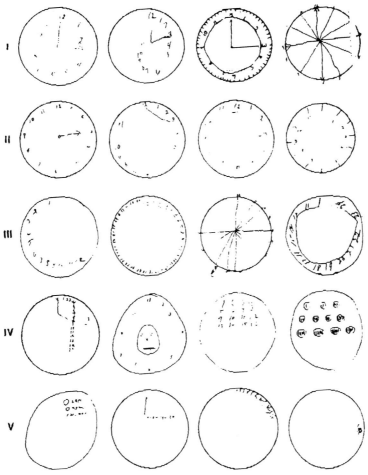

Clinical examples of clock errors

Classification of clock errors

I   Visuospatial
     (a)   Mildly impaired spacing of times
     (b)   Draws times outside circle
     (c)   Turns page while writing numbers so that some numbers appear upside down
     (d)   Draws in lines (spokes) to orient spacing

II   Errors in denoting the time as 3 o'clock
     (a)   Omits minute hand
     (b)   Draws a single line from 12 to 3
     (c)   Writes the words '3 o'clock'
     (d)   Writes the number 3 again
     (e)   Circles or underlines 3
     (f)   Unable to indicate 3 o'clock

III Visuospatial
     (a)   Moderately impaired spacing of times (so that 3 o'clock cannot be accurately denoted)
     (b)   Omits numbers
     Perseveration
     (a)   Repeats the circle
     (b)   Continues on past 12 to 13, 14, 15, etc.
     Right–left reversal – numbers drawn counterclockwise
     Dysgraphia – unable to write numbers accurately

IV   Severely disorganized spacing
     (a)   Confuses 'time' – writes in minutes, times of day, months or seasons
     (b)   Draws a picture of human face on the clock
     (c)   Writes the word 'clock'

V   Unable to make any reasonable attempt at a clock
     (excludes severe depression or other psychotic state)

Scale continued overleaf

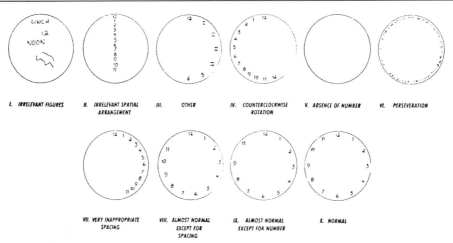

The 10 clock patterns

Sources: Sunderland T, Hill JL, Mellow AM, Lawlor BA, Gundersheimer J, Newhouse PA, Grafman JH (1989) Clock drawing in Alzheimer's disease; and Wolf-Klein GR, Silverstone FA, Levy AP, Brod MS, Breuer J (1989) Screening for Alzheimer's disease by clock drawing, *Journal of American Geriatrics Society*. Vol. 37, no. 8. pp 725–9 and 730–4, respectively; also Brodaty H, Moore CM (1997) The Clock Drawing Test for dementia of the Alzheimer's type: a comparison of three scoring methods in a memory disorders clinic; and Shulman K, Shedleksky R, Silver I (1986) The challenge of time. Clock drawing and cognitive function in the elderly, *International Journal of Geriatric Psychiatry*. Vol. 12, pp. 619–27 and Vol. 1, pp. 135–40, respectively (Copyright John Wiley & Sons Limited. Reproduced with permission).

The Ten-Point Clock Test

Reference: **Manos PJ, Wu R (1994) The Ten Point Clock Test: a quick screen and grading method for cognitive impairment in medical and surgical patients.** *International Journal of Psychiatry in Medicine* **24: 229–44**

Time taken 3–5 minutes

Rating by experienced interviewer

Main indications

The Ten-Point Clock Test is used to screen for dementia.

Commentary

A 4.5 inch diameter circle is traced using a template and the patient is asked to put the numbers in the face of the clock. The numbers are put in and the patient is then asked to make the clock say 10 minutes after 11. The clock is scored in a standardized way using a plastic transparent template. The test shows good test/retest and inter-rater reliability.

Address for correspondence

J Mark Baar
275 Burnett Ave #8
San Francisco
CA 94131
USA

Scoring: (A) Score = 0. (B) The number 1 is in the correct position; score = 1. (C) Numbers 1 and 11 are in the correct positions; score = 2. (D) Numbers 7, 8, 10 and 11 are in the correct positions; score = 4. (E) Numbers 1, 2, 4, 5, 7, 8, 10 and 11 are in the correct positions; score = 8. No points for hands of equal length regardless of position. (F) Numbers 1, 2, 4, 5, 7, 8, 10 and 11 are in correct position for 8 points. The little hand is on the 11 (1 point) and the big hand is on the 2 (1 point); score = 10 points.

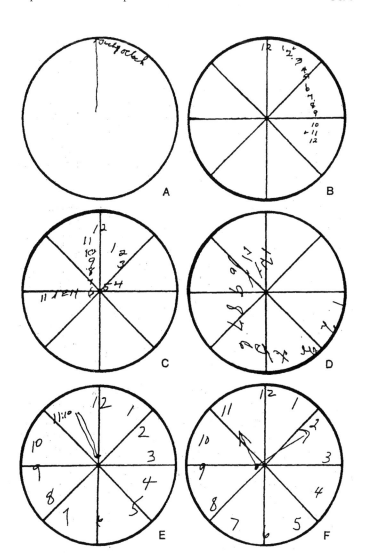

Clifton Assessment Procedures for the Elderly (CAPE)

Reference: **Pattie AH, Gilleard CJ (1979)** *Manual of the Clifton Assessment Procedures for the Elderly (CAPE).* **Sevenoaks: Hodder & Stoughton Educational**

Time taken 15–25 minutes (both scales)

Rating by trained interviewer

Main indications

Assessment of mental and physical functioning in elderly people.

Commentary

The Clifton Assessment Procedures for the Elderly (CAPE) consists of two related scales: the Cognitive Assessment Scale (CAS), which itself comprises the questionnaires exploring information and orientation, mental ability and a psychomotor test (the Gibson Maze; Gibson, 1977), and the Behaviour Rating Scale (BRS). The BRS grew out of the Stockton Geriatric Rating Scale (page 250). Some 18 items were derived from the original scale by dropping those with an inter-rater reliability of less than 0.4, and two items from inappropriate settings outside hospital were also dropped (Gilleard and Pattie, 1977). Measures of sensory deficits were added, but not included in the total score. Normative data on 400 subjects over the age of 60 are available (Gilleard and Pattie, 1977). Pattie and Gilleard (1975) reported the results of the Psychogeriatric Assessment Schedule and Stockton Geriatric Rating Scale in 100 consecutive admissions to a psychiatric hospital, showing that the information/orientation subtest of the CAS correctly classified 92% of patients. The scale successfully discriminated those patients who at follow-up were still in hospital and those who had been discharged (Pattie and Gilleard, 1978). A survey version of the CAPE has been described (Pattie, 1981).

The BRS has essentially the same principal areas as the Stockton Geriatric Rating Scale (physical disability, apathy, communication difficulties and social disturbance). Inter-rater reliability of the BRS is consistently above 0.8. The communication difficulties and social disturbance scales have slightly lower inter-rater reliabilities. Test/retest reliability on the CAS is high. Validity of the two instruments has been demonstrated in terms of correlations with other neuropsychological tests and with longitudinal studies. The scales tend to intercorrelate, but the pattern is suggestive of overlapping disabilities rather than simply reflecting one single dimension (Pattie and Gilleard, 1979).

Additional references

Gibson H (1977) *Manual of the Gibson Spiral Maze* (2nd edition). London: Hodder & Stoughton.

Gilleard C, Pattie A (1977) The Stockton Geriatric Rating Scale: a shortened version with British nominative data. *British Journal of Psychiatry* **131**: 90–4.

Pattie A (1981) A survey version of the Clifton Assessment Procedures for the Elderly. *British Journal of Clinical Psychology* **20**: 173–8.

Pattie A, Gilleard C (1975) A brief psychogeriatric assessment schedule: validation against psychiatric diagnosis and discharge from hospital. *British Journal of Psychiatry* **127**: 489–93.

Pattie A, Gilleard C (1978) The two year predictive validity of the Clifton Assessment Schedule and the Shortened Stockton Geriatric Rating Scale. *British Journal of Psychiatry* **133**: 457–60.

Clifton Assessment Procedures for the Elderly (CAPE) – Cognitive Assessment Scale (CAS)

Date of birth: **Occupation:**

Information/Orientation

Name: Hospital Address: Colour of British Flag:

Age: City: Day:

DoB: PM: Month:

Ward/Place: US President: Year:

I/O Score

Mental Ability

Count 1–20 Time: Errors:		Alphabet: Time: Errors:	
≤10 secs no errors	3	≤10 secs no errors	3
≤30 secs no errors	2	≤30 secs no errors	2
≤30 secs 1 error	1	≤30 secs 1 error	1
	0		0

Write name:		Reading: (See overleaf)	
Correct and legible	2	10 words or more	3
Can write but not correctly	1	6–9 words	2
Not able to	0	1–5 words	1
		0 words	0

MAb Score

Psychomotor Time		Errors	**Pm Score**
Scoring			

Score 1 point for each correct answer. The psychomotor test is the Gibson Spiral Maze.

Scale continued overleaf

Clifton Assessment Procedures for the Elderly (CAPE) – Behaviour Rating Scale (BRS)

Please ring the appropriate number for each item

1. WHEN BATHING OR DRESSING, HE/SHE REQUIRES:

    no assistance — 0
    some assistance — 1
    maximum assistance — 2

2. WITH REGARD TO WALKING, HE/SHE:

    shows no signs of weakness — 0
    walks slowly without aid, or uses a stick — 1
    is unable to walk, or if able to walk, needs frame, crutches or someone by his/her side — 2

3. HE/SHE IS INCONTINENT OF URINE AND/OR FAECES (day or night):

    never — 0
    sometimes (once or twice per week) — 1
    frequently (3 times per week or more) — 2

4. HE/SHE IS IN BED DURING THE DAY (bed does not include couch, settee, etc.):

    never — 0
    sometimes — 1
    almost always — 2

5. HE/SHE IS CONFUSED (unable to find way around, loses possessions, etc.):

    almost never confused — 0
    sometimes confused — 1
    almost always confused — 2

6. WHEN LEFT TO HIS/HER OWN DEVICES, HIS/HER APPEARANCE (clothes and/or hair) IS:

    almost never disorderly — 0
    sometimes disorderly — 1
    almost always disorderly — 2

7. IF ALLOWED OUTSIDE, HE/SHE WOULD:

    never need supervision — 0
    sometimes need supervision — 1
    always need supervision — 2

8. HE/SHE HELPS OUT IN THE HOME/WARD:

    often helps out — 0
    sometimes helps out — 1
    never helps out — 2

9. HE/SHE KEEPS HIM/HERSELF OCCUPIED IN A CONSTRUCTIVE OR USEFUL ACTIVITY (works, reads, plays games, has hobbies, etc):

    almost always occupied — 0
    sometimes occupied — 1
    almost never occupied — 2

10. HE/SHE SOCIALISES WITH OTHERS:

    does establish a good relationship with others — 0
    has some difficulty establishing good relationships — 1
    has a great deal of difficulty establishing good relationships — 2

11. HE/SHE IS WILLING TO DO THINGS SUGGESTED OR ASKED OF HIM/HER:

    often goes along — 0
    sometimes goes along — 1
    almost never goes along — 2

12. HE/SHE UNDERSTANDS WHAT YOU COMMUNICATE TO HIM/HER (you may use speaking, writing, or gesturing):

    understands almost everything you communicate — 0
    understands some of what you communicate — 1
    understands almost nothing of what you communicate — 2

13. HE/SHE COMMUNICATES IN ANY MANNER (by speaking, writing or gesturing):

    well enough to make him/herself easily understood at all times — 0
    can be understood sometimes or with some difficulty — 1
    can rarely or never be understood for whatever reason — 2

14. HE/SHE IS OBJECTIONABLE TO OTHERS DURING THE DAY (loud or constant talking, pilfering, soiling furniture, interfering with affairs of others):

    rarely or never — 0
    sometimes — 1
    frequently — 2

cont.

15. HE/SHE IS OBJECTIONABLE TO OTHERS DURING THE NIGHT (loud or constant talking, pilfering, soiling furniture, interfering in affairs of others, wandering about, etc.):

rarely or never	0
sometimes	1
frequently	2

16. HE/SHE ACCUSES OTHERS OF DOING HIM/HER BODILY HARM OR STEALING HIS/HER PERSONAL POSSESSIONS – If you are sure the accusations are true, rate zero, otherwise rate one or two:

never	0
sometimes	1
frequently	2

17. HE/SHE HOARDS APPARENTLY MEANINGLESS ITEMS (wads of paper, string, scraps of food, etc.):

never	0
sometimes	1
frequently	2

18. HIS/HER SLEEP PATTERN AT NIGHT IS:

almost never awake	0
sometimes awake	1
often awake	2

EYESIGHT: (tick which applies)

can see (or can see with glasses)
partially blind
totally blind

HEARING: (tick which applies)

no hearing difficulties, without hearing aid
no hearing difficulties, though requires hearing aid
has hearing difficulties which interfere with communication
is very deaf

The Mini-Cog

Reference: Scanlan J, Borson S (2001) The Mini-Cog: receiver operating characteristic with expert and naive raters. *International Journal of Geriatric Psychiatry* 16: 216–22

Time taken approximately 5 minutes

Raters untrained raters

Main indications

The Mini-Cog was developed as a brief test for discriminating demented from non-demented persons in community samples.

Commentary

In this paper the authors describe the development of the Mini-Cog's scoring algorithm, its receiver operating characteristics and generalizability of its clock drawing scoring system. To assess the clock drawing test scoring generalizability, 20 naïve raters without explicit instructions or prior CDT exposure scored 80 randomly selected clocks as normal or abnormal. The CDT concordance between naïve and trained raters was greater than 98% for normal, moderately and severely impaired clocks but lower (60%) for mildly impaired clocks. The recalculation of the Mini-Cog's performance, assuming that a naïve rater would score all mildly impaired clock drawing tests and a full sample as normal, retained high sensitivity (97%) and specificity (95%).

Additional references

Borson S, Scanlan J, Brush M, Vitaliano P, Dokmak A (2000) The mini-cog: a cognitive 'vital signs' measure for dementia screening in multi-lingual elderly. *International Journal of Geriatric Psychiatry.* 15: 1021–7.

Address for correspondence

J Scanlan
Box 356560
University of Washington School of Medicine
1959 NE Pacific Street
Seattle
WA 98195-6560
USA

jscanlan@u.washington.edu

Brief Cognitive Rating Scale (BCRS)

Reference: **Reisberg B, Ferris SH (1988) Brief Cognitive Rating Scale (BCRS). Psychopharmacology Bulletin 24: 629–36**

Time taken about 15 minutes (reviewer's estimate)

Rating by clinician

Main indications

The assessment of cognitive symptoms.

Commentary

The Brief Cognitive Rating Scale (BCRS) is part of the triad of assessments with the Global Deterioration Scale (GDS; page 236) and the Functional Assessment Staging (FAST; page 235). It is divided into five axes: concentration, recent memory, past memory, orientation and function/self-care. The scales on the five axes correlate approximately to the GDS. The validity of the scale has been assessed in a number of studies (Reisberg et al, 1983, 1985), and the validity was measured against the clinical syndrome of age-associated memory impairment and progressive degenerative dementia as well as a number of different psychometric tests. Reliability is generally about 0.9 for all the five axes in the three reliability studies published (Foster et al, 1988; Reisberg et al, 1989).

Additional references

Foster JR, Sclan S, Welkowitz J et al (1988) Psychiatric assessment in medical longterm care facilities: reliability of commonly used rating scales. *International Journal of Geriatric Psychiatry* **3**: 229–35.

Reisberg B, Schneck MK, Ferris SH et al (1983) The Brief Cognitive Rating Scale (BCRS). Findings in primary degenerative dementia (PDD). *Psychopharmacology Bulletin* **19**: 47–50.

Reisberg B, Ferris SH, Anand R et al (1985) Clinical assessment of cognitive decline in normal and aging and primary degenerative dementia: concordant ordinal measures. In Pinchot P et al, eds. *Psychiatry*. Vol. 5. New York: Plenum Press, 333–8.

Reisberg B, Ferris SH, Steinberg G et al (1989) Longitudinal study of dementia patients and aged controls. In Lawton MP, Herzog AR, eds. *Special research methods for gerontology*. Amityville, NY: Baywood, 195–231.

Address for correspondence

Barry Reisberg
Department of Psychiatry
Aging and Dementia Research Center
NYU Medical Center
550 First Avenue
NY 10016
USA

e-mail: barry.reisberg@med.nyu.edu

Brief Cognitive Rating Scale (BCRS)

Axis	Rating (Circle Highest Score)	Item
Axis I: **Concentration**	1 =	No objective or subjective evidence of deficit in concentration.
	2 =	Subjective decrement in concentration ability.
	3 =	Minor objective signs of poor concentration (e.g. on subtraction of serial 7s from 100).
	4 =	Definite concentration deficit for persons of their background (e.g. marked deficit on serial 7s; frequent deficit in subtraction of serial 4s from 40).
	5 =	Marked concentration deficit (e.g. giving months backwards or serial 2s from 20).
	6 =	Forgets the concentration task. Frequently begins to count forward when asked to count backwards from 10 by 1s.
	7 =	Marked difficulty counting forward to 10 by 1s.
Axis II: **Recent Memory**	1 =	No objective or subjective evidence of deficit in recent memory.
	2 =	Subjective impairment only (e.g. forgetting names more than formerly).
	3 =	Deficit in recall of specific events evident upon detailed questioning. No deficit in the recall of major recent events.
	4 =	Cannot recall major events of previous weekend or week. Scanty knowledge (not detailed) of current events, favorite TV shows, etc.
	5 =	Unsure of weather; may not know current President or current address.
	6 =	Occasional knowledge of some recent events. Little or no idea of current address, weather, etc.
	7 =	No knowledge of any recent events.
Axis III: **Past Memory**	1 =	No subjective or objective impairment in past memory.
	2 =	Subjective impairment only. Can recall two or more primary school teachers.
	3 =	Some gaps in past memory upon detailed questioning. Able to recall at least one childhood teacher and/or one childhood friend.
	4 =	Clear-cut deficit. The spouse recalls more of the patient's past than the patient. Cannot recall childhood friends and/or teachers but knows the names of most schools attended. Confuses chronology in reciting personal history.
	5 =	Major past events sometimes not recalled (e.g. names of schools attended).
	6 =	Some residual memory of past (e.g. may recall country of birth or former occupation).
	7 =	No memory of past.
Axis IV: **Orientation**	1 =	No deficit in memory for time, place, identity of self or others.
	2 =	Subjective impairment only. Knows time to nearest hour, location.
	3 =	Any mistake in time > 2 hrs; day of week > 1 day; date > 3 days.
	4 =	Mistakes in month > 10 days of year > 1 month.
	5 =	Unsure of month and/or year and/or season; unsure of locale.
	6 =	No idea of date. Identifies spouse but may not recall name. Knows own name.
	7 =	Cannot identify spouse. May be unsure of personal identity.
Axis V: **Functioning and Self-Care**	1 =	No difficulty, either subjectively or objectively.
	2 =	Complains of forgetting location of objects. Subjective work difficulties.
	3 =	Decreased job functioning evident to co-workers. Difficulty in traveling to new locations.
	4 =	Decreased ability to perform complex tasks (e.g. planning dinner for guests, handling finances, marketing, etc.).
	5 =	Requires assistance in choosing proper clothing.
	6 =	Requires assistance in feeding, and/or toileting, and/or bathing, and/or ambulating.
	7 =	Requires constant assistance in all activities of daily life.

Concentration: test for concentration and attentiveness directly e.g. serial 7s
Recent memory: index of cognitive deficiency
Orientation: in time, place and person

Cambridge Neuropsychological Test Automated Battery (CANTAB)

Reference: **Sahakian BJ, Morris RG, Evenden JL, Heald A, Levy R, Philpot M, Robbins TW (1988) A comparative study of visual/spatial memory and learning in Alzheimer type dementia and Parkinson's disease. Brain 111: 695–718**

Time taken varies with each subscale. Total battery, *c.* 90 minutes

Rating by trained neuropsychologists or assistant nurse, technician or equivalent.

Main indications

A computerized battery of tests for neuropsychological evaluation.

Commentary

The Cambridge Neuropsychological Test Automated Battery (CANTAB) is a neuropsychological battery which is of proven sensitivity and specificity in differentiating patients with a number of neurological conditions from each other and from normal controls. Various sub-tests provide assessment of different cognitive functions, including learning, memory, attention (including sustained, divided and selective forms) and tests of executive function (including problem solving and planning). As a computerized battery, it can control for movement disability, it is tailored to the individual, and the tests are graded in difficulty – avoiding floor and ceiling effects. Specific batteries include separate Alzheimer and Parkinson's disease batteries, an attention battery, visual memory battery, and working memory and planning battery, also available in parallel forms. The tests are administered via a touch-screen, and are largely language- and culture-free.

Additional references

Eagger SA, Levy R, Sahakian BJ (1991) Tacrine in Alzheimer's disease. *Lancet* **337**: 989–92.

Fowler KS et al (1997) Computerized neuropsychological tests in the early detection of dementia: prospective findings. *Journal of the International Neuropsychological Society* **3**: 139–46.

Sahakian B et al (1988) A comparative study of visual/ spatial memory and learning in Alzheimer type dementia and Parkinson's disease. *Brain* **111**: 695–718.

Sahakian BJ, Coull JT (1994) Nicotine and tetrahydroaminoacradine – evidence for improved attention in patients with dementia of the Alzheimer-type. *Drug Development Research* **31**: 80–8.

Sagal A et al (1991) Detection of visual memory and learning deficits in Alzheimer's disease using CANTAB. *Dementia* **2**: 150–8.

Address for correspondence

Professor Ken Wilson
Consultant in Old Age Psychiatry
Wirral Community Healthcare NHS Trust
Elderly Mental Health Directorate
St Catherine's Hospital
Church Road
Birkenhead L42 0LQ
UK

e-mail: Kw500505@liverpool.ac.uk

Short Portable Mental Status Questionnaire (SPMSQ)

Reference: **Pfeiffer E (1975) A Short Portable Mental Status Questionnaire for the assessment of organic brain deficit in elderly patients.** *Journal of the American Geriatrics Society* **23: 433–41**

Time taken 2 minutes

Rating by clinical interview

Main indications

To assess organic brain function in the elderly.

Commentary

The Short Portable Mental Status Questionnaire (SPMSQ) is a short 10-question reliable instrument to detect the presence of intellectual impairment and to determine the degree. It is particularly useful for clinicians whose practice includes the elderly. Validity studies were performed using a clinical diagnosis of organic brain syndrome, so it appears to be subjective. Test/retest reliability was over 0.82. The questionnaire explores short-term memory, long-term memory, orientation and the ability to conduct serial operations.

Address for correspondence

E Pfeiffer, MD
USF Suncoast Gerontology Center
12901 Bruce B Downs Boulevard
MDC 50
Tampa
FL 33612
USA

http://nncf.unl.edu/alz/manual/sec1/portable.html

Short Portable Mental Status Questionnaire (SPMSQ)

Instructions: Ask questions 1–10 in this list and record all answers. Ask question 4a only if patient does not have a telephone. Record total number of errors based on ten questions.

Allow one more if subject has had only a grade school education.
Allow one less error if subject has had education beyond high school.
Allow one more error for black subjects, using identical educational criteria.

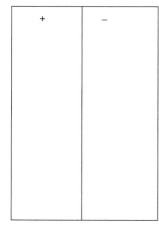

+	–

1. What is the date today? _____
                  Month   Day   Year
2. What day of the week is it? _____
3. What is the name of this place? _____
4. What is your telephone number? _____
4a. What is your street address? _____
   (Ask only if patient does not have a telephone)
5. How old are you? _____
6. When were you born? _____
7. Who is the President of the US now? _____
8. What was President just before him? _____
9. What was your mother's maiden name? _____
10. Subtract 3 from 20 and keep subtracting 3 from each new number, all the way down.

TOTAL NUMBER OF ERRORS

    0–2   Errors   Intact Intellectual Functioning
    3–4   Errors   Mild Intellectual Impairment
    5–7   Errors   Moderate Intellectual Impairment
    8–10 Errors   Severe Intellectual Impairment

To be completed by interviewer

Patient's Name: _____   Date: _____

    Sex: 1. Male   Race: 1. White
           2. Female   2. Black
                                                3. Other

Years of education: _____   1. Grade School
                                           2. High School
                                         3. Beyond High School

Interviewer's name: _____

Reproduced from Pfeiffer E (1975) Short Portable Mental Status Questionnaire for the assessment of organic brain deficit in elderly patients. *Journal of the American Geriatrics Society*, Vol. 23, no. 10, pp. 433–41.

SET Test

Reference: **Isaacs B, Akhtar AJ (1972) The SET Test: a rapid test of mental function in old people.** *Age and Ageing* **1: 222–6**

Time taken 5 minutes, often 2

Rating by interviewer

Main indications

Assessment of mental function in older people.

Commentary

The object of the SET Test was to provide a brief test of mental function in older people which was not perceived as a threat. The test is essentially a variant of verbal fluency. The original paper described the results of the test in 64 elderly people over the age of 65 who were seen in their own homes by a doctor who also carried out the Mill Hill Vocabulary Test, Raven's Progressive Colour Matrices and a modified version of the Crichton Royal Behavioural Rating Scale (page 241). There were highly significant correlations between the SET Test and the scores on these scales.

The SET Test

The test is introduced to the subject as a challenge rather than a threat, the appropriate words being 'let's see how good your memory is', or some variant of this. The subject is then asked 'I want you to tell me all the colours you can think of'. The examiner may repeat the instructions as often as required, but should offer no other help. There is no time limit, this part of the test being complete when the subject has offered ten different colours, in which case he is awarded a score of ten; or when he cannot think of any more, or begins to repeat himself, in which case his score is the number of different colours he has given. The end-point is usually clear, the subject coming to an abrupt stop with an admission of failure such as 'That's all I can think of', or a defensive rationalization like 'There are lots more'.

The test is then repeated three times more by asking in turn for animals, fruits and towns. A maximum of 10 points is awarded for each of the four sets and a maximum of 40 for the total.

Source: Isaacs B, Akhtar AJ (1972) The SET Test: a rapid test of mental function in old people. *Age and Ageing* 1: 222–6. By kind permission of Oxford University Press.

Short Mental Status Questionnaire

Reference: **Robertson D, Rockwood K, Stolee P (1982) A Short Mental Status Questionnaire.** *Canadian Journal on Aging* **1: 16–20**

Time taken about 5 minutes

Rating by interviewer

Main indications

Assessment of mental status in elderly people.

Commentary

The justification for the development of another scale measuring cognitive function was on the need to develop a short questionnaire for use in the Saskatchewan Health Survey where questions such as 'Who is the President of the United States?' were felt to be less relevant to elderly Canadians compared with Americans, and the validity of asking the patient to recall his or her mother's maiden name was of doubtful significance in view of the inability to verify that information. The questions about monarchs and presidents were replaced by asking the name of the Prime Minister of Canada and recalling three words instead of a fictitious name and address, and, as calculations appear to have a high error rate, counting from 20 down to 1 was suggested. Fifty elderly subjectes were examined with a test/retest correlation of 0.89. While the questioner identified moderate and severe cognitive impairment satisfactorily it was difficult, on the basis of the test alone, to differentiate those with mild impairment from normal controls.

Short Mental Status Questionnaire

1.	What is your full name?	Correct forename and surname
2.	What is your address?	Correct street address and municipality
3.	What year is this?	Correct year
4.	What month is this?	Correct month
5.	What day of the week is this?	Correct day of week (not date)
6.	How old are you?	Correct age, verified by another person, or from date of birth
7.	What is the name of the Prime Minister of Canada?	Correct answer to include surname of current Prime Minister
8.	When did the First World War start?	Year 1914
9.	Remember these three items. I will ask you to recall them in a few minutes . . . **bed, chair, window**. Have subject repeat items correctly before proceeding.	
10.	Count backwards from 20 to 1 (If necessary like this, 20, 19 and so on)	No error. Any uncorrected error = 0
11.	Repeat the three items I asked you to remember	All items correct = 1 Any uncorrected error = 0

Short Orientation–Memory–Concentration Test

Reference: **Katzman R, Bown T, Fuld P, Peck A, Schechter R, Schimmel H (1983) Validation of a Short Orientation–Memory–Concentration Test of cognitive impairment.** *American Journal of Psychiatry* **140: 734–9**

Time taken less than 5 minutes (reviewer's estimate)

Rating by clinician

Main indications

A brief six-item cognitive test developed from the longer Blessed Information and Concentration test.

Commentary

The Short Orientation–Memory–Concentration Test is a six-item test that was developed out of the larger 26-item Mental Status Questionnaire, which was carried out on a group of people in a nursing facility (322 subjects in total). When post-mortems were carried out on 38 subjects, the 26 questions were subject to multivariant analyses and the six items most correlated with senile plaque counts in the cerebral cortex were described – year, time of day, counting backwards from 20 to 1, months backwards, the memory phase (name and address) and month. The scale, once developed, was tested on three additional populations: 170 subjects admitted to the same nursing facility on whom the original study was performed, 42 subjects in a dementia ward and 52 subjects at a senior citizens day centre. The shorter scale stood up statistically very well in comparison with the longer scale. The correlation between the scores and plaque counts at post-mortem was highly significant (0.52) and very similar to the correlation of the 26-item test.

www.strokecenter.org/trials/somct.html

Short Orientation–Memory–Concentration Test

Items	Maximum error	Score		Weight
1 What year is it now?	1	___ ×	4	= ___
2 What month is it now?	1	___ ×	3	= ___
Memory phrase	Repeat this phrase after me: John Brown, 42 Market Street, Chicago			
3 About what time is it? (within 1 hour)	1	___ ×	3	= ___
4 Count backwards 20 to 1	2	___ ×	2	= ___
5 Say the months in reverse order	2	___ ×	2	= ___
6 Repeat the memory phrase	5	___ ×	2	= ___

Score of 1 for each incorrect response; maximum weighted error score = 24

Syndrom Kurztest (SKT)

Reference: **Erzigkeit H (1989) The SKT: a short cognitive performance test as an instrument for the assessment of clinical efficacy of cognition enhancers. In Bergener M, Reisberg B, eds.** *Diagnosis and treatment of senile dementia.* **Berlin: Springer-Verlag, 164–74**

Time taken 10–15 minutes

Rating by anyone trained in the use of the test

Main indications

The Syndrom Kurztest (SKT) is a short cognitive performance test to assess memory and attention. The SKT was specially designed to be a brief and practicable measure of cognitive function.

Commentary

The test is available in five parallel forms to allow repeated administration. There are nine subtests: object naming, object recall, learning, reading numbers from blocks, arranging the blocks, replacing them in their original position, simple recognition and interference task, and two memory performance tasks. Reliability of the test is between 0.6 and 0.8, face validity has been shown and significant correlations occur between the SKT results and other psychometric tests as well as neuroimaging parameters – CT and EEG. The SKT has also been shown to be sensitive to the effects of drugs.

Additional references

Erzigkeit H (1991) The development of the SKT project. In Hindmarch I, Hippius H, Wilcox J, eds. *Dementia: molecules, methods and measures.* Chichester: Wiley, 101–8.

Lehfeld H, Erzigkeit H (1997) The SKT – a short cognitive performance test for assessing deficits of memory and attention. *International Psychogeriatrics* **9** (suppl 1): 115–21

Overall J, Schaltenbrand R (1992) The SKT neuropsychological test battery. *Journal of Geriatric Psychiatry and Neurology* **5**: 220–7.

Address for correspondence

H Lehfeld
Psychiatrische Universitätsklinik Erlangen
Schwabachanlage 6
91054 Erlangen
Germany

Cognitive Abilities Screening Instrument (CASI)

Reference: **Teng EL, Hasegawa K, Homma A, Imai Y, Larson E, Graves A, Sugimoto K, Yamaguchi T, Sasaki H, Chiu D, White LR (1994) The Cognitive Abilities Screening Instrument (CASI): a practical test for cross-cultural epidemiological studies of dementia.** *International Psychogeriatrics* **6: 45–58**

Time taken 15–20 minutes

Rating by trained interviewer

Main indications

A cognitive test providing a quantitative assessment (from 0 to 100) for a wide range of cognitive skills.

Commentary

The Cognitive Abilities Screening Instrument (CASI) consists of items similar to those used in a number of existing scales such as the Hasegawa Dementia Screening Scale (Hasegawa, 1983), and the Mini-Mental State Examination (MMSE; page 36), according to DSM-III-R criteria, is included. A number of different versions of the CASI are available, in English and in Japanese, and the study has been described in the USA and in Japan (Teng et al, 1994). Training is required (provided by the authors).

Additional references

Hasegawa K (1983) The clinical assessment of dementia in the aged: a dementia screening scale for psychogeriatric patients. In Bergener M, Lehr U, Lang E et al, eds. *Ageing in the eighties and beyond.* New York: Springer, 207–18.

Teng EL, Chui HC (1987) The Modified Mini-Mental State Examination. *Journal of Clinical Psychiatry* **48**: 314–18.

Address for correspondence

EL Teng, c/o L White
EDB Program, National Institute on Ageing
Gateway Building, Room 3C309
National Institute of Health
Bethesda
MD 20892
USA

Main items of the Cognitive Abilities Screening Instrument (CASI)

Where were you born?
When were you born?
How old are you?
How many minutes are there in an hour?
In what direction does the sun set?
Registration and recall of 3 words
Repeating words backwards
Serial 3s
Today's date
Day of the week
Season
Orientation to place

Number of animals with 4 legs
A comparison of objects, e.g. an orange and a banana are both fruit
What action would you take if you saw you neighbour's house catching fire?
Repeat 'He would like to go home?'
Obey command 'raise your hand'
Write 'he would like to go home'
Copy 2 interlocking pentagons
Three-stage command
Recognition of body parts
Recognition of objects
Recall of objects

Cognitive Drug Research Assessment System (COGDRAS)

Reference: **Simpson PM, Surmon DJ, Wesnes KA, Wilcock GK (1991) The Cognitive Drug Research computerized Assessment System for demented patients: a validation study.** *International Journal of Geriatric Psychiatry* **6: 95–102**

Time taken approximately 30 minutes

Rating by trained personnel

Main indications

A computerized battery to assess the effects of drugs on cognitive functions in dementia.

Commentary

The Cognitive Drug Research Assessment System (COG-DRAS) was developed to assess the effects of drugs on cognitive function. The version presented is validated for use in patients suffering from dementia. Refinements of the system included: avoidance of negative feedback; larger presentation of words and digits; the presence of trained technical support; and the ability to modify the programme if the patient is distracted. The following tests were used in the study: immediate verbal recognition; picture presentation; number vigilance task; choice reaction time; memory scanning task; delayed word recognition and picture recognition. The COGDRAS-D was administered to 51 patients attending a memory clinic and validated by other neuropsychological tests such as the Mini-Mental State Examination (MMSE; page 36) and the Kew Cognitive Test (page 73). Patients with dementia showed impairments in speed of choice reaction and in all the memory tests. Test/retest reliability was good, and the results showed that the system had comparable properties to the previous versions.

Additional reference

Simpson PM, Wesnes KA, Christmas L (1989) A computerised system for the assessment of drug-induced performance changes in young, elderly and demented populations. *British Journal of Clinical Pharmacology* **27**: 711–12P.

Address for correspondence

Dr Keith Wesnes
Chief Executive
Cognitive Drug Research Ltd
Reading and Human Cognitive Neuroscience Unit
University of Northumbria
Newcastle upon Tyne
NE1 5ST
UK

Cognitive Drug Research Assessment System (COGDRAS)

Immediate verbal recognition
A series of 12 words is presented visually at the rate of one every three seconds. Immediately after, the 12 words are presented in random order with 12 different words and the patient required to press a button each time to signal whether or not the word was from the originally presented list.

Picture presentation
A series of 14 pictures is presented on the monitor at the rate of one every three seconds.

Number vigilance task
A number is constantly displayed just to the right of the centre of the screen. A series of 90 digits is presented in the centre at the rate of 80 per minute. The patient has to press the YES button every time the digit in the centre matches the one constantly displayed.

Choice reaction time
Either the word YES or the word NO is presented in the centre of the monitor. The patient is instructed to press the YES or NO button as appropriate as quickly as possible. There are 20 trials and the intertrial interval varies randomly between one and 2.5 seconds.

Memory scanning task
Three digits are presented singly at the rate of one every 1.2 seconds for the patient to remember. A series of 18 digits is then presented and for each one the patient must press the YES button if he/she believes it was one of three presented or NO if not.

Delayed word recognition
The 12 words originally presented are presented again with 12 new distractors. Again the patient must decide whether or not each word was from the original list, pressing the YES or NO button accordingly.

Picture recognition
The 14 pictures presented earlier are presented again with 14 new ones in a randomized order. The patient signals recognition by pressing the YES or NO button as appropriate.

Reproduced from Simpson PM, Surmon DJ, Wesnes KA, Wilcock GK (1991) The Cognitive Drug Research computerized Assessment System for demented patients: a validation study. *International Journal of Geriatric Psychiatry* **6**: 95–102. Copyright John Wiley & Sons Limited. Reproduced with permission.

Kew Cognitive Test

Reference: **Hare M (1978) Clinical checklist for diagnosis of dementia.** *British Medical Journal* **2: 266–7**

Time taken 5–10 minutes (reviewer's estimate)

Rating by clinical interview

Main indications

Assessment of memory, speech and parietal function in dementia.

Commentary

The Kew Cognitive Test assesses cognitive function in the three areas of memory, aphasia and parietal signs using a simple 15-item questionnaire, five in each category. Two studies have used a modified version of the test, the study by Hare (1978) and McDonald (1969). Hare (1978)

examined 200 people admitted to a psychogeriatric assessment unit, repeated 4 or 6 weeks later. Patients with deficits in language ability or praxis had a significantly poorer outcome than those with memory deficits alone. McDonald used the test (among others) to divided patients into two groups showing that heterogeneity existed in terms of age and mortality with an older group who did not have parietal lobe signs and a better prognosis compared with a younger group with parietal dysfunction and higher mortality.

Additional reference

McDonald C (1969) Clinical heterogeneity in senile dementia. *British Journal of Psychiatry* **115**: 267–71.

Kew Cognitive Test

Memory
What year are we in?
What month is it?
Can you tell me two countries we fought in the Second World War?
What year were you born?
What is the capital city of England?

Aphasia
What do you call this (a watch)?
What do you call this (a wrist strap or band)?
What do you call this (a buckle or clasp)?

What is a refrigerator for?
What is a thermometer for?
What is a barometer for?

Parietal signs
Show me your left hand
Touch your left ear with your right hand
Name the coin in hand named (as 10p or two shillings)
No tactile inattention present
Normal two point discrimination
Draw a square

This table was first published in the *BMJ* (Hare M, Clinical checklist for diagnosis of dementia, 1978, Vol. 2, pp. 266–7) and is reproduced by permission of the *BMJ*.

Severe Impairment Battery (SIB)

Reference: **Saxton J, McGonigle-Gibson K, Swihart A, Miller M, Boller F (1990) Assessment of severely impaired patients: description and validation of a new neuropsychological test battery.** *Psychological Assessment* **2: 298–303**

Time taken 30–40 minutes (reviewer's estimate)

Rating by trained interviewer

Main indications

Assessment of cognitive function, particularly in severe dementia.

Commentary

The Severe Impairment Battery (SIB) has the strength of assessing cognitive function in patients with moderate to severe dementia. Items are single words or one-step commands combined with gestures. Nine areas are assessed

(see below), and the score is between 0 and 100. It appears sensitive to change. Panisset et al (1994) examined 69 patients with severe dementia using the SIB and found it to be a helpful neuropsychological measure in people with severe dementia.

Additional references

Albert M, Cohen C (1992) The Test for Severe Impairment, an instrument for the assessment of patients with severe cognitive dysfunction. *Journal of American Geriatric Society* **40**: 449–53.

Panisset M, Roudier M, Saxton J et al (1994) Severe Impairment Battery: a neuropsychological battery for severely impaired patients. *Archives of Neurology* **51**: 41–5.

www.tvtc.com/tvtc/tvtcpage/sib.html

Severe Impairment Battery Domains	
Domain	Questions
Orientation	Name
	Place (town)
	Time (month and time of day)
Attention	Digit span
	Counting to visual and auditory stimuli
Language	Auditory and reading comprehension
	Verbal fluency (food and months of the year)
	Naming from description, pictures of objects, objects, colors and forms
	Repetition
	Reading
	Writing
	Copying of written material
Praxis	How to use a cup, a spoon
Visuospatial	Discrimination of colors and forms
Construction	Spontaneous drawing, copying and tracing a figure
Memory	Immediate short- and long-term recall for examiner's name, objects, colors, forms and a short sentence
Orientation to name	When the patient's name is called from behind
Social interaction	Shaking hands, following general direction

Source: Panisset M, Roudier M, Saxton J et al (1994) Severe Impairment Battery: a neuropsychological battery for severely impaired patients. *Archives of Neurology* **51**: 41–5.

Mental Status Questionnaire (MSQ)/Face–Hand Test (FHT)

Reference: **Kahn RL, Goldfarb AI, Pollack M, Peck A (1960) Brief objective measures for the determination of mental status in the aged.** *American Journal of Psychiatry* 117: 326–8

Time taken MSQ – 5 minutes, FHT – 5 minutes (reviewer's estimate)

Rating by trained interviewer

Main indications

Assessment of cognitive function.

Commentary

These tests reflect an early attempt to describe a quantative measure of cognitive function. The Mental Status Questionnaire (MSQ) consists of ten questions, the point being made that the questions themselves are well known but the difference is that they are administered in a standardized way and the method of marking the number of errors gives a quantitative measure of mental functioning. The Face–Hand Test (FHT) was based on a test described by Fink et al (1952) and used because it is culture-free and can be used with patients who have impaired communication. As the response to the FHT is the same in 90% of cases whether the eyes are open or not, it was given with eyes open. It is said to be sensitive to brain damage. The paper reported the results on 1077 residents of nursing homes and mental hospitals. Diagnostic categories were assigned by psychiatric interview within a month of the assessment. Some 94% of patients scoring full marks on the MSQ and 70% scoring as negative on the FHT were rated as having none or mild chronic brain syndrome (CBS). The results were similar for patients with CBS and psychosis and those rated as having management problems.

Additional reference

Fink M, Green MA, Bender MB (1952) The Face–Hand test as a sign of organic mental syndrome. *Neurology* 1: 46–58.

Mental Status Questionnaire (MSQ)/Face–Hand Test (FHT)

1. What is the name of this place?
2. Where is it located (address)?
3. What is today's date?
4. What is the month now?
5. What is the year?
6. How old are you?
7. When were you born (month)?
8. When were you born (year)?
9. Who is the president of the United States?
10. Who was the president before him?

The Face–Hand Test: This test was first described by Fink et al (1952) as a diagnostic procedure for brain damage. The test consists of touching the patient simultaneously on the cheek and on the dorsum of the hand, and asking him to indicate where he was touched. Ten trials are given: 8 face–hand combinations divided between 4 contralateral (e.g. right cheek and left hand) and 4 ipsilateral (e.g. right cheek and right hand) stimuli, and 2 interspersed symmetric combinations of face–face and hand–hand. After the second trial, if the patient only reports one stimulus, he is asked, 'Were you touched any place else?' in order to give him the concept of twoness. If the patient fails consistently to locate both stimuli correctly within the 10 trials, he is classed as positive. The main types of errors are extinction, in which only 1 stimulus is indicated (almost always the face), and displacement, in which 2 stimuli are indicated but 1 of them, generally the hand stimulus, is displaced to another part of the body (e.g. if the person indicates both cheeks when the face and hand were actually touched). A patient is rated negative if he is consistently correct within the 10 trials. Frequently he makes an error on the first 4 trials, but is consistently correct after perceiving the 2 symmetric stimuli.

Cognitive Capacity Screening Examination

Reference: **Jacobs JW, Bernhard MR, Delgado A, Strain JJ (1977) Screening for organic mental syndromes in the medically ill.** *Annals of Internal Medicine* **86: 40–6**

Time taken 5 minutes

Rating by clinician

Main indications

Assessment of mental status in medically ill patients.

Commentary

The Cognitive Capacity Screening Examination was produced with the express intention of overcoming the difficulties in assessing mental function in medical patients. Standard examinations were considered inadequate because of the time taken for their administration, their lack of sensitivity and the need to give the whole test – taking into consideration the patients' education and cultural background and the variability of symptoms. The Mini-Mental State Examination (MMSE; page 36) was felt to have the shortcoming of having the specific purpose of screening psychiatric patients. The 30-item questionnaire was administered to different groups of patients to assess validity and reliability: 24 medical patients, 29 psychiatric patients, a further 69 medical patients and 25 normal controls. These groups revealed that a score of 20 or above was unlikely in the presence of an organic brain syndrome. The majority of psychiatric patients scored above that score, one third of medical admissions scored below 20 and only one of the normal controls scored below that score. Inter-rater reliability was 100%.

Cognitive Capacity Screening Examination

1.	What day of the week is this?	____
2.	What month?	____
3.	What day of month?	____
4.	What year?	____
5.	What place is this?	____
6.	Repeat the numbers 8 7 2.	
7.	Say them backwards.	
8.	Repeat these numbers 6 3 7 1.	____
9.	Listen to these numbers 6 9 4. Count 1 through 10 out loud, then repeat 6 9 4. (Help if needed. Then use numbers 5 7 3.)	____
10.	Listen to these numbers 8 1 4 3. Count 1 through 10 out loud, then repeat 8 1 4 3.	____
11.	Beginning with Sunday, say the days of the week backwards.	____
12.	9 + 3 is	____
13.	Add 6 (to the previous answer or 'to 12').	____
14.	Take away 5 ('from 18').	____
	Repeat these words after me and remember them, I will ask for them later: HAT, CAR, TREE, TWENTY-SIX.	
15.	The opposite of fast is slow. The opposite of up is	____

16.	The opposite of large is	____
17.	The opposite of hard is	____
18.	An orange and a banana are both fruits. Red and blue are both	____
19.	A penny and a dime are both	____
20.	What were those words I asked you to remember? (HAT)	____
21.	(CAR)	____
22.	(TREE)	____
23.	(TWENTY-SIX)	____
24.	Take away 7 from 100, then take away 7 from what is left and keep going: 100 − 7 is	____
25.	Minus 7	____
26.	Minus 7 (write down answers; check correct subtraction of 7)	____
27.	Minus 7	____
28.	Minus 7	____
29.	Minus 7	____
30.	Minus 7	____

Total correct (maximum score = 30)   ____

7-Minute Neurocognitive Screening Battery

Reference: **Solomon PR, Hirschoff A, Kelly B et al (1998) A 7 minute neurocognitive screening battery highly sensitive to Alzheimer's disease.** *Archives of Neurology* **55: 349–55**

Time taken Mean 7 minutes 42 seconds (range 6–11 minutes)

Rating by trained interviewer

Main indications

A screening test for cognitive impairment to distinguish patients with dementia and normal controls.

Commentary

The 7 Minute Neurocognitive Screening Battery consists of four tests representing four cognitive areas affected by Alzheimer's disease. These are: memory, verbal fluency, visuospatial and visioconstruction and orientation for time. The screening instrument was designed so that it could be rapidly administered by a technician, requiring no clinical judgement or training in its use. It was capable of distinguishing patients with Alzheimer's disease from those with normal ageing, and it was based on recent understanding of the fundamental differences between Alzheimer's disease and normal ageing. Sixty patients with Alzheimer's disease and 30 controls were examined. Test/retest reliability was evaluated in 25 of each, with overall test/retest reliability of the scale being between 0.83 and 0.92. Inter-rater reliability was 0.93 using logistic regression. Each of the four tests was able to detect patients with Alzheimer's disease in 92% of cases and to detect 96% of healthy subjects, as high sensitivity was apparent with patients with very mild, mild and moderate disease. Age, sex and education do not appear to affect the results. The results are presented in a way which does not make it easy to extract exact cut-off points on the various tests. The entire battery seems better predicted than any individual scale.

Address for correspondence

Paul R Solomon PhD
Bronfman Science Center
Williams College
Williamstown MA 01267
USA

e-mail: psolomon@williams.edu

---

7 Minute Neurocognitive Screening Battery

The four tests used were:

Enhances Cued Recall

Category Fluency
Benton Orientation Test
Clock Drawing

Revised Hasegawa's Dementia Scale (HDS-R)

Reference: Imai Y, Hasegawa K (1994) The revised Hasegawa's dementia scale (HDS-R) – evaluation of its usefulness as a screening test for dementia. *Journal of Hong Kong College of Psychiatry* 4: 20–4

Time taken 5 minutes (reviewer's estimate)

Rating by interview

Main indications

Assessment of cognitive function as a means of screening for dementia.

Commentary

The Revised Hasegawa's Dementia Scale was developed from the original Hasegawa scale, published in 1983, which comprised 11 questions. Five questions were deleted (place of the subject's birth, the last year of World War II, the number of days in a year, the Prime Minister of Japan, and the length of time the individual has been at the place of interview). Immediate and delayed recall of 3 words and list generating fluency were added. The revised version consists of 9 questions with a maximum score of 30. Imai and Hasegawa (1994) reported on the results of 157 subjects, 95 of whom had dementia. Cronbach's alpha was 0.90. Using a cut-off point of 20/21, a sensitivity of 0.90 and a specificity of 0.82 were achieved in discriminating people with dementia from controls. A correlation with the Mini-Mental State Examination (MMSE; page 36) was 0.94. The scale was able to distinguish between stages of dementia rated on the Global Deterioration Scale (GDS; page 236).

Address for correspondence

Yukimichi Imai
Department of Psychiatry
St Marianna University
School of Medicine
2-16-1 Sugao Miyamae-Ku
Kawasaki 216
Japan

Revised Hasegawa's Dementia Scale (HDS-R)

1.	How old are you? (+/– 2 yrs.)		0	I	
2.	Year, month, date, day?	Year	0	I	
	I point each.	Month	0	I	
		Date	0	I	
		Day	0	I	
3.	What Is this place?				
	Correct answer in 5 sec: 2 points.		0	2	
	Correct choice between 'hospital? office?'		0	I	
4.	Repeating 3 words. I point each. (To use only one version per test.)	a)	0	I	
	Version A: 'a) cherry blossom b) cat c) tram'.	a)	0	I	
	Version B: 'a) plum blossom b) dog c) car'.	b)	0	I	
5.	100 − 7=? If correct, I point.	93	0	I	
	If not: skip to item #6.				
	−7 again=? If correct, I point.	86	0	I	
6.	Repeat 6-8-2 backwards.		0	I	
	If not: skip to item #7.				
	Repeat 3-5-2-9 backwards.		0	I	
7.	Recall 3 words. For each word	a)	0	I	2
	2 points for spontaneous recall.	b)	0	I	2
	I point for correct recall after category cue.	c)	0	I	2
8.	Show live unrelated common object, then take them back and ask for recall.		0	I	2
	I point each.		3	4	5
9.	Name all vegetables that come to mind.				
	No time limit. May remind once.		0	I	2
	Terminate when there is no further answer after a 10 sec Interval. For each vegetable name after the 5th one: I point.	3	4	5	
	1. ___ 2. ___ 3. ___ 4. ___ 5. ___				
	6. ___ 7. ___ 8. ___ 9. ___ 10. ___				
	Total score				/30

Reproduced, with permission, from Imai Y and Hasegawa K (1994) The revised Hasegawa's dementia scale (HDS-R) – evaluation of its usefulness as a screening test for dementia. *Journal of Hong Kong College of Psychiatry* **4**: 20–24.

The Time and Change Test: a Simple Screening Test for Dementia

Reference: **Inouye SK, Robinson JT, Groehlich TE, Richardson ED (1998) The Time and Change Test: a simple screening test for dementia.** *Journal of Gerontology* **54A: M281–M286**

Time taken 25 seconds (yes, 25 seconds!)

Rating by experienced rater

Main indications

To have a simple standardized performance-based test incorporating real world activities as an adjunct to screening tests developed for dementia.

Commentary

In the original study 770 people were examined, 14% of whom had a diagnosis of dementia. Ratings on the Time and Change Test were validated using the Blessed Dementia Rating Scale and the Mini-Mental State Examination. The test had 86% sensitivity and 71% specificity, with a negative predictive value of 97%. Test/retest and inter-rater agreement rates were 88% and 78%, respectively. Education effects were about a quarter of what they were on the MMSE. The authors concluded that the Time and Change Test is a simple, accurate and reliable performance-based tool for the detection of dementia and can be used as a screening test in older people.

Telling time test A large clock-face diagram with the hands set at 11.10 is held 14 inches from the participant's eyes. The participant is cued: 'Please tell me what time it says on this clock'. For study purposes, the participant's response time is measured with a stopwatch that is started immediately after the cue is given. The participant is allowed two tries within a 60-second period. If they fail to respond correctly after two tries, the task is terminated and an error is recorded. Response time and any difficulties with the testing (e.g. vision, tremor, weakness and pain) are also recorded.

Making change task A standard amount of change (three quarters, seven dimes and seven nickels) is placed on a well-lit tabletop. The participant is cued: 'Please give me a dollar's worth of change'. For study purposes, the participant's response time is measured with a stopwatch that is started immediately after the cue is given. The participant is allowed two tries within a 180-second period. If they fail to respond correctly after two tries, the task is terminated and an error is recorded. As above, response time and any difficulties with the testing are also recorded.

Scoring If the responses were incorrect on either or both the telling time and making change tasks, then the T & C Test was scored as indicating dementia, a positive result. Correct responses on both the telling time and making change tasks were considered correct, a negative result.

Address for correspondence

Dr Sharon K Inouye
Yale University School of Medicine
20 York Street
Tompkins 15
New Haven
CT 06504
USA

Memory Impairment Screen

Reference: Buschke H, Kuslansky G, Katz M, Stewart WF, Sliwinski MJ, Eckholdt HM, Lipton RB (1999) Screening for dementia with the memory impairment screen. *Neurology* 52: 231–8

Time taken 4 minutes

Rating by experienced interviewer

Main indications

To develop and validate a sensitive and specific screening test for Alzheimer's disease and to improve the discrimination in screening between Alzheimer's disease and other dementias.

Commentary

The Memory Impairment Screen (MIS) was devised using a 4-minute, four-item delayed free and cued recall test of memory impairment using controlled learning to ensure attention, induce specific semantic processing, and optimising coding specificity to improve the detection of dementia. A total of 483 older people were assessed, 50 of whom had dementia. Reliability was found by administering one of two forms of the MIS and showed an intraclass correlation of 0.69 and an internal consistency (alpha value) of 0.67. Construct validity was assessed by the Free and Cued Selective Reminding Test, and discriminant validity was assessed showing the ability of the scale to differentiate between dementia and Alzheimer's disease. Normative values are provided to show the sensitivity, specificity and positive predictive value for each score on the MIS.

Address for correspondence

Dr Herman Buschke
Department of Neurology
Kennedy 912
Albert Einstein College of Medicine
Bronx, NY 10461
USA

Structured Telephone Interview for Dementia Assessment (STIDA)

Reference: **Go RCP, Duke LW, Harrell LE, Cody H, Bassett SS, Folstein MF, Albert MS, Foster JL, Sharrow NA, Blacker D (1997) Development and validation of a Structured Telephone Interview for Dementia (STIDA): the NIMH Genetics Initiative.** *Journal of Geriatric Psychiatry and Neurology* 10: 161–7

Time taken 30 minutes for the full version, 10 minutes for shortened version

Rating by experienced interviewer

Main indications

As part of the National Institute for Mental Health Genetics Initiative Alzheimer's Disease Study Group, a brief structured telephone interview was used to distinguish individuals with normal cognitive function from those with changes in cognition and daily functioning suggestive of early Alzheimer's disease (the Structured Telephone Interview for Dementia Assessment, STIDA).

Commentary

The score yielded a numerical value between 0 and 81 (higher scores indicating greater impairment) and subscales correlated with the subscales of the Clinical Dementia Rating (see p. 238) when a score of 10 or more was used to identify people with mild impairment. The STIDA has a sensitivity of 0.93 and a specificity of 0.92 for a CDR score of 0.5. An abbreviated version comprising six questions was able to detect possible cognitive impairment with a sensitivity of 0.93 and a specificity of 0.77. The results confirmed that the shortened version provides a sensitive and fairly specific telephone screen for dementia, whereas the full version, which consists of an interview with a knowledgeable informant and subject testing, is approximately the same as a face-to-face clinical interview and provides a reliable and balanced screening and staging assessment.

As part of the study 28 subjects and their knowledgeable informants were examined.

Address for correspondence

Dr Rodney CP Go
720 S 20th Street
TH 202A
Birmingham
AL 35294-0008
USA

Structured Telephone Interview for Dementia Assessment (STIDA)

The screening instrument, known as the Structured Telephone Interview for Dementia Assessment (STIDA), was designed to reduce the educational bias associated with measures based solely on cognitive testing by including questions about functional decline. It includes three sections: 1) an initial section on relevant medical history, used to identify potential medical causes of dementia; 2) a section on reported current cognitive abilities and functional status; and 3) a cognitive screening test consisting of the oral response items from the Mini-Mental State Examination (MMSE) and the short form of the Blessed Dementia Scale known as the Blessed-Orientation-Memory-Concentration Test (BOMC). In the present study, the first two sections of the interview were given in two versions, one administered to each potentially affected subject and the other administered to a knowledgeable informant to compare the utility of these two approaches. The first part of the interview reviews a number of relatively emotionally, neutral medical issues, and serves as a good means to establish a rapport with the subject or informant prior to beginning a discussion of the more sensitive questions regarding functional and cognitive status. This first section is not required for the assessment of dementia per se, but instead serves to screen for possible causes of dementia. All questions in sections 2 and 3 – the current cognitive abilities and functional status, and cognitive testing portions of the interview – yield a dementia score ranging from 0 to 81 possible points, with higher scores indicating greater impairment. The current cognitive abilities and functional status includes items from an interview about cognition and functional status, the Telephone Interview About Cognition and Health, developed for use in the multicenter study mentioned above (38 points). The cognitive testing section consists of the abbreviated MMSE (22 points, with each point indicating an item missed) and the BOMC (21 points, with each point indicating an item missed). These 81 points were allocated among four STIDA subscales corresponding roughly to the four domains evaluated by the Clinical Dementia Rating (CDR) Scale (see Figure below).

Score sheet for STIDA Score and Clinical Dementia Rating (CDR)

Family Name _____   Date _____

Subject Name _____   Informant Name _____

Interviewer _____   Evaluated by _____

CDR/STIDA Subscale	STIDA Subscore	Possible points	Actual points	0	.5	1	2	3
MEMORY	Expressive language	4						
	Other language	8						
	Memory	5						
	Mini-Mental	12						
	Short Blessed	18						
Sub-total	Circle CDR	47		0	.5	1	2	3
				0–7	8–10	11–30	31–40	41–47
ORIENTATION	Mini-Mental	10						
	Short Blessed	3						
	Spatial functions	5						
Sub-total	Circle CDR	18		0	.5	1	2	3
				0–3	4–6	7–10	11–17	18
JUDGMENT	Calculation	6						
	Conceptualization	4						
	Problem solving	1						
Sub-total	Circle CDR	11		0	.5	1	2	3
				0	1	2–6	7–10	11
PERSONAL CARE	Community	1						
	Home	1						
	Personal	3						
Sub-total	Circle CDR	5		0	.5	1	2	3
				0	1	2–3	4	5
STIDA SCORE		81						

Source: Reproduced by permission from Go RCP *et al. J Geriatr Psychiatry Neurol* 1997; **10:** 161–7.

Détérioration de Cognition Observée (DECO)

Reference: Ritchie K, Fuhrer R (1996) The validation of an Informant Screening Test for Irreversible Cognitive Decline in the Elderly: performance characteristics within a general population sample. *International Journal of Geriatric Psychiatry* 11: 149–56

Time taken 11–15 minutes (reviewer's estimate)

Rating by experienced interviewer

Main indications

The informant questionnaire Détérioration de Cognition Observée (DECO) was developed to assess the performance of a Brief Informant Screening Test. The test was included as part of a general population study of brain ageing, a prospective study of a representative sample of 3777 people over the age of 65 selected from the electoral register in Aquitaine, France. Receiver operating characteristics of the scale showed a specificity of 90% and a sensitivity of 79% for the detection of senile dementia, using a cut-off score of 24/25. The discriminability of the test was not affected by level of education.

Address for correspondence

Dr Karen Ritchie
Directeur de Recherche
INSERM E0361
Pathologies du Système Nerveux
Recherche Epidémiologique et Clinique
Hôpital la Colombière, 39 Ave Charles Flahault
34093 Montpellier Cedex 5, France
e-mail: Ritchie@montp.inserm.fr

DECO

We would like you to tell us how your relative was a year ago. The following questions ask about a number of everyday situations. We would like you to tell us whether in these situations he/she is doing about the same, not as well or much worse, than a year ago. Put a cross in the square to show your reply.

	Better or about the same	Not as well	Much worse
Does he/she remember as well as before which day of the week and which month it is?	☐	☐	☐
When he/she goes out of the house, does he/she know the way as well as before?	☐	☐	☐
Have there been changes in his/her ability to remember her own address or telephone number?	☐	☐	☐
In the house, does he/sher remember as well as before where things are usually kept?	☐	☐	☐
And when an object isn't in its usual place, is he/she capable of finding it again?	☐	☐	☐
In comparison with a year ago, how well is he/she able to use household appliances (washing machine, etc. . . .)?	☐	☐	☐
Has his/her ability to dress or undress changed at all?	☐	☐	☐
How well does he/she manage his/her money, for example doing the shopping?	☐	☐	☐
Apart from difficulties due to physical problems, has there been a reduction in his/her activity level?	☐	☐	☐
How well can he/she follow a story on television, in a book or told by someone?	☐	☐	☐
And writing letters for business or to friends, does he/she do this as well as a year ago?	☐	☐	☐
How well does he/she recall a conversation you have had with him/her a few days ago? Has this changed over the past year?	☐	☐	☐
And if you remind him/her of this conversation, does he/she still have difficulty remembering it in comparison with a year ago?	☐	☐	☐
Does he/she forget what he/she wanted to say in the middle of a conversation? Has this changed over the past year?	☐	☐	☐
In a conversation, does he/she sometimes have difficulty finding the right word?	☐	☐	☐
In comparison with a year ago, how well does he/she recognize the faces of people he/she knows well?	☐	☐	☐
And how well does he/she remember the names of these people?	☐	☐	☐
In comparison with a year ago, how well does he/she remember other details concerning people he/she knows well: where they live, what they do?	☐	☐	☐
Over the past year, have there been changes in his/her ability to remember what has happened recently?	☐	☐	☐

Source: Ritchie K *et al. Int J Geriatr Psychiatry* 1996; 11: 149–56. Reprinted by permission of John Wiley & Sons, Inc. © 1996.

Objective Assessment of Praxis

Reference: **Connelly PJ, Jamieson FE (1991) Objective Assessment of Praxis – the OPA Diagram – Simply testing for dementia.** *International Journal of Geriatric Psychiatry* **6: 667–72**

Time taken 1 minute

Rating the simplicity of the diagram suggests it can be used by untrained interviewers

Main indication

The Objective Assessment of Praxis (OAP) is a simple, quick test which is easy to administer and score. It identifies cognitively impaired subjects by focusing on visual constructive ability in the form of copying a task.

Commentary

A 10-line asymmetrical figure is used. A trial involving 60 female patients compared the Cognitive Assessment Schedule (CAS), the Behaviour Rating Scale (BRS) of the Clifton Assessment Procedure for the Elderly (CAPE), the Parietal Signs Scale of the Kew Cognitive Map, the copying task from the Mini-Mental State Examination (MMSE) and the OAP diagram. Each rater randomly undertook cognitive or drawing assessment on each patient while remaining blind to the ratings from the other categories. There were 25 functional patients and 35 demented patients. There was a high correlation between the CAS scores and the number of lines of the OAP diagram drawn correctly. High inter-rater reliability suggests the scoring system is easy to use. The OAP diagram proved to be significantly better than the MMSE diagram at differentiating organic and functional groups. The specificity of the OAP is 0.84 at cut-off ≥9, and that of the OAP is 0.8 at cut-off ≥8. Non-demented patients do not tend to make mistakes.

Additional references

Schulman KI, Shedletsky R, Silver IL (1986) The challenge of time: clock drawing and cognitive function in the elderly. *International Journal of Geriatric Psychiatry* **1**: 135–40.

McPherson FM, Gamsu CV, Cockran LL, Cooke D (1986a) Use of the CAPE Pm test with disabled patients. *British Journal of Clinical Psychology* **25**: 145–6.

McPherson FM, Gamsu CV, Cockran LL, Cooke D (1986b) Inter-scorer agreement in scoring errors in the Pm (Maze) test of the CAPE. *British Journal of Clinical Psychology* **25**: 255–6.

Address for correspondence

Dr Peter J Connelly
Consultant Psychiatrist
Murray Royal Hospital
Perth PH2 7BH
UK

Lay Person-Based Screening for Early Detection of Alzheimer's Disease

Reference: **Mundt JC, Freed DM, Greist JH (2000) Lay person-based screening for early detection of Alzheimer's disease; development and validation of an instrument.** *Journal of Gerontology, Psychological Sciences* **55B: 163–70**

Time taken approx. 10–15 minutes

Rating by lay persons with minimal clinical training or expertise

Main indications

A validated short dementia screening questionnaire that can be used widely in general populations for screening by non-trained raters.

Commentary

This short dementia screening questionnaire has been empirically devised from neuropsychological research data and can be administered either by telephone or via a paper and pencil questionnaire. The validity of the instrument was evaluated on 103 patients, all of whom had received a complete neuropsychological assessment. The telephone interviewers did not know the research diagnosis of the patients. Applied to the validation sample, the simple short scale indicated potential sensitivity and specificity of 98.4% and 81%, respectively, with positive and negative predictive values of 88.2% and 97.1%, respectively. These correlated with Mini-Mental State scores.

Additional reference

Mundt JC, Ferber K, Greist JH (2000) Development of a short informant based screening instrument for dementias. (Poster) 40th Annual meeting of New Clinical Drug Evaluation Unit. 31 May 2000. Boca Raton, Florida, USA

Address for correspondence

James C Mundt
Healthcare Technology Systems
LLC 7617 Mineral Point Road
Suite 300
Madison
WI 53717
USA

mundj@healthtechsys.com

The Telephone Interview for Cognitive Status

Reference: **Brandt J, Spencer M, Folstein M (1988) The telephone interview for cognitive status.** *Neuropsychiatry, Neuropsychology and Behavioural Neurology* **1: 111–17**

Time taken approx. 10 minutes

Rating by trained interviewer

Main indications

A cognitive screening test that does not require face-to-face interaction between the patient and the examiner and can be administered over the telephone. Application is for large-scale field studies of cognitive impairment.

Commentary

The Telephone Interview for Cognitive Status (TICS) correlates very highly with the Mini-Mental Test Examination. It has high test/retest reliability and high sensitivity and specificity for cognitive impairment in a clinic sample of Alzheimer's disease. The sample consisted of 100 patients with a diagnosis of Alzheimer's disease compared to 33 individuals who served as a normal control group. The TICS is composed of 11 items with a maximum score of 41; two of the items are identical to the Mini-Mental Test items. In the sample of 16 mild Alzheimer's disease patients and 33 normal controls the TICS had a sensitivity of 94% and a specificity of 100%.

Additional reference

Nelson A, Fogel BS, Faust D (1986) Bedside cognitive screening instruments. *Journal of Nervous and Mental Disease* 174: 73–83.

Address for correspondence

Dr J Brandt
Department of Psychiatry and Behavioural Sciences
Mery 218
Johns Hopkins University School of Medicine
600 North Wolfe Street
Baltimore
MD 21205
USA

e-mail: jbrandt@welch.jhu.edu

Telephone Interview for Cognitive Status (TICS)

Name: _____   Date: _____

Directions: (1) Explain exam to subject (or patient's caregiver). (2) Get address. (3) Be sure distractions are minimal (e.g. no TV or radio on, remove pens and pencils from reach). (4) Be sure sources of orientation (e.g. newspapers, calendars) are not in subject's view. (5) Caregivers may offer reassurance, but not assistance. (6) Single repetitions permitted, except for items 5 and 8.

Instruction	Scoring criteria	Score
1. 'Please tell me your full name?'	1 pt. for first name, 1 pt. for last name.	_____
2. 'What is today's date?'	1 pt. each for month, date, year, day of week, and season. If incomplete, ask specifics (e.g. 'What is the month?' 'What season are we in?')	_____
3. 'Where are you right now?'	1 pt. each for house number, street, city, state, zip. If incomplete, ask specifics (e.g. 'What street are you on right now?')	_____
4. 'Count backwards from 20 to 1.'	2 pts. if completely correct on the first trial; 1 pt. if completely correct on second trial; 0 pts. for anything else.	_____
5. 'I'm going to read you a list of ten words. Please listen carefully and try to remember them. When I am done, tell me as many words as you can, in any order. Ready? The words are: cabin, pipe, elephant, chest, silk, theatre, watch, whip, pillow, giant. Now tell me all the words you can remember.'	1 pt. for each correct response. No penalty for repetitions or intrusions.	_____
6. 'One hundred minus 7 equals what?' 'And 7 from that?', etc.	Stop at 5 serial subtractions. 1 pt. for each correct subtraction. Do not inform the subject of incorrect responses, but allow subtractions to be made from his/her last response (e.g. '93–85–78–71–65' would get 3 points).	_____
7. 'What do people usually use to cut paper?'	1 pt. for 'scissors' or 'shears' only.	_____
'How many things are in a dozen?'	1 pt. for '12'.	_____
'What do you call the prickly green plant that lives in the desert?'	1 pt. for 'cactus' only.	_____
'What animal does wool come from?'	1 pt. for 'sheep' or 'lamb' only.	_____
8. 'Say this: "No ifs, ands or buts".' 'Say this: "Methodist episcopal".'	1 pt. for each complete repetition on the first trial. Repeat only if poorly presented.	_____
9. 'Who is the President of the United States right now?'	1 pt. for correct first and last name.	_____
'Who is the Vice-President?'	1 pt. for correct first and last name.	_____
10. 'With your finger, tap 5 times on the part of the phone you speak into.'	2 pts. if 5 taps are heard; 1 pt. if subject taps more or less than 5 times.	_____
11. 'I'm going to give you a word and I want you to give me its opposite. For example, the opposite of hot is cold. What is the opposite of "west"?'	1 pt. for 'east'.	_____
'What is the opposite of "generous"?'	1 pt. for 'selfish', 'greedy', 'stingy', 'tight', 'cheap', 'mean', 'meager', 'skimpy', or other good antonym.	_____
	Total	_____

Source: Brandt J *et al. Neuropsychiatry Neuropsychology Behav Neurol* 1988; 11: 111–17. Reproduced by permission.

Observation List for Early Signs of Dementia (OLD)

Reference: **Hopman-Rock M, Tak ECPM, Staats PGM (2001) Development and validation of the Observational List for Early Signs of Dementia (OLD).** *International Journal of Geriatric Psychiatry* **15: 406–14**

Time taken 5 minutes

Rating by general practitioners (GPs)

Main indications

A short list of possible early signs of dementia for use in general practice. Can indicate when it may be useful to use other existing screening instruments.

Commentary

The Observational List for Early Signs of Dementia (OLD) can be used in unselected elderly populations and can be administered without unduly alarming patients and relatives. Initially 29 signs were identified, and this was later reduced to 12. The GPs administered the test on 5 working days to the first two patients over 75 years old seen by them. Exclusion criteria included psychiatric treatment, a known diagnosis of dementia or severe depression, or acute illness with confusion. The reliability of the OLD was measured using internal consistency and factor analysis. Test/retest was not possible because patients were observed during real-life consultation. The OLD score did not correlate with the Global Deterioration Scale (GDS) score for depression, indicating good discriminant validity.

Additional reference

Hopman-Rock M, Tak ECPM, Staats PGM (1998) Checklist Alzheimer Dementie. Fase a; de Ontwikkeling. TNO PG: Leiden 73

Address for correspondence

Dr Marijke Hopman-Rock
TNO Prevention and Health
PO Box 2215
2301 CE Leiden
The Netherlands
m.hopman@pg.tno.nl

Early Signs of Dementia Checklist

Reference: **Visser FE, Aldenkamp AP, van Huffelen AC, Kuilman M, Overweg J, van Wijk J (1997) Prospective study of the prevalence of Alzheimer-type dementia in institutionalized individuals with Down syndrome.** *American Journal of Mental Retardation* 101: 400–12

Time taken 15 minutes (reviewer's estimate)

Main indications

To detect dementia in people with learning disability.

Commentary

The questionnaire was developed retrospectively in institutionalized people with Down's syndrome.

The current study involved a longitudinal follow-up of 307 individuals with Down's syndrome over 5–10 years. Cognitive functioning, clinical signs and EEG changes were assessed and post-mortem examination carried out where possible. The mean age of onset of dementia was 56 years – 11% of those between the ages of 40 and 49 had dementia, 77% between the ages of 60 and 69 and everyone over the age of 70 years. The early signs of dementia checklist aims to score the first clinical signs of change and consists of 37 questions. The checklist is completed by a nurse who knows the individual well. Internal consistency was 0.82 and inter-rater reliability was 0.80.

Additional references

Visser FE, Kuilman M (1990) A study of dementia in Down's syndrome of an institutionalized population. *Nederlands Tijdschrift voor Geneeskunde* 134: 1141–5.

Questions from the Early Signs of Dementia Checklist by Category

General
1. Does resident show decrease in interest in work, hobby, objects, certain events, or social contacts?
2. Does resident show decrease in general pace or initiative?

Personality Changes
3. Does resident show exaggeration of character traits?
4. Does resident show changes in mood?
5. Does resident show increased excitability?
6. Does resident show emotional instability, anxiety, or nervousness?

Decrease in Performance
7. Does resident show a decrease in quality of work or a decrease in working pace?
8. Has resident lost the ability to work?
9. Does resident show a deterioration in performance of household chores?
10. Does resident need assistance in domestic jobs?
11. Has resident become dependent on supervision for daily living activities?
12. Has resident become dependent on assistance for daily living activities?
13. Has resident become dependent on nursing care?

Deterioration of Language Skills
14. Does resident show a deterioration of speech or speech fluency?
15. Has resident lost speech completely?
16. Does resident show decreased reactivity when spoken to?

Deterioration of Gait
17. Does resident show a decrease in quality of gait or does resident stumble more often?

18. Has resident become dependent on support for walking?
19. Has resident become unable to walk?

Disorientation
20. Does resident lose his or her way in the neighborhood, the group home, or his or her own room?
21. Has resident become afraid to go to bed?
22. Does resident reverse day/night rhythm?
23. Is resident anxious at night?
24. Does resident want to eat, go to work at the wrong moment?
25. Does resident no longer recognize members of the nursing staff?
26. Does resident bo longer recognize family?

Incontinence
27. Does resident occasionally show urinary incontinence during the day?
28. Does resident show continuous urinary incontinence during the day?
29. Does resident occasionally show urinary incontinence at night?
30. Does resident always show urinary incontinence at night?
31. Does resident show fecal incontinence?

Epilepsy
32. Has resident developed epilepsy?

Loss of School-Acquired Skills
33. Has resident's ability to read deteriorated?
34. Has resident's writing worsened?
35. Has resident's ability to cipher deteriorated?
36. Has there been a decrease in the playing ability of a patient who plays an instrument?
37. Has resident's ability to do arts and crafts deteriorated?

Source: Reproduced with permission from Visser FE *et al.* Am J Ment Retard 1997; **101**: 400–12.

A Cognitive Screening Battery for Dementia in the Elderly

Reference: Jacqmin-Gadda H, Fabrigoule C, Commenges D, Letenneur L, Dartignes JF (2000) A Cognitive Screening Battery for Dementia in the Elderly. *Journal of Clinical Epidemiology* 53: 980–7

Time taken less than 20 minutes

Rating by trained interviewer

Main indications

A screening instrument for dementia based on neuropsychological tests that can be used in multicentric studies.

Commentary

Paquid research programme is a prospective cohort study of normal and pathological cerebral ageing. The aim was to find a screening test for dementia that has a sensitivity of 1 and the best specificity possible. In this study data from five visits were pooled and the authors tried to improve the specificity by adding another four neurological tests. A major finding was a combination of the Mini-Mental State Examination, the Isaacs Set Test of verbal fluency and the Benton Visual Retention Test. With the MMSE subscores, orientation to time and recall were the most discriminating between demented and non-demented subjects. Results showed a specificity of 0.8 and a sensitivity of 1. It is less associated with educational level among demented subjects than are other screening tests.

Additional reference

Commenges D, Gagnon M, Letenneur L et al (1992) Improving screening for dementia in the elderly using Mini-Mental State Examination subscores, Benton's Visual Retention Test and Isaacs Set Test. *Epidemiology* 3:185–8.

Address for correspondence

Helene.jacqumin-gadda@bordeaux.inserm.fr

Test Battery for the Diagnosis of Dementia in Individuals with Intellectual Disability

Reference: **Burt DB, Aylward EH (2000) Test Battery for the Diagnosis of Dementia in Individuals with Intellectual Disability.** *Journal of Intellectual Disability Research* **44: 175–80**

Time taken lengthy

Rating by trained interviewers

Main indications

A comprehensive battery of tests for the diagnosis of dementia in individuals with intellectual disability recommended for international use, as part of both ongoing and new longitudinal research in clinical practice.

Commentary

Members of the Working Group for the Establishment of Criteria for the Diagnosis of Dementia in Individuals with Intellectual Disability proposed this comprehensive battery of tests to increase the overlap of tests used to assess dementia at research and clinical sites. It includes 17 instruments, of which six are administered to the informant and 11 to the individual. To meet the diagnostic criteria for dementia, documented declines on at least one memory test and at least one of the tests of other cognitive ability are required. It is therefore recommended that it should be administered at least once before 40 years of age to all adults with Down's syndrome, and before 50 years of age to other adults with intellectual disability in order to establish baseline levels of performance when healthy. It should then be administered periodically between 1 and 5 years depending on age and risk for dementia, and as soon as possible when dementia is suspected.

Address for correspondence

Dr Diana B Burt
6509 Gettysburg Drive
Madison WI 53705
USA
dbburt@aol.com

The Test for Severe Impairment (TSI)

Reference: **Albert M, Cohen C (1992) The Test for Severe Impairment: an instrument for the assessment of patients with severe cognitive dysfunction.** *Journal of the American Geriatrics Society* **40: 449–53**

Time taken 10 minutes

Rating by trained interviewer

Main indications

To assess cognitive function in patients with advanced dementia.

Commentary

The Test for Severe Impairment consists of 24 items which assess eight cognitive domains: memory (immediate and recall), general knowledge, language (verbal, comprehensive and production), social interactiveness, conceptionalization and motor performance. The test can be administered without the need for intact speech and is independent of age and education. Its test/retest and inter-rater reliability were satisfactory and comparable to the highest mean values reported in the literature for the Severe Impairment Battery (SIB). However, the TSI remains unhelpful for subjects who are uncooperative and/or unresponsive.

Additional reference

Appollonio I, Gori C, Riva GP et al (2001) Cognitive Assessment of Severe Dementia: The Test for Severe Impairment (TSI). *Archives of Gerontology* Suppl **7**: 25–31

Address for correspondence

Dr I Appollonio
Istituto Protetto
Mons L Biraghi Nursing Home
via Videmari 2
1-20063 Cernusco
Milan
Italy

The Frontal Behavioral Inventory

Reference: **Kertesz A, Nadkarni N, Davidson W, Thomas AW (2000) The Frontal Behavioral Inventory in the differential diagnosis of frontotemporal dementia.** *Journal of the International Neuropsychological Society* **6: 460–8**

Time taken 15–30 minutes

Rating by trained interviewer with caregiver

Main indications

A behavioural inventory specific for the diagnosis of frontal lobe dementia.

Commentary

The Frontal Behavioral Inventory (FBI) is a 24-item scoreable questionnaire. It consists of deficit behaviours such as apathy, lack of spontaneity, indifference, inflexibility, concreteness, personal neglect, disorganization, inattention, loss of insight, logopenia, verbal apraxia and alien hand. Positive groups of behaviour contain perseveration, irritability, excessive of childish jocularity, irresponsibility, inappropriateness, impulsivity, restlessness, aggression, hyperorality, hypersexuality, utilization behaviour and incontinence. The FBI has been successful in discriminating between other causes of dementia, although high scores are also achieved in vascular dementia. The total score above a conservative cut-off point of 30 is suggestive of frontal lobe dementia. The high scores on indifference, perseveration and utilization behaviour, when present, are useful to discriminate frontal lobe dementia. It has a high inter-rater reliability and content validity and is easy to administer.

Additional reference

Kertesz A, Davison W, Fox H (1997) Frontal behaviour inventory: diagnostic criteria for frontal lobe dementia. *Canadian Journal of Neurological Sciences* **24**: 29–36.

Address for correspondence

Dr Andrew Kertesz
St Joseph's Health Centre
Department of Neurology
268 Grosvenor Street
London, Ontario
N6A 4V2
Canada

The Frontal Behavioral Inventory (FBI)

Explain to the caregiver that you are looking for a change in behavior and personality. Ask the caregiver these questions in the absence of the patient. Elaborate if necessary. At the end of each question, ask about the extent of the behavioral change, and then score it according to the following: 0 = none, 1 = mild, occasional, 2 = moderate, 3 = severe, most of the time.

1. *Apathy:* Has s/he lost interest in friends or daily activities? _____

2. *Aspontaneity:* Does s/he start things on his/her own, or does s/he have to be asked? _____

3. *Indifference, Emotional Flatness:* Does s/he respond to occasions of joy or sadness as much as ever, of has s/he lost emotional responsiveness? _____

4. *Inflexibility:* Can s/he change his/her mind with reason or does s/he appear stubborn or rigid in thinking lately? _____

5. *Concreteness:* Does s/he interpret what is being said appropriately or does s/he choose only the concrete meanings of what is being said? _____

6. *Personal Neglect:* Does s/he take as much care of his/her personal hygiene and appearance as usual? _____

7. *Disorganization:* Can s/he plan and organize complex activity or is s/he easily distractible, impersistent, or unable to complete a job? _____

8. *Inattention:* Does s/he pay attention to what is going on or does s/he seem to lose track or not follow at all? _____

9. *Loss of Insight:* Is s/he aware of any problems or changes, or does s/he seem unaware of them or deny them when discussed? _____

10. *Logopenia:* Is s/he talkative as before or has the amount of speech significantly decreased? _____

11. *Verbal Apraxia:* Has s/he been talking clearly or has s/he been making errors in speech? Is there slurring or hesitation? _____

12. *Perseveration:* Does s/he repeat or perseverate actions or remarks? _____

13. *Irritability:* Has s/he been irritable or short-tempered, or is s/he reacting to stress or frustration as s/he always had? _____

14. *Excessive Jocularity:* Has s/he been making jokes excessively or offensively or at the wrong time? _____

15. *Poor Judgment:* Has s/he been using good judgment in decisions or in driving, or has s/he acted irresponsibly, neglectfully, or in poor judgment? _____

16. *Inappropriateness:* Has s/he kept social rules or has s/he said or done things outside of what is acceptable? Has s/he been rude or childish? _____

17. *Impulsivity:* Has s/he acted or spoken without thinking about the consequences, on the spur of the moment? _____

18. *Restlessness:* Has s/he been restless or hyperactive, or is the activity level normal? _____

19. *Aggression:* Has s/he shown aggression, or shouted at anyone or hurt them physically? _____

20. *Hyperorality:* Has s/he been drinking more than usual, eating excessively anything in sight, or even putting objects in his/her mouth? _____

21. *Hypersexuality:* Has his/her sexual behavior been unusual or excessive? _____

22. *Utilization:* Does s/he seem to need to touch, feel, examine, or pick up objects within reach and sight? _____

23. *Incontinence:* Has s/he wet or soiled him/herself (excluding physical illness, such as urinary infection or immobility)? _____

24. *Alien Hand:* Does s/he have any problem using a hand, and does it interfere with the other hand (excluding arthritis, trauma, paralysis, etc.)? _____

Total Score: _____

Source: Reprinted with permission from Kertesz A *et al. Can J Neurol Sci* 1997; **24:** 29–36.

The General Practitioner Assessment of Cognition (GPCOG)

Reference: **Brodaty H, Pond D, Kemp NM, Luscombe G, Harding L, Berman K, Huppert FA (2000) The GPCOG: A new screening test for dementia designed for general practice.** *Journal of the American Geriatrics Society* **50: 530–4**

Time taken 5–6 minutes

Rating by experienced interviewer

Main indications

Screening test for dementia in general practice.

Commentary

This is a screening test for dementia designed specifically for general practice. There are two parts, a patient cognitive testing section and a brief informant interview. The instrument has been validated and shown satisfactory sensitivity and specificity, and has been found to be accept- able to both patients and general practitioners. It has been found to be superior to the Abbreviated Mental Test and possibly the MMSE as a screening test for dementia. The novel aspect of the screening instrument is the fact that it includes an informant interview.

Address for correspondence

Professor Henry Brodaty
Academic Department for Old Age Psychiatry
Prince of Wales Hospital
Randwick
NSW 2031
Australia
h.brodaty@unsw.edu.au

GPCOG Patient Examination

Unless specified, each question should only be asked once.

Name and address for subsequent recall test

1. *'I am going to give you a name and address. After I have said it, I want you to repeat it. Remember this name and address because I am going to ask you to tell it to me again in a few minutes: John Brown, 42 West Street, Kensington.'* (Allow a maximum of 4 attempts but do not score yet)

	Correct	Incorrect
Time orientation		
2. *What is the date?* (exact only)	☐	☐
Clock Drawing (visuospatial functioning) – use page with printed circle		
3. *Please mark in all the numbers to indicate the hours of a clock* (correct spacing required)	☐	☐
4. *Please mark in hands to show 10 minutes past eleven o'clock* (11:10)	☐	☐
Information		
5. *Can you tell me something that happened in the news recently?* (recently = in the last week)	☐	☐
Recall		
6. *What was the name and address I asked you to remember?*		
John	☐	☐
Brown	☐	☐
42	☐	☐
West (St)	☐	☐
Kensington	☐	☐

Scoring guidelines

Clock drawing: For a correct response to question 3, the numbers 12, 3, 6, and 9 should be in the correct quadrants of the circle and the other numbers should be approximately correctly placed. For a correct response to question 4, the hands should be pointing to the 11 and the 2, but do not penalize if the respondent fails to distinguish the long and short hands.

Information: Respondents are not required to provide extensive details, as long as they demonstrate awareness of a recent news story. If a general answer is given, such as 'war', 'a lot of rain', ask for details – if unable to give details, the answer should be scored as incorrect.

GPCOG Informant Interview

Ask the informant: *Compared to a few years ago,*

	Yes	No	Don't Know	N/A
I. Does the patient have more trouble remembering things that have happened recently?	☐	☐	☐	
II. Does he or she have more trouble recalling conversations a few days later?	☐	☐	☐	
III. When speaking, does the patient have more difficulty in finding the right word or tend to use the wrong words more often?	☐	☐	☐	
IV. Is the patient less able to manage money and financial affairs (e.g. paying bills, budgeting)?	☐	☐	☐	☐
V. Is the patient less able to manage his or her medication independently?	☐	☐	☐	☐
VI. Does the patient need more assistance with transport (either private or public)?	☐	☐	☐	☐

Source: Brodaty H *et al. J Am Geriatr Soc* 2000; **50**: 530–4. Reproduced by permission.

Computerized Cognitive Examination of the Elderly (ECO)

Reference: Ritchie K, Allard M, Huppert FA, Nargeot C, Pinek B, Ledesert B (1993) Computerized cognitive examination of the elderly (ECO). The development of a neuropsychological examination for clinical and population use. *International Journal of Geriatric Psychiatry* 8: 899–914

Time taken 30–45 minutes. The same battery of tests administered by paper and pencil takes over 90 minutes

Rating by experienced interviewer

Main indications

This is a computerized test battery (Examen Cognitif par Ordinateur, ECO) which was developed to be of use in epidemiological studies, combining 'friendly' software with a portable computer system.

Commentary

The test selection for the programme was based on a literature review regarding information processing models of intellectual function in normal adults. Four areas are examined: memory, visuospatial analysis, language and attention. The subtests of the ECO are as follows: simple reaction time; auditory attention with and without interference; visual attention with and without interference; dual task performance; word comprehension; sentence comprehension and reading; articulation and immediate verbal recall; visuospatial span; visuospatial matching; visuospatial reasoning; mime construction; delayed verbal and non-verbal recall; paired associate learning; verbal fluency; narrative recall; implicit memory.

A total of 335 elderly people between the ages of 60 and 100 were examined. The examination was very acceptable to older people – many found the procedures so enjoyable that they asked to repeat it. Means and standard deviations by 10-year age group are available.

Address for correspondence

Dr Karen Ritchie
Directeur de Recherche
INSERM E0361
Pathologies du Système Nerveux
Recherche Epidémiologique et Clinique
Hôpital la Colombière
39 Ave Charles Flahault
34093 Montpellier Cedex 5
France

e-mail: Ritchie@montp.inserm.fr

The Neuropsychological Impairment Scale – Senior (NIS–S)

Reference: O'Donnell WE (2001) The Neuropsychological Impairment Scale – Senior: a procedure for evaluating awareness disturbance in geriatric patients. *Journal of Clinical Psychology* 57: 423–7

Time taken 5–7 minutes

Rating by experienced interviewer

Main indications

To evaluate an elderly person's awareness of their cognitive functioning.

Commentary

This is a 30-item questionnaire administered to geriatric patients about symptoms of cognitive impairment, affective disturbance and defensiveness. The items are read to the patient using a three-choice response format ('not at all, a little bit, quite a bit'). The purpose of this scale is to assess the patient's awareness of their cognitive functioning. Of the 30 questions, 18 enquire about cognitive deficits, five gauge defensiveness and seven measure affective disturbance.

The NIS–S should not be used on its own. Data do not replace performance measures of cognitive ability. It should be used in the context of a comprehensive assessment of all factors that might be contributing to the patient's condition.

Address for correspondence

William E O'Donnell
PO Box 1541
Annapolis
MD 21404
USA

Senior Items*

	I	II	III	IV	V
Defensiveness Items					
3. Like everyone	0.01	−0.13	0.69	0.02	−0.04
8. Always happy	−0.02	−0.33	0.70	0.03	−0.07
12. Always do right	−0.08	0.11	0.68	0.02	−0.04
16. Always tell truth	−0.07	0.13	0.70	−0.13	−0.03
25. Always good mood	−0.10	−0.31	0.78	−0.03	0.04
Affective Disturbance Items					
5. Sad or blue	0.19	0.77	−0.10	0.04	0.04
10. Lonely/isolated	0.03	0.78	−0.01	0.17	0.16
15. Depressed	0.14	0.77	−0.16	0.12	0.15
18. Anxious/afraid	0.27	0.59	−0.03	0.35	0.13
20. Tense/upset	0.22	0.73	−0.04	0.08	0.22
23. Life stressful	0.35	0.62	−0.11	−0.10	0.01
28. Worry	0.21	0.70	−0.04	0.11	0.05
Global Measure of Impairment Items					
1. Forgetful	0.43	0.05	−0.06	−0.02	0.52
9. Forget/saying	0.44	0.12	−0.02	0.33	0.47
13. Lose things	0.25	0.14	−0.07	0.12	0.78
21. Remember/important	0.43	0.16	0.01	0.23	0.60
22. Lost easily	0.32	0.16	0.06	0.33	0.45
26. Forget/put things	0.24	0.13	−0.09	0.00	0.83
17. Speech worse	0.26	0.18	−0.05	0.77	0.08
19. Trouble talking	0.24	0.14	−0.02	0.75	0.17
2. Mind/slow	0.74	0.07	−0.06	0.21	0.03
4. Words/mix	0.67	0.13	−0.10	0.19	0.16
6. Serious/memory	0.52	0.23	0.02	0.22	0.37
7. Thinking/blocked	0.56	0.22	−0.10	0.14	0.42
11. Confused easily	0.62	0.25	−0.01	0.24	0.29
14. Difficulty/decisions	0.49	0.32	−0.11	0.24	0.28
24. Difficulty/attention	0.68	0.24	−0.04	0.02	0.21
27. Trouble/concentrating	0.72	0.24	−0.05	0.02	0.27
29. Trouble/thinking	0.69	0.27	−0.04	0.18	0.22
30. Do things slowly	0.39	0.08	−0.03	0.31	0.28

*n = 373

Summary

The NIS–S has adequate reliability (internal consistency and stability) and validity (concurrent, structural, and discriminant) with appropriate clinical and non-clinical normative references. The relatively small sample of patients and non-clinical subjects used for test development warrants replication of these findings in different settings with a larger pool of subjects. It should be cautioned, however, that the NIS–S should not be used as a stand-alone instrument: it does not replace performance measures of cognitive ability. Also, it does not measure cognitive impairment as such, but whether the patient believes that he or she has cognitive difficulties. Its proper use is within the context of a comprehensive assessment of all factors that might be contributing to the patient's condition. Its relative ease of administration, scoring and interpretation suggests that it could be a practical ancillary tool for psychologists in geriatric settings.

Source: O'Donnell WE. *J Clin Psychol* 2001; **57**: 423–7. Reproduced by permission of John Wiley & Sons, Inc. © 2001.

Short and Sweet Screening Instrument (SAS–SI)

Reference: **Belle SH, Mendelsohn AB, Seaberg EC, Ratcliff G (2000) A Brief Cognitive Screening Battery for Dementia in the Community.** *Neuroepidemiology* 19: 43–50

Time taken approx. 10 minutes

Main indications

Screening for dementia in the community.

Commentary

This is a brief battery consisting of three standard cognitive tests: the MMSE, category fluency for animals, and temporal orientation test.

Using these three tests provides high sensitivity and specificity for the diagnosis of dementia in the community and showed substantially higher specificity than the MMSE alone.

Address for correspondence

Steven H Belle
Epidemiology Data Center
Graduate School of Public Health
University of Pittsburgh
127 Parran Hall, 130 DeSoto Street
Pittsburg
PA 15261
USA

Middlesex Elderly Assessment of Mental State (MEAMS)

Reference: **Golding E (1989)** *The Middlesex Elderly Assessment of Mental State.* England: **Thames Valley Test Company**

Time taken 10 minutes

Rating by experienced interviewer

Main indications

A brief screening test which aims to distinguish between organic and functional impairment in older people.

Commentary

There are 12 subtests which give rise to a total score depending on whether each individual test is passed or failed. Parallel forms are available for retesting.

A test/retest study of the MEAMS (Powell et al, 1993) showed that reliability was good.

Additional reference

Powell T, Brooker DJR, Papadopolous A (1993) Test–retest reliability of the MEAMS: a preliminary investigation in people with probable dementia. *British Journal of Clinical Psychology* **32**: 224–6

Address for correspondence

Thames Valley Test Company
Unit 22, The Granary
Station HIll
Thurston, Bury St Edmunds
Suffolk IP31 3QU
England

http://www.tvtc.com/tvtc/tvtcpage/meams.html

The Executive Interview

Reference: **Royall DR, Mahurin RK, Gray KF (1992) Bedside Assessment of Executive Cognitive Impairment: the Executive Interview.** *Journal of the American Geriatrics Society* **40: 1221–6**

Time taken 10–15 minutes

Rating by experienced interviewer

Main indications

A clinical tool to assess executive function.

Commentary

Executive cognitive functions are those processes which control simple ideas, movements or actions into complex goal-directed behaviour. In their absence, activities such as cooking, dressing or self-care tend to break down into their component parts. Clinically, executive dysfunction can often be inferred from the results of 'frontal lobe' tests but this often requires extensive formal neuropsychological testing which is impracticable for routine use. Clinically based bedside screening for executive function, (The Executive Interview) was developed. A pool of 50 test items was developed after a review of the literature and the following were considered for inclusion: frontal release, motor or cognitive perseveration, verbal intrusions, disinhibitions, loss of spontaneity, imitation behaviour, environmental dependency and utilization behaviour. Others included the SNOUT reflex, word fluency, go/no go task,

echopraxia and griptask. Each item is scored on a three point scale: 0=intact, 1=specific partial error or equivocal response, 2=specific incorrect response or failure to perform the task. The final set of items was decided excluding those with low clinical utility or item-class correlations. The final form, the EXIT contains 25 items requiring 10 minutes to administer, the scores ranging from 0 to a maximum of 50. In the original paper, 40 subjects were recruited and administered the EXIT. A Mini Mental State Examination, the Wisconsin Card Sorting Task, Trail Making Tests A and B and the Serial Attention Test were also administered as was the Nursing Home Behaviour Problem Rating Scale. Good correlations were found between EXIT scores and the other scales.

Address for correspondence

Dr Donald Royall
Department of Psychiatry
The University of Texas Health Science Center
at San Antonio
7703 Floyd Curl Drive
San Antonio
TX 78284-7792
USA

e-mail: royall@uthscsa.edu

Short Cognitive/Neuropsychological Test Battery for First-Tier Fitness-to-Drive Assessment of Older Adults

Reference: **De Raedt R, Ponjaert-Kristoffersen I (2001) Short Cognitive/Neuropsychological Test Battery for First-Tier Fitness-to-Drive Assessment of Older Adults.** *Clinical Neuropsychologist* 15: 329–36

Time taken varies with each subscale

Main indications

The aim was to identify the predictive power of a short neuropsychological test battery in relation to the judgement of expert driving instructors in an official Fitness to Drive Assessment Centre.

Commentary

The problems faced by the older car driver with cognitive impairment are significant and, as the population ages, many more drivers will receive a diagnosis of dementia. The authors developed a general practice-based screening battery to evaluate the necessity for further referral to specialized centres. Eighty-four subjects between the ages of 65 and 96 came to the Belgian Road Safety Institute for Fitness to Drive Evaluation. The predictive power of a battery consisting of the Trail Making Test, Part A, a visual acuity test, a clock-drawing test, the Mini-Mental State Examination and age was analysed. The judgement of an independent driving instructor (fit to drive versus not unconditional fit to drive) based on a real-world road test, was used as the dependent variable. A specificity score of 85% (subjects fit to drive correctly classified) and a sensitivity score of 80% (subjects not fit to drive correctly classified) was achieved. The instrument may be seen as a useful first step in what is a complex assessment.

Items included in the battery:

1. 'Ergovision' testing device – used to assess static visual acuity on a scale from 0 to 10. It is a regular acuity test in which digits of different sizes have to be perceived correctly (further information: Essilor, 1 Rue Thomas Edison, 94028 Créteil Cedex, France). Each test score is multiplied by 60.
2. The Trail Making Test. During this task a paper with randomly distributed circled numbers is presented and subject is asked to draw lines between the numbers in the correct order. Time needed to complete the test (in seconds) was subtracted from 200 and multiplied by three. (Times greater than 200 were scored as 0.)
3. The Mini-Mental State Examination. The score out of 30 was multiplied by 20.
4. Clock-drawing test. People were asked to draw a clock and asked to put 10 past 11 as the time. Four points were scored: clock face complete (max. 10% missing), all digits present; axes 12–6 and 9–3 must be placed at right-angles (max. 20 difference); hands correctly placed (they must be placed closer to 11 and 2 than to the neighbouring digits). The total score (max. = 4) was multiplied by 150. Finally, the age of each person was subtracted from 105 and multiplied by 15 (the minimum age in the population to assess is 65 years).

The total maximum score on the whole battery was therefore 3000 (5 × 600), which was divided by 100 to yield a transformed maximum score of 30.

Address for correspondence

Rudi De Raedt
Department of Developmental and Lifespan Psychology
Free University of Brussels
Pleinlaan 2 (3C247)
B-1050 Brussels
Belgium
Rudi-de-raedt@vub.ac.be

Neuropsychological Tests   Robert Coen

This section contains brief descriptions of a selection of the most commonly used neuropsychological tests likely to be encountered by health professionals working in old age psychiatry. A huge variety of tests are available for use in neuropsychological assessment. The specific tests used will depend on the individual characteristics of the person being evaluated (e.g. age, education, presenting syndrome, current mental status, premorbid intellect, gender, ethnicity), the specific referral question to be addressed, and the neuropsychologist's familiarity with, or preference for, specific tests. Localization of brain damage is often assumed to be a primary goal of neuropsychological assessment, but has been superseded by a range of superior neurodiagnostic technologies. However, although these can provide information on brain structure, metabolic and electrophysiological activity, they cannot tell us what the individual is or is not actually capable of doing, and here neuropsychological assessment makes a unique contribution. Three issues commonly addressed by neuropsychological assessment in old age settings are (i) differential diagnosis, (ii) early detection of dementia, and (iii) monitoring change, including progressive decline or response to intervention. Tests that are excellent for one purpose may be inappropriate for another. For example, a test that is useful for the early detection of dementia may quickly 'floor' and be insensitive to progressive decline. Test batteries therefore need to be flexibly tailored to the client and referral question, and different tests will be appropriate for different applications.

Neuropsychological assessment is increasingly recognized as a crucial component in dementia evaluation, and is, for example, a requirement in the NINCDS/ADRDA criteria for Alzheimer's disease. However, for purposes of diagnosis neuropsychological assessment alone is not sufficient, and must be combined with clinical, laboratory and neuroimaging findings, ideally using a multidisciplinary consensus approach. With regard to differential diagnosis, over time it has become clear that, at least in the earlier stages, many brain disorders have characteristic neuropsychological profiles of deficits and preserved abilities, e.g. Alzheimer's disease, dementia with Lewy bodies, frontotemporal dementias and subcortical dementias. As these signature profiles have become more clearly defined, neuropsychological assessment can be particularly useful in distinguishing between different forms of dementia. Highlighting retained abilities is important, as this can contribute to the development of management or rehabilitation programmes. Neuropsychological assessment can also assist in discriminating dementia from depression or from age-related decline. Neuropsychological markers, particularly measures of delayed free recall, are among the best predictors of subsequent progression to dementia among individuals with 'mild cognitive impairment', or

even in individuals who are initially asymptomatic. There are also areas in which neuropsychological assessment is less successful. Some test batteries were originally devised to distinguish between 'organic' and 'functional' disorders, but neuropsychological tests are generally limited in their ability to discriminate between individuals with deficits due to organic brain damage and those with deficits due to cerebral dysfunction such as psychosis. Detailed assessment is also of very limited benefit in individuals with severe cognitive impairment.

In contrast to mental status evaluation, which typically produces a single index of general cognitive functioning, a comprehensive neuropsychological assessment will evaluate a wide range of cognitive abilities across a number of cognitive domains. The specific test used is perhaps less important than the domain evaluated, with the proviso of course that the test is valid, reliable, and appropriate to the client and referral question. Domains typically assessed include orientation, attention/concentration, various aspects of verbal and visual memory, including acquisition, retention, retrieval and recognition, expressive and receptive language, visuospatial and visuoperceptual function, construction/praxis, and executive functions such as planning, problem solving, mental flexibility and abstraction. Specific domains can be further subdivided (e.g. episodic memory, semantic memory, working memory, autobiographical memory, prospective memory, explicit versus implicit memory), and the extent to which different aspects are evaluated again depends on the question being addressed.

Two issues which are important in understanding the interpretation of performance on neuropsychological tests are norm-referencing and qualitative evaluation. Whereas the commonly used tests are well standardized in terms of administration and scoring, and have generally adequate norms up to early old age, norms for the older elderly are generally less well developed, although this has been improving over time. Given that many of these tests are age sensitive and that longevity is increasing, the development of robust norms stratified by age, education and gender remains a priority. With regard to norm-based interpretation authorities differ a little, but generally a score greater than 2 standard deviations below the mean (<5th percentile) is considered significant and abnormal, whereas scores below the 10th percentile are considered borderline and moderately suggestive of brain damage.

It is also important to consider not just the quantitative aspects of performance (norm-referenced speed and/or accuracy) but also the quality of performance. Few, if any, neuropsychological tests evaluate a single cognitive function in isolation, and all can fail for a variety of reasons. For example, drawing a clock may sound simple but is a highly complex task from a neuropsychological perspective, requiring intact language comprehension, semantic representation (visuospatial features of a clock; time conceptualization), visuoperceptual, visuospatial and visuomotor processing (to translate mental representation into motor programme), hemiattentional processing (representing both sides of space), executive control (planning, simultaneous processing, monitoring and correcting motor output), and linguistic system input (graphomotor representation of the clock numbers). Deficits in any of these areas could contribute to failure on the clock-drawing test, or the patient might simply have been too poorly motivated to bother in the first place, maybe due to frustration, boredom, or a dysexecutive syndrome.

Observation of the qualitative aspects of performance provides crucial information as to why a test was poorly performed, which complements the quantitative evaluation and can direct attention to other aspects of behaviour and cognition that warrant consideration. Neuropsychological assessment therefore goes beyond the simple quantification of test performance, and tests such as those described in the following pages should ideally be administered and/or interpreted by an experienced specialist.

Recommended reading

Spreen O, Strauss E (1998) A compendium of neuropsychological tests. Administration, norms, and commentary, 2nd edn. New York: Oxford University Press.

Spreen O, Strauss E (1996) Assessment: Neuropsychological testing of adults. Considerations for neurologists. Report of the Therapeutics and Technology Assessment Subcommittee of the American Academy of Neurology. *Neurology* **47**: 592–9.

Lezak MD (1995) Neuropsychological assessment, 3rd edn. New York: Oxford University Press.

Golden CJ, Espe-Pfeifer P, Wachsler-Felder J (2000) Neuropsychological interpretations of objective psychological tests. New York: Kluwer Academic.

Buschke Selective Reminding Test

References: **Buschke H (1973) Selective reminding for analysis of memory and learning.** *Journal of Verbal Learning and Verbal Behaviour* **12: 543–50**

Buschke H, Fuld PA (1974) Evaluating storage, retention and retrieval in disordered memory and learning. *Neurology* **24: 1019–25**

Time taken varies depending on number of words and trials – 5–15 minutes. If delayed free recall/recognition is incorporated this takes about 5 minutes, and the delay interval varies (typically 30 minutes, but can be as short as 5 minutes)

Main indications

Simultaneous analysis of several components of memory and learning in verbal free recall, with emphasis on storage, retention and retrieval.

Commentary

Description

This word-list learning procedure is more a paradigm than a test per se, and a number of different versions exist, varying in number of words (typically 12, though this varies from six to 20) and number of trials (typically up to 12, but may be as few as six). Four equivalent forms (12 words × 12 trials) developed by Hannay and Levin (1985) are widely used. Though not part of the original procedure, it is common practice also to evaluate delayed free recall and recognition, and cued recall procedures (e.g. prompting with the first two letters of each word) are sometimes incorporated. Selective reminding basically involves selectively presenting on each recall trial only those words that were not recalled on the immediately preceding trial, and this is the crucial difference between this paradigm and standard word list learning tasks (where *all* words are re-presented on every trial). Using this procedure a number of different scores can be derived, including total recall, short-term recall (STR), long-term storage (LTS), long-term retrieval (LTR), and list learning or consistent long-term retrieval (CLTR).

Norms for the different versions have been compiled by Spreen and Strauss (1998) – see page 107 for reference.

The test purports to distinguish between retrieval from long-term storage and recall from short-term storage, based on the assumption that if an item is only ever recalled on those trials in which it was presented (selective reminding) then that item is not in long-term storage. This central assumption has drawn critical comment, as retrieval failure from long-term storage could produce the same pattern of performance and the short-term/long-term distinction becomes blurred (as is seen when individuals free recall words that were not in LTS). Reliability of the various scores derived from the selective reminding procedure varies, with total recall being the most stable and STM the least. LTR and CLTR have been found useful for distinguishing mild dementia from normal ageing, whereas total recall and delayed recall scores were useful preclinical predictors of the development of dementia (Masur et al, 1990).

Additional references

Hannay HJ, Levin HS (1985) Selective Reminding Test: an examination of the equivalence of four forms. *Journal of Clinical and Experimental Neuropsychology* **7**: 251–63.

Masur DM, Fuld PA et al (1990) Predicting development of dementia in the elderly with the Selective Reminding Test. *Journal of Clinical and Experimental Neuropsychology* **12**: 529–38.

Address for correspondence

Dr. Herman Buschke
Department of Neurology
Kennedy 912
Albert Einstein College of Medicine
Bronx
NY 10461
USA

Rey Auditory Verbal Learning Test

References: **Rey, A (1964) L'examen clinique en psychologie. Paris: Presses Universitaires de France**

Lezak MD (1976) Neuropsychological assessment. New York: Oxford University Press

Time taken acquisition, interference and immediate recall about 10–15 minutes. Typical delay interval 20 minutes. Delayed recall and recognition about 5 minutes

Main indications

Immediate memory, new learning, proactive and retroactive interference, delayed recall, delayed recognition

Description

There are many variations of this word list learning test. Lezak (1976) popularized an adapted English version. In the most commonly used version (see Spreen and Strauss 1998) a list of 15 words is read aloud to the client, who then free recalls them in any order. The whole list is then read out again, the client free recalls them, and this procedure is repeated for five trials. After the fifth trial a new list of 15 words is presented, and the client has to free recall these new words. Immediately following this, the client is asked to free recall the words from the first (repeated) list. After a 20-minute delay the client is again asked to free recall the words from the first (repeated) list. This is followed by a recognition trial in which the words from both lists and 20 new (not previously presented) words are combined, and the client has to specify whether each word is new or from one of the lists (specifying which one).

Commentary

The introduction of a second (interference) word list sets this test apart from standard serial word list learning tests such as that used in the CERAD neuropsychological test battery. As a consequence, a number of different aspects of learning and memory can be investigated using this procedure. Recall on the first trial reflects immediate memory span. A learning curve can be established by evaluating acquisition across the five consecutive trials. Comparing new list and initial list first trial recall evaluates proactive interference (old learning affecting new learning). Subsequent recall of the initial list evaluates retroactive interference (new learning affecting old learning). Delayed free recall and recognition are also evaluated. Norms are available from many sources and have been compiled by Spreen and Strauss (1998), who also provide copies of alternative forms for repeat assessment to reduce practice effects. Age significantly affects performance, education and gender less so. Two widely used variants warrant mention. In the California Verbal Learning Test (Delis et al, 1987), a crucial difference is the use of 16 words, each belonging to one of four categories, which introduces an interaction between verbal memory and conceptual ability/semantic memory. The WMS-III Word Lists subtest is also based on the Rey Auditory Verbal Learning Test.

Additional references

Delis DC, Kramer JH et al (1987) The California Verbal Learning Test. San Antonio, TX: Psychological Corporation.

Spreen O, Strauss E (1998) A compendium of neuropsychological tests. Administration, norms, and commentary, 2nd edn. New York: Oxford University Press, 326–40.

Rey Osterrieth Complex Figure

References: **Corwin J, Bylsma FW (1993) Translations of excerpts from Andre Rey's Psychological examination of traumatic encephalopathy and PA Osterrieth's The Complex Figure Copy Test.** *Clinical Neuropsychologist* **7: 3–15**

Spreen O, Strauss E (1998) A compendium of neuropsychological tests. Administration, norms, and commentary, 2nd edn. New York: Oxford University Press, 341–63

Time taken although untimed, copying the figure is typically completed within 5 minutes. The delayed recall interval varies from 3 minutes to 45 minutes (typically 30 minutes)

Main indications

Assessment of visuospatial constructional ability and visual memory.

Description

This test was originally developed by Rey and elaborated by Osterrieth in the 1940s. Over time a wide variety of administration and scoring procedures have been developed (see Spreen and Strauss, 1998 for review). The figure is complex and not easily verbally encoded. In the copy condition (visuoconstruction) the client is asked to draw the figure, which remains in view. This taps perceptual, visuospatial and organizational skills. To assess visual memory, without warning the client is asked to reproduce the figure from memory after a delay. Two of the most common variations are either reproduction after 30 minutes or reproduction after 3 and 30 minutes, and norms vary accordingly. A recognition format has been developed by Meyers and Meyers (1995). Alternative figures include the Taylor figure and four developed by the Medical College of Georgia (MCG). The most commonly used scoring system is an 18-point system proposed by Osterrieth and adapted by Taylor, who provided detailed scoring instructions (see Spreen and Strauss, 1998).

Commentary

Obviously, if the client has difficulties copying the figure this visuoconstructional component will also influence performance when reproducing it from memory. In such cases retention is best evaluated by calculating savings (the delayed reproduction score expressed as a percentage of the original copy score). Norms for the different versions have been compiled by Spreen and Strauss (1998). Performance is affected by intellectual level, and a significant age effect has been a consistent finding. Variations in the delay interval from 15 to 60 minutes appear to have little effect on overall recall performance. Although the different forms of the complex figure are equally difficult when copied, the Rey Osterrieth form is more difficult to reproduce from memory than either the Taylor or the four MCG forms, which are of equivalent difficulty. Strictly specified scoring systems yield high (>0.90) inter-rater reliability. Test/retest reliability has ranged from moderate to high across studies. Evaluation of the quality of the client's approach and performance when copying the drawing can yield important additional information. For example, clients with posterior pathology are more likely to have problems with the spatial organization aspect, whereas those with anterior pathology are more likely to have difficulties with planning, approach or application.

Additional references

Lezak MD (1995). Neuropsychological assessment, 3rd edn. New York: Oxford University Press, 475–480.

Meyers J, Meyers K (1995) The Meyers Scoring System for the Rey Complex Figure and the Recognition Trial: professional manual. Odessa, FL: Psychological Assessment Resources.

Trail Making Test

References: **Reitan RM (1958) Validity of the Trail Making Test as an indicator of organic brain damage.** *Perceptual and Motor Skills* **8: 271–6**

Spreen O, Strauss E (1998) A compendium of neuropsychological tests. Administration, norms, and commentary, 2nd edn. New York: Oxford University Press, 533–47

Time taken 5–10 minutes

Main indications

Processing speed, attention, sequencing, mental flexibility, visual search, motor function

Description

Part of the Halstead–Reitan neuropsychological test battery, the Trail Making Test has two parts. In Part A the client has to draw lines to join 25 consecutively numbered circles randomly arranged on a page. In Part B some of the circles are numbered, others are lettered, and the client has to alternate between consecutive numbers and letters (1, A, 2, B ...). Administration and scoring procedures have changed over the years, the most widely used being those of Reitan, in which errors are pointed out for correction as they occur and the score is time taken to completion, with errors reflected in increased time. Subtracting time for Part A from time for Part B essentially removes the psychomotor speed element. Variations on the Trail Making Test include an oral version, and the Color Trails Test (D'Elia et al, 1996). The latter was designed to minimise the language component (knowledge of the English alphabet) by using colour. In Part 1 even-numbered circles have a yellow background and odd-numbered ones have a pink background, the task being to join the numbers sequentially. Part 2 shows the numbers 1–25 twice, with yellow backgrounds for one set and pink for the other. Here the task requires alternating between the colours while joining the numbers sequentially.

Commentary

These may look like very simple tasks, but in fact the Trail Making Test is highly sensitive to brain dysfunction. Observation of the qualitative aspects of the client's performance during the test can be helpful in identifying the nature of the deficit(s), for example visual search, psychomotor speed, or the mental flexibility (set shifting) requirement on Part B. Sequencing and set shifting difficulties are more characteristic of frontal lobe pathology. Although Part B is the more sensitive part, both A and B are highly sensitive to progressive cognitive decline even early in dementia. The test is also strongly influenced by age and education. A variety of age- and education-stratified norms have been published, but as there is notable variation between some sources, particularly as age increases, the Spreen and Strauss compilation of available norms is recommended. The Color Trails Test norms are stratified by age (18–89) and education.

Additional references

D'Elia L, Satz P et al (1996) Color Trails Test. Odessa, FL: Psychological Assessment Resources.

Rasmusson DX, Zonderman AB et al (1998) Effects of age and dementia on the Trail Making Test. *Clinical Neuropsychology* 12: 169–78.

Address for correspondence

Reitan Neuropsychology Laboratory
2920 South 4th Avenue
South Tucson
AZ 85713-4819
USA

Wechsler Adult Intelligence Scale (WAIS-III)

References: Wechsler D (1997) Wechsler Adult Intelligence Scale, 3rd edn. San Antonio, TX: The Psychological Corporation

Wechsler D (1998) Wechsler Adult Intelligence Scale, 3rd edn. London: The Psychological Corporation

Time taken 60–90 minutes

Main indications

Comprehensive evaluation of intellectual ability.

Description

Although originally designed to measure intelligence, the Wechsler Adult Intelligence Scale forms a core instrument in clinical neuropsychological assessment, where the emphasis is on the individual subtests and intra-test scatter. Kaplan et al (1991) published supplementary process information and adjunctive techniques for the Wechsler Adult Intelligence Scale – Revised (WAIS-R as a Neuropsychological Instrument), some of which have been incorporated into the WAIS-III, or can readily be applied. The WAIS-III retains the same basic structure as the WAIS-R, with 11 revised subtests and 3 new subtests:

Picture completion	visual detail (parts omitted in pictures)
Vocabulary	defining words
Digit symbol – coding	psychomotor processing speed
Similarities	abstract verbal reasoning
Block design	block visuoconstruction
Arithmetic	mental calculations
Matrix reasoning	abstract visual reasoning
Digit span	repeating digit sequences forwards and backwards.
Information	general knowledge
Picture arrangement	planning/sequencing (rearrange pictures in logical order)
Comprehension	of social rules and concepts, and everyday reasoning
Symbol search	detection of target symbols embedded in symbol groups
Letter–number sequencing	resequencing numbers and letters (working memory)
Object assembly	puzzles of common objects which require assembly

Commentary

In addition to providing measures of verbal IQ, performance IQ, and full-scale IQ, the WAIS-III permits calculation of index scores based on more refined domains of cognitive functioning, namely verbal comprehension, perceptual organization, working memory and processing speed. The norms cover the age range 16–89. As the WAIS-III has been co-normed with the Wechsler Memory Scale, 3rd edition (WMS-III), an individual's intellect and memory can be directly compared and various aspects of expected memory performance can be predicted on the basis of intellect. An additional test, the Wechsler Test of Adult Reading (co-normed with the WAIS-III and WMS-III), can be used to predict premorbid intellectual and memory abilities. To reduce administration time a number of abbreviated forms have been developed over the years. One of the best validated is Ward's seven-subtest short form, originally for the WAIS-R but recently validated also for the WAIS-III (Pilgrim et al, 1999). It permits reliable estimation of VIQ, PIQ, and FSIQ, and has been further validated for estimation of the additional index scores.

Additional references

Kaplan E, Fein D et al (1991) WAIS-R as a neuropsychological instrument. San Antonio, TX: The Psychological Corporation.

Pilgrim BM, Meyers JE, et al (1999) Validity of the Ward seven-subtest WAIS-III Short Form in a neuropsychological population. *Applied Neuropsychology* **6**: 243–6.

The Psychological Corporation (1997) The WAIS-III WMS-III Technical Manual. San Antonio, TX: Psychological Corporation.

Address for correspondence

The Psychological Corporation
PO Box 9954
San Antonio
TX 78204-0954
USA

Wechsler Memory Scale (WMS-III)

References: Wechsler D (1997) Wechsler Memory Scale, 3rd edn. San Antonio, TX: The Psychological Corporation

Wechsler D (1998) Wechsler Memory Scale, 3rd edn. London: The Psychological Corporation

Time taken 60–90 minutes

Main indications

Comprehensive evaluation of multiple aspects of memory.

Description

This is a major revision of the preceding Wechsler Memory Scale – Revised (WMS-R), itself an extensive revision of the original Wechsler Memory Scale first published in 1945. They are the most commonly used memory scales in both clinical and neuropsychology. The WMS-III version provides a far more comprehensive evaluation of multiple aspects of auditory and visual memory, both immediate and delayed. It contains 11 subtests (four new, seven revised from WMS-R):

Information and orientation	autobiographical, historical and current information
Logical memory	story recall (immediate, delayed, and recognition)
Faces (recognition)	24 presented faces, 24 distractors (immediate and delayed)
Verbal paired associates	eight word pairs (immediate, delayed, and recognition)
Family pictures	four scenes: who, where, doing what (immediate and delayed)
Word lists (akin to RAVLT*)	12 words, two lists (immediate, delayed, recognition)
Visual reproduction	five designs (immediate, delayed, recognition, copy, match)
Letter–number sequencing	resequencing numbers and letters (working memory)
Digit span	repeating digit sequences forwards and backwards
Spatial span	tapping block sequences forwards and backwards
Mental control	control during performance of overlearned tasks

*Rey Auditory Verbal Learning Test

Commentary

The WMS-III has a number of significant advantages over its predecessors. First and foremost, it has been co-normed with the Wechsler Adult Intelligence Scale, 3rd edition (WAIS-III), which permits direct comparison of an individual's memory and intellect so that relative strengths and weaknesses can be profiled. The norms cover the age range 16–89. Primary indices (mean 100, SD 15) can be computed for immediate and delayed auditory and visual memory, delayed auditory recognition, working memory and general memory. The latter is an amalgam of delayed measures considered to be 'the best overall measure of the types of abilities that are critical to effective memory in day-to-day tasks'. In addition to the primary indices, additional information on a variety of memory processes can be derived, including single-trial learning, learning slope, retention, and retrieval, which may be of assistance in identifying different forms of memory failure. The entire battery is lengthy, but only six of the subtests are required for calculation of the primary indices, the remaining five being optional. Therefore the administration time can be substantially reduced when fatigue or compliance is an issue.

Additional references

The Psychological Corporation (1997) The WAIS-III WMS-III Technical Manual. San Antonio, TX: Psychological Corporation.

Tulsky DS, Ledbetter MF (2000) Updating to the WAIS-III and WMS-III: considerations for research and clinical practice. *Psychological Assessment* **12**: 253–62.

Address for correspondence

The Psychological Corporation
PO Box 9954
San Antonio
TX 78204-0954
USA

Wisconsin Card Sorting Test (WCST)

References: Heaton RK, Chelune GJ et al (1993) Wisconsin Card Sorting Test Manual. Revised and expanded. Odessa, FL: Psychological Assessment Resources

Nelson HE (1976) A modified card sorting test sensitive to frontal lobe defects. *Cortex* 12: 313–24

Time taken standardized version about 20–30 minutes. Nelson modified version about 10–15 minutes

Main indications

Assessment of problem solving, concept formation, set maintenance, cognitive flexibility/set shifting, and feedback utilization.

Description

This is a complex task, first developed by Berg and Grant in the 1940s. In the standardized version (Heaton et al, 1993) there are four stimulus cards and 128 response cards depicting different forms (crosses, circles, triangles or stars), colours (red, blue, yellow or green) and number of figures (one, two, three or four). The client is required to match the response cards, one by one, with one of the four stimulus cards, and is told whether each response is right or wrong (no further feedback given). After 10 consecutive correct responses the tester changes the sorting category (colour, form or number) without telling the client (this becomes evident as 'right' responses now become 'wrong'). The task continues until the client successfully completes six categories or until all 128 cards have been used. A number of scores can be derived, among which number of categories achieved and number of perseverative errors (persisting with a 'wrong' category) are the most clinically useful. A large number of abbreviated and modified versions have been developed, the most widely used in clinical settings being that of Nelson (1976), in which all response cards sharing more than one attribute with a stimulus card are removed (Modified WCST). This shortens the test to 48 cards and significantly reduces ambiguity in scoring responses. More controversially, in Nelson's version respondents are explicitly told each time the target category is changed.

Commentary

Although the WCST has earned a reputation as a 'frontal lobe test' it is neither as sensitive nor as specific to frontal pathology as tends to be assumed. Patients with frontal lobe damage may perform normally, and patients with non-frontal or diffuse lesions may perform badly, as may depressed patients. Both the standardized and the Modified versions are influenced by age and education. Norms for the former cover the age range 6.5–89, and Obonsawin et al (1999) provide norms for the Modified version (ages 16–75). Nelson considered that her modifications not only reduced administration time and response ambiguity, but also made the test simpler and less stressful, thereby reducing fatigue and distress. Some authorities argue that making the category changes explicit crucially alters the nature of the test, but others have reported both versions to be highly sensitive to reasoning or set shifting difficulties, recommending that the choice of version be guided by the client's ability level. Bondi et al (1993) verified the utility of the Modified WCST for the early detection of Alzheimer's disease.

Additional references

Bondi MW, Monsch AU et al (1993) Utility of a modified version of the Wisconsin Card Sorting Test in the detection of dementia of the Alzheimer type. *Clinical Neuropsychologist* **7**: 161–70.

Obonsawin MC, Crawford JR et al (1999) Performance on the Modified Card Sorting Test by normal, healthy individuals: relationship to general intellectual ability and demographic variables. *British Journal of Clinical Psychology* **38**: 27–41.

Address for correspondence

Psychological Assessment Resources Inc.
PO Box 998
Odessa
FL 33556-0998
USA

National Adult Reading Test (NART)

Reference: **Nelson HE, Willison J (1991) National Adult Reading Test (NART): Test Manual, 2nd edn. Windsor: NFER-Nelson**

Time taken about 10 minutes

Main indications

Estimation of premorbid intellect.

Description

The NART was designed to provide an estimate of pre-morbid intellectual ability and in this it differs crucially from most other tests, which evaluate current ability level. It consists of a written list of 50 short 'irregular' words of increasing difficulty. 'Irregular' words do not follow the normal rules of pronunciation, and therefore cannot be correctly pronounced unless they are known and recognised (e.g. the correct pronunciation of 'demesne' cannot be guessed). Reading ability and intelligence are highly correlated, and as reading recognition is less sensitive to brain damage than many other cognitive measures it provides a means of estimating premorbid intellect. The client simply reads out loud each word, guessing when unsure, and the number of errors are recorded. The original NART provided regression equations for estimation of WAIS verbal, performance, and full-scale IQ, and the second edition (NART-2, Nelson and Willison, 1991) provides WAIS-R estimates. It has not been revised for WAIS-III, as a new test, the Wechsler Test of Adult Reading (WTAR), itself styled on the NART and its American counterparts, has been co-normed with the WAIS-III and WMS-III to provide estimates of premorbid intellect and aspects of memory.

Commentary

Reliability and validity have been well established, and Spreen and Strauss (1998) suggest that, despite its limitations, the NART is the method of choice for estimating premorbid intellect – see page 107 for reference. This may change with the increasing use of WTAR, WAIS-III and WMS-III. NART estimation is superior to estimation based on demographic variables, alone or in combination (Bright et al, 2002). An important but overlooked point is that test administrators need to familiarize themselves with the acceptable pronunciations prior to testing. Clinical judgement is required concerning the suitability of NART for individual clients (e.g. history of reading disability or language disorder, first language not English). Caution is required when dealing with individuals of high or low premorbid intellect, as a ceiling effect leads to underestimation of IQ in those of superior intellect, whereas a floor effect may lead to a false conclusion of cognitive decline in low IQ individuals. Age does not appear to have a strong bearing on performance. However, contrary to popular belief, dementia does affect performance, and this becomes more pronounced with increasing severity. Patterson et al (1994) found a dramatic decrease in NART performance as a function of the severity of dementia in Alzheimer's disease, which they attributed primarily to semantic memory impairment. Premorbid IQ was underestimated by about 15 IQ points in moderate-stage patients. In a useful extension, Crawford et al (1992) have published NART equations for the estimation of premorbid verbal fluency (FAS test).

Additional references

Bright P, Jaldow E et al (2002) The National Adult Reading Test as a measure of premorbid intelligence: a comparison with estimates derived from demographic variables. *Journal of the International Neuropsychological Society* **8**: 847–54.

Crawford JR, Moore JW, Cameron IM (1992) Verbal fluency: a NART-based equation for estimation of premorbid performance. *British Journal of Clinical Psychology* **31**: 327–9.

Patterson K, Graham N et al (1994) Reading in dementia of the Alzheimer type: a preserved ability? *Neuropsychology* **8**: 395–407.

Psychological Corporation (2001) Wechsler Test of Adult Reading. Psychological Corporation: San Antonio, TX.

Address for correspondence

NFER-Nelson
Darville House
2 Oxford Road East
Windsor
Berkshire SL4 1DF
UK

Verbal Fluency: FAS Test/Category Fluency

References: **Spreen O, Strauss E (1998) A compendium of neuropsychological tests. Administration, norms, and commentary, 2nd edn. New York: Oxford University Press, 447–64**

Lezak MD (1995) Neuropsychological assessment, 3rd edn. New York: Oxford University Press, 545–8

Time taken about 5 minutes for three letters or three categories

Main indications

Spontaneous verbal production of words beginning with a particular letter, or exemplars from a particular category.

Description

The FAS test is the most common form of the Controlled Oral Word Association test (alternative letters include CFL and PRW, Benton et al, 1994). The client is asked to say as many words as he/she can beginning with a particular letter, excluding proper nouns, numbers, and the same word with different endings. Category fluency differs in that the client is asked to say as many exemplars as he/she can from a particular category, for example, 'tell me the names of as many animals as you can'. The category 'animals' is very widely used and is incorporated in the CERAD neuropsychological battery (Morris et al, 1989), with norms collated by Spreen and Strauss. However, the use of several categories improves sensitivitiy and specificity in dementia, and the categories 'animals', 'fruits' and 'vegetables' are frequently used (Monsch et al, 1994).

Commentary

Converging lines of evidence, including experimental, neuropsychological and neuroimaging studies, indicate that letter fluency is relatively more dependent on strategic search processes mediated by left frontal lobe regions, whereas category fluency is more dependent on left temporal lobe-mediated semantic knowledge. Depending on bias, some authors conceptualize category fluency as a test of executive functioning, whereas others consider it primarily a test of semantic memory. Contrasting both types of fluency can be informative. In Alzheimer's disease category fluency tends to be more impaired than letter fluency, whereas with frontal lobe pathology the reverse pattern predominates. Subcortical conditions tend to reduce both types equally, as performance also depends on rate of verbal production. Of course, the relative levels of performance depend critically on the specific letters and categories used, which accounts at least partly for discrepancies in the literature. The FAS test is affected more by education than by age, whereas category fluency is more sensitive to age than education, and so norm-based evaluation is important.

Additional references

Benton AL, Hamsher K de S et al (1994) Multilingual Aphasia Examination, 3rd edn. Iowa City IA: AJA Associates.

Monsch AU, Bondi MW et al (1994) A comparison of category and letter fluency in Alzheimer's disease and Huntington's disease. *Neuropsychology* **8**: 25–30.

Morris JC, Heyman A et al (1989) The Consortium to Establish a Registry for Alzheimer's disease (CERAD). Part 1. Clinical and neuropsychological assessment of Alzheimer's disease. *Neurology* **39**: 1159–65.

Stroop Colour–Word Test

References: **Stroop JR (1935) Studies of interference in serial verbal reaction.** *Journal of Experimental Psychology* **18: 643–62**

Trenerry MR, Crosson B et al (1989) Stroop Neuropsychological Screening Test Manual. Odessa, FL: Psychological Assessment Resources

Time taken less than 10 minutes

Main indications

Selective attention and cognitive flexibility.

Description

This is one of the oldest paradigms in experimental psychology, predating Stroop's publication (Stroop, 1935). There are numerous versions, some of which are commercially available (see Spreen and Strauss, 1998 – see page 107 for reference). The version described here is that of Trenerry et al (1989), which was designed as a standardized version for use as a neuropsychological screening measure. In this version there are two stimulus sheets. The first (Form C) consists of 112 colour names (red, green, blue, tan) arranged in four columns of 28. The names are printed in one of four colours (red, green, blue, tan) but the colour name and the ink colour are never the same (e.g. the name 'red' is never printed in red ink). The second sheet (Form C-W) is the same except for the order of the colour names. The client is first asked to read out the colour names on Form C as quickly and accurately as possible for 2 minutes. They are then asked to name the ink in which the colour names are printed on Form C-W as quickly and accurately as possible for 2 minutes. On the latter task interference slows performance. In this version, the main score is the number of correct responses on Form C-W minus the number of errors, and norms are provided for two age ranges, 19–49 and 50+, including the probability of brain damage associated with each score.

Commentary

The Trenerry et al version omits a third condition which is frequently included in other versions: reading the colour names printed in black ink. Reading words and naming colours are relatively automatic overlearned tasks, whereas naming the colour of dissonant print requires active response inhibition (ignoring the word) and shifting between conflicting verbal response modes. Depending on orientation, the Stroop test is conceptualized as a test of attention or of executive functioning, which is understandable given that the crucial response inhibition aspect of selective attention is dependent on frontal lobe-mediated attention control systems. Interference tends to be greatest in patients with left frontal lobe damage, but the Stroop test is not specific to frontal lobe pathology. In mild Alzheimer's disease the interference effect is very high. In contrast, more severely impaired cases are slower on colour naming but show little interference, probably owing to diminished awareness of their defective performance (Koss et al, 1984). Performance is affected by age more than by education.

Additional references

Koss E, Ober BA et al (1984) The Stroop Color–Word Test: indicator of dementia severity. *International Journal of Neuroscience* **24**: 53–61.

Address for correspondence

Psychological Assessment Resources Inc.
PO Box 998
Odessa
FL 33556-0998
USA

Boston Naming Test

References: **Goodglass H, Kaplan E (1983) Boston Naming Test. Philadelphia: Lea & Febiger**

Goodglass H, Kaplan E et al (2001) Boston Diagnostic Aphasia Examination, 3rd edn (BDAE-3). San Antonio, TX: The Psychological Corporation

Time taken about 10–15 minutes

Main indications

Ability to name pictured objects.

Description

The Boston Naming Test, an addition to the Boston Diagnostic Aphasia Examination, is also available separately. Both have been recently revised (Goodglass et al, 2001). The 60-item version (Goodglass and Kaplan, 1983) continues to be the most widely used test of confrontation naming. It consists of 60 line-drawn pictures of objects with names ranging from high-frequency ('bed') to low-frequency ('abacus'). As each picture is presented the client is asked to name it, and up to 20 seconds is allowed for a response. If the response indicates that the client has misperceived the object then a stimulus cue is given (e.g. 'a piece of furniture'). After every failure to respond or incorrect response a phonemic (first sound in name) cue is given. A number of short forms (15 or 30 items) have been developed. White Williams et al (1989) validated Odd and Even 30-item versions for use in Alzheimer's disease. Acknowledging its continuing use in differential diagnosis of dementia, Saxton et al (2000) developed two equivalent 30-item forms based on item difficulty, with norms for the full and 30-item versions.

Commentary

The Boston Naming Test has been well standardized across ages, with norms from various sources collated by Spreen and Strauss (1998), and ranging from 25 to 97.

Performance is affected by both age and education, with the age effect being most evident over 70 years. A cultural bias is likely for some items, particularly when used outside the USA, and it is important to consider regional variations in acceptable names. The Boston Naming Test has been found to be highly sensitive to very mild Alzheimer's disease, and may aid in differential diagnosis. The test lends itself to additional qualitative analysis, as errors may be semantic/anomic or visually based, with the former being more prominent early in Alzheimer's disease (probably reflecting semantic memory impairment), whereas visually based errors are more common in subcortical conditions (Hodges et al, 1991).

Additional references

Hodges JR, Salmon DP et al (1991) The nature of the naming deficit in Alzheimer's disease and Huntington's disease. *Brain* 114: 1547–58.

Saxton J, Ratcliff G et al (2000) Normative data on the Boston Naming Test and two equivalent 30-item short forms. *Clinical Neuropsychologist* 14: 526–34.

White Williams B, Mack W et al (1989) Boston Naming Test in Alzheimer's disease. *Neuropsychologia* 27: 1073–9.

Address for correspondence

The Psychological Corporation
PO Box 9954
San Antonio
TX 78204-0954
USA

Stepwise Comparative Status Analysis (STEP)

Reference: **Wallin A, Gottfries C-G, Karlsson I, Regland B, Sjogren M (1996) Stepwise comparative status analysis (STEP): a tool for identification of regional brain syndromes in dementia.** *Journal of Geriatric Psychiatry and Neurology* **9: 185–99**

Time taken 30 minutes (reviewer's estimate)

Rating by experienced interviewer

Main indications

The STEP was developed to act as a complement to clinical and ADL assessment in the evaluation of a person with suspected dementia.

Commentary

The Stepwise Comparative Status Analysis (STEP) is used to assess symptoms of dementia in identifying patients with regional brain syndrome (i.e. the predominating syndrome among those referable to a specific brain region). A number of primary variables are related to compound variables (general symptoms of dementia, delirium, personality change, instrumental difficulties, dementia, extrapyramidal symptoms, bipyramidal symptoms and pseudobulbar symptoms) which are then related to complex variables (global brain syndrome, fronto-brain syndrome, subcortical brain syndrome, parietal brain syndrome, frontosubcortical brain syndrome, frontoparietal brain syndrome and other complex brain syndromes). The STEP was developed from clinical experience and combines neurological and psychiatric status examination methods. Measures from other scales have been drawn. The manual and the protocol are required along with a box containing five common objects, a piece of paper with a cube drawn on it, an envelope and a reflex hammer.

Wallin et al (1996) described 96 patients with dementia who underwent the assessment. Descriptions of the various syndromes present were related to diagnosis in terms of vascular dementia, Alzheimer's disease and other dementias. The inter-rater reliability of the STEP has been shown (Edman et al, 2001) and it has also been used to assess the prevalence of dementia in people with Parkinson's disease (Wallin et al, 1999). The assessment is available in Swedish (Edman and Wallin, 1998).

Additional references

Edman A, Mahnfeldt M, Wallin A (2001) Inter-rater reliability of the STEP protocol. *Journal of Geriatric Psychiatry and Neurology* **14**: 140–4.

Wallin A, Edman A, Blennow K, Gottfies C-G, Karlsson I, Regland B, Sjogren M (1996) Stepwise comparative status analysis (STEP): a tool for identification of regional brain syndromes in dementia. *Journal of Geriatric Psychiatry and Neurology* **9**: 185–99.

Wallin A, Jennersjo C, Granerus A-K (1999) Prevalence of dementia and regional brain syndromes in long-standing Parkinson's disease. *Parkinsonism and Related Disorders* **5**: 103–10.

Address for correspondence

Dr Anders Wallin
Goteborg University
Institute of Clinical Neuroscience
Department of Psychiatry and Neurochemistry
Molndal Hospital
S-431, 80 Molndal
Sweden

PRIMARY VARIABLES

The scores on the primary variables reflect *observations* of single dementia symptoms.

1. **Reduced wakefulness** refers to reduction of the degree of wakefulness, as reflected in facial expressions, posture and speech; a quantitative reduction of consciousness; should be distinguished from delirium
9   not assessed/not assessable
0   wide-awake
1   dozes, yawns occasionally
2   fluctuating microsleep; tends to fall asleep when left in peace
3   falls asleep during the examination or is difficult to wake

2. **Concentration difficulties** refer to disturbance of attention, manifest as impaired ability to retain or switch attention to external or internal stimuli
9   not assessed/not assessable
0   adequate attention
1   occasionally distracted by irrelevant stimuli
2   markedly distractible
3   distracted by various stimuli to such an extent that proper examination is impossible

3. **Hallucinatory behaviour** refer to behavioural disturbance that indicates hallucinations (or delusions, which in this context may be difficult to distinguish from hallucinations) (e.g. the patient talks with invisible people (voices) or appears to be frightened by visual hallucinations); should be distinguished from visual agnosia
9   not assessed/not assessable
0   no hallucinatory behaviour
1   single episodes of suspected hallucinatory behaviour not disturbing the examination
2   obvious signs of hallucinatory behaviour not disturbing the examination
3   frequent episodes of hallucinatory behaviour disturbing the examination

4. **Paranoid symptoms** refer to symptoms suggesting suspiciousness or delusions of influence and/or persecution
9   not assessed/not assessable
0   no evidence for paranoid symptoms
1   signs of a tendency towards paranoid behaviour (e.g. suspiciousness)
2   signs of delusions of influence and/or persecution, yet without appreciable consequences for daily living
3   signs of pronounced paranoid delusions of influence and/or persecution disturbing daily living

5. **Restless movements** refer to aimless motor activity, such as fiddling with objects and wringing one's hands, and inability to sit still
9   not assessed/not assessable
0   no restless movements
1   has difficulty in keeping hands still, repeatedly changes position, fiddles with objects
2   wrings hands and fiddles frenetically with various objects, makes efforts to rise during the examination
3   can only sit still for a little while; paces up and down

6. **Depressed mood** refers to an observed decline in the basal emotional state (as distinct from affects released by the situation or spontaneously); includes gloominess, melancholy, and low-spiritedness, as manifest in facial expressions, posture and movement pattern; should be distinguished from apathy, mental slowness, poverty of language, and hypokinesia
9   not assessed/not assessable
0   no depressed mood
1   low-spirited during the examination, but occasionally displays a more cheerful mood
2   low-spirited and unhappy all the time irrespective of subject of discussion
3   displays extreme gloominess, melancholy or despair throughout the examination

7. **Elevated mood** refers to observed elevation of the basal emotional state (as distinct from affects released by the situation or spontaneously); it includes enhanced well-being, self-assurance, merriness, and elation, as manifest in speech, choice of subject of discussion, facial expressions, posture and pattern of movement; should be distinguished from disinhibition
9   not assessed/not assessable
0   no elevated mood
1   merry and self-assured, but changes without difficulty to a more serious mood, adequate to the situation
2   clearly elated, excessively self-assured; displays merriness that is not divertible
3   displays extreme elation and self-esteem all the time

8. **Apathy** refers to lack of motivation and impaired ability to experience and/or express emotional nuances, as manifest in shallowness, indifference, lack of initiative; should be distinguished from depressed mood, mental slowness, poverty of language and hypokinesia
9   not assessed/not assessable
0   no evidence for apathy
1   displays signs of emotional functioning but the more subtle emotional nuances are lacking
2   expresses joy, sorrow, etc., but in a shallow manner
3   complete lack of emotional functioning; unable to show sorrow, joy, hate, fear, anger, etc.

9. **Disinhibition** refers to impaired ability to experience and/or express emotional nuances, as manifest in casualness, lack of distance and lack of feeling for other people's needs and reactions; should be distinguished from elevated mood
9   not assessed/not assessable
0   no evidence for disinhibition
1   subtle emotional nuances are lacking
2   expresses joy, sorrow, etc., but in an uninhibited manner
3   constantly displays signs of uninhibited behaviour and lack of distance

10. **Vulnerability to stress** refers to anxiety induced by cognitive or practical tasks
9   not assessed/not assessable
0   no evidence for vulnerability to stress
1   slight vulnerability, not interfering with the ability to perform new tasks
2   moderate vulnerability, causing some difficulty performing new tasks
3   pronounced vulnerability, causing great difficulty performing new tasks

11. **Perseveration** refers to maintenance of a particular behavioural response to a stimulus, manifest as purposeless repetition of this behaviour even in response to new stimuli; should be distinguished from delirium
9   not assessed/not assessable
0   no evidence for perseveration
1   slight perseveration
2   moderate perseveration
3   pronounced perseveration

12. **Mental slowness** refers to a slowing down of the speed at which the patient gives verbal answers or performs simple tasks, such as the five-object test (see below item 13); should be distinguished from depressed mood, apathy, poverty of language, and hypokinesia
9   not assessed/not assessable
0   no evidence for mental slowness   *cont.*

1 slight mental slowness, causing no impairment of ADL functioning
2 moderate mental slowness, causing intermittent impairment of ADL functioning
3 pronounced mental slowness, causing constant impairment of ADL functioning

13. Memory disturbance refers to impaired ability to pass the five-object test (ask the patient to name and to remember five selected objects, e.g. a paper clip, a screw, a thimble, a coin, and a match-box); cover them up for 5 minutes and then ask what the five objects (or their functions) were; two or more errors indicate impairment)

9 not assessed/not assessable
0 no memory disturbance (remembers 4 or 5 objects)
1 remembers 3 objects
2 remembers 2 objects
3 remembers 0 or 1 object

14. Disorientation refers to disorientation to time and place

9 not assessed/not assessable
0 fully orientated
1 is not orientated to day of the week and/or month, but to place; finds the way on the ward
2 is not orientated to day of the week and/or month, nor to place; finds the way on the ward
3 is not orientated to year and cannot find the way in a room

15. Reduced capacity for abstract thinking refers to impaired ability to solve problems; suitable test tasks are interpretation of a proverb (e.g. 'People who live in glass houses should not throw stones'), presenting similarity between two verbally named objects (e.g. orange and banana), and simple numerical calculations (e.g. detracting 3 at a time from 100 down to 73, with not more than 1 error); in case of inconclusive answers, new analogous questions are given

9 not assessed/not assessable
0 normal capacity for abstract thinking
1 manages 2 tasks of 3
2 manages 1 task of 3
3 manages no task (i.e. interprets a proverb in a concrete way, does not recognise similarities between words, and fails on simple numerical calculations)

16. Visuospatial disturbance refers to impaired ability to think and orientate oneself in three dimensions; test task: to copy a cube

9 not assessed/not assessable
0 no visuospatial disturbance
1 manages to draw a cube with only minor defects; from the drawing one can see that the model is 3-dimensional
2 fails to draw a cube from which one can see that the model is 3-dimensional; the object drawn looks mainly 2-dimensional
3 fails to draw a cube that looks 3- or 2-dimensional; just draws a few strokes

17. Poverty of language refers to reduction of the flow of speech and to poor language and meagre vocabulary; the patient expresses himself by means of a few significant words; can be considered to be a variant of motor aphasia; should be distinguished from depressed mood, mental slowness, and apathy

9 not assessed/not assessable
0 no functional disturbance
1 takes his time to answer a question and gives short answers; can say things spontaneously
2 often gives monosyllable answers; says nothing spontaneously
3 may be prompted to give a few monosyllable answers, but does it reluctantly; mutism

18. Sensory aphasia refers to inability to understand spoken language (one's own and other people's); the flow of speech is normal; should be distinguished from delirium

9 not assessed/not assessable
0 no sensory aphasia
1 slight signs of deficient understanding of speech; it is relatively easy to carry on a conversation

2 obvious signs of deficient understanding of speech, e.g. inappropriate words, phrases, or sounds (paraphasia) and/or nonsense words (neologisms); it is difficult to carry on a conversation
3 marked signs of deficient understanding of speech; gives answers that are completely nonsequitur from what is asked; no conversation is possible

19. Visual agnosia refers to inability to interpret primary visual impressions despite good function of the primary sensory organ; test: place all the objects from the 5-object test in front of the patient, give the correct name of one of the objects and ask the patient to pick it up; this test may be given before the 5-object test; should be distinguished from defect of the visual field and hallucinatory behaviour

9 not assessed/not assessable
0 no visual agnosia
1 has some difficulty finding the object, but manages
2 has obvious difficulty finding the object, fumbles for it but eventually manages
3 fumbles for the object without finding it

20. Apraxia refers to difficulty in performing intentional movements despite the absence of paresis/tactile disturbances, e.g. difficulty in dressing and undressing or eating with a knife and fork; test: ask the patient to put a sheet of paper of the A4 size in a smaller envelope; for a normal result, the sheet should be folded correctly and be put in the envelope so that it fills up the whole envelope, and the envelope should be sealed

9 not assessed/not assessable
0 no apraxia
1 has difficulty folding the sheet so it fits the envelope, but manages
2 has difficulty folding the sheet so it fits the envelope, makes unsuccessful efforts to put the sheet in the envelope or puts it there without filling up the envelope
3 fumbles with the sheet without folding it, makes no efforts to put it in the envelope

21. Dysarthria refers to difficulty in articulating speech; should be distinguished from aphasia

9 not assessed/not assessable
0 not present
1 mild dysarthria without communication difficulties
2 moderate dyarthria with slight communication difficulties
3 pronounced dysarthria with obvious communication difficulties

22. Dysphagia refers to paresis of tongue or pharynx

9 not assessed/not assessable
0 not present
1 mild dysphagia without significant functional impairment
2 moderate dysphagia with intermittent tendency to choke
3 pronounced dysphagia; the patient constantly chokes or is unable to swallow

23. Positive masseter reflex: There is a positive masseter reflex if the patient shows a tendency to close his half-open mouth after a slight blow of a reflex hammer on the investigator's index finger, which is placed on the patient's chin just under his lower lip

9 not assessed/not assessable
0 not present
1 present

24. Tremor refers to 'parkinsonian' rhythmic (5/s) tremor of the pill-rolling type; occurs when the patient is at rest, disappears when he is in motion, increases with tension, is absent during sleep

9 not assessed/not assessable
0 not present
1 mild tremor causing no impairment of ADL functioning
2 moderate impairment causing intermittent impairment of ADL functioning
3 pronounced tremor causing constant impairment of ADL functioning (e.g., the patient cannot dress himself or eat by himself)

cont.

25. **Rigidity** refers to increased tonus in connection with both rapid and slow movements; should be distinguished from spasticity, which brings about increased tonus only in connection with rapid movements, and paratonia
9   not assessed/not assessable
0   not present
1   mild rigidity causing no impairment of ADL functioning
2   moderate rigidity causing intermittent impairment of ADL functioning
3   pronounced rigidity causing constant impairment of ADL functioning (e.g. the patient cannot dress himself, eat by himself, or walk without support)

26. **Paratonia** refers to inability to alternate between agonists and antagonists (muscle groups) in connection with passive movement; gegenhalten, pseudovoluntary resistance; should be distinguished from rigidity and spasticity
9   not assessed/not assessable
0   not present
1   mild paratonia causing no impairment of ADL functioning
2   moderate paratonia causing intermittent impairment of ADL functioning
3   pronounced paratonia causing constant impairment of ADL functioning (e.g. the patient cannot eat by himself or walk without support)

27. **Hypokinesia** refers to paucity of facial expressions, flattened facial expressions, retarded movement pattern; should be distinguished from depressed mood, apathy, mental slowness, and marche à petits pas
9   not assessed/not assessable
0   not present
1   mild hypokinesia causing no impairment of ADL functioning
2   moderate hypokinesia causing intermittent impairment of ADL functioning
3   pronounced hypokinesia causing constant impairment of ADL functioning (e.g. the patient cannot dress himself, eat by himself, or walk without support)

28. **Marche à petits pas** refers to a gait with very short steps and/or to hyperadduction of both lower extremities (scissor gait); signs of paraparesis; should be distinguished from hypokinesia
9   not assessed/not assessable
0   not present
1   pace 30–45 cm
2   pace 15–30 cm
3   pace less than 15 cm

29. **Increased reflexes** refers to *bilaterally* increased reflexes (spasticity) in arms and/or legs
9   not assessed/not assessable
0   not present
1   slightly increased reflexes
2   markedly increased reflexes
3   subclonus/clonus

30. **Babinski's phenomenon** refers to *bilateral* disturbance
9   not assessed/not assessable
0   not present
1   suspected to be bilaterally positive
2   definitely bilaterally positive

31. **Ataxia** refers to *bilateral* coordination disturbance of the cerebellar type, as evident from the finger-nose and knee-heel test and/or the gait; should be distinguished from body agnosia
9   not assessed/not assessable
0   not present
1   mild ataxia causing no walking difficulties
2   moderate ataxia causing walking difficulties, but the patient can walk without support

3   pronounced ataxia causing difficulty walking without support

32. **Body agnosia** refers to reduced awareness of bodily postures; the basis of the assessment is the way the patient lies down on a couch/performs the finger-nose test; to lie down in a deviant manner, e.g. with the body across the short side of the couch, and/or to fumble for the nose without finding it are signs of body agnosis; right-left delirium may be an early form of body agnosia; should be distinguished from ataxia
9   not assessed/not assessable
0   not present
1   mild deficiency causing, e.g. right-left delirium
2   moderate deficiency causing fumbling movements at the finger-nose test
3   pronounced deficiency causing inability to adequately sit down on a chair or lie down on a couch

33. **Myoclonus** refers to sudden rapid muscle twitches, preferentially of brachial flexors and leg extensors, causing movements of the joints
9   not assessed/not assessable
0   not present
1   occasionally present
2   intermittently present
3   constantly or almost constantly present

34. **Focal neurologic symptoms** refer to the kind of symptoms of neurologic decline that could be associated with circumscribed brain lesions; often manifest as a right-left difference (e.g. hemiparesis, facial paresis, sensibility disturbance, and visual field deficiency)
9   not assessed/not assessable
0   not present
1   present
    (What symptoms?)_____

35. **Other emotional, cognitive, or neurologic symptoms**
9   not assessed/not assessable
0   not present
1   present
    (What symptoms?) _____

COMPOUND VARIABLES

The scores on the primary variables for the basis for the *assessment/evaluation* of the compound variables. The primary variables that are included in the definition of a compound variable are marked in bold type.

36. **General symptoms of dementia** refer to the presence of **concentration difficulties, memory disturbances, disorientation**, and **reduced capacity for abstract thinking**; cf dementia (item 40)
9   not assessed/not assessable
0   no evidence for general symptoms of dementia
1   presence of 1 general symptom of dementia
2   presence of 2 general symptoms of dementia
3   presence of 3 or 4 general symptoms of dementia

37. **Delirium** refers to a qualitative change of consciousness (clouding of sensorium) involving **concentration difficulties** in conjunction with **restless movements** or **hallucinatory behaviour/paranoid symptoms**, often occurring as episodes; should be distinguished from sensory aphasia
9   not assessed/not assessable
0   no evidence for delirium
1   occurs intermittently on certain days, often in connection with stressful events
2   occurs daily during a limited part of the day or the night
3   occurs more or less constantly

38. **Personality change ('frontal-lobe symptoms')** refers to a condition that includes **apathy/disinhibition, perseveration**,

cont.

and **poverty of language**; should be distinguished from depressed/elevated mood

9   not assessed/not assessable
0   no evidence of personality change
I   slight signs of personality change but no disturbed behaviour
2   obvious signs of personality change occasionally resulting in disturbed behaviour
3   pronounced signs of personality change resulting in more or less constant behaviour disturbance

39. Instrumental difficulties ('parietal-lobe symptoms') refer to the presence of **sensory aphasia, visual agnosia, apraxia**, and/or **body agnosia**

9   not assessed/not assessable
0   no signs of instrumental difficulty
I   slight signs of instrumental difficulty, but without appreciable consequences for daily living
2   obvious signs of instrumental difficulty, resulting in partial impairment of daily living
3   pronounced signs of instrumental difficulty, resulting in more or less total impairment of daily living.

40. Dementia refers to a dementia syndrome (symptom constellation) including **memory disturbance** (obligate) + at least I of the following disturbances: **reduced capacity for abstract thinking, visuospatial disturbance**, language disturbance (anomia, motor aphasia, **poverty of language, sensory aphasia), apraxia, apathy/disinhibition**; the dementia syndrome or its constituent symptoms have been present for a longer period (at least 6 months) and cause occupational and/or social adaptation difficulties; the syndrome must not mainly be a manifestation of delirium or depression; the grading of the severity of the dementia below is in agreement with DSM-III-R; cf General symptoms of dementia (item 36)

9   not assessed/not assessable
0   not dementia
I   the patient is demented but can manage alone
2   the patient is demented, cannot manage alone, needs intermittent supervision
3   the patient is demented, cannot manage alone, needs constant supervision

41. Extrapyramidal symptoms refer to the presence of *bilateral* extrapyramidal symptoms, such as **rigidity, tremor, hypokinesia**, chorea, and dyskinesia

9   not assessed/not assessable
0   not present
I   presence of I bilateral extrapyramidal symptom
2   presence of 2 bilateral; extrapyramidal symptoms
3   presence of at least 3 bilateral extrapyramidal symptoms

42. Bipyramidal symptoms refer to the presence of *bilateral* signs of disturbed pyramidal pathways (e.g. **marche à petits pas**/paraparesis (group I), **increased reflexes**/spasticity (group 2), and **Babinski's phenomenon** (group 3))

9   not assessed/not assessable
0   not present
I   presence of symptoms from I of the groups
2   presence of symptoms from 2 of the groups
3   presence of symptoms from all 3 groups

43. Pseudobulbar symptoms refer to the presence of pseudobulbar symptoms, such as **dysarthria, dysphagia, positive masseter reflex**, and compulsive laughter

9   not assessed/not assessable
0   not present
I   presence of I pseudobulbar symptom
2   presence of 2 pseudobulbar symptoms
3   presence of 3 or 4 pseudobulbar symptoms

COMPLEX VARIABLES

The outcome of the analysis of the primary and compound variables forms the basis for the *evaluation* of the complex variables. In the explanatory text for a complex status variable, the primary (only mental slowness) and compound status variables that are included in the definition of the complex variable are marked in bold type. Only one regional brain syndrome should be indicated (only one positive score). When a syndrome preponderates over another, it means that this syndrome has greater negative impact on the patient's ability to perform every-day-life activities

44. Global (nonregional) brain syndrome refers to a condition in which **general symptoms of dementia** preponderate over **personality change, instrumental difficulties**, and **mental slowness**/basal motor symptoms (**extrapyramidal, bipyramidal**, and **pseudobulbar**)

9   not evaluated/not possible to evaluate
0   no evidence of a global brain syndrome
I   evidence of a global brain syndrome

45. Frontal brain syndrome refers to a condition in which **personality change** preponderates over **instrumental difficulties** and **mental slowness**/basal motor symptoms (**extrapyramidal, bipyramidal**, and **pseudobulbar**), *and the* predominant brain syndrome is not global

9   not evaluated/not possible to evaluate
0   no evidence of a frontal brain syndrome
I   evidence of a frontal brain syndrome

46. Subcortical brain syndrome refers to a condition in which **mental slowness**/basal motor symptoms (**extrapyramidal, bipyramidal**, and **pseudobulbar**) preponderate over **personality change** and **instrumental difficulties**, *and the* predominant brain syndrome is not global

9   not evaluated/not possible to evaluate
0   no evidence of a subcortical brain syndrome
I   evidence of a subcortical brain syndrome

47. Parietal brain syndrome refers to a condition in which **instrumental difficulties** preponderate over **personality change** and **mental slowness**/basal motor symptoms (**extrapyramidal, bipyramidal**, and **pseudobulbar**), *and the* predominant brain syndrome is not global

9   not evaluated/not possible to evaluate
0   no evidence of a parietal brain syndrome
I   evidence of a parietal brain syndrome

48. Frontosubcortical brain syndrome refers to a condition in which **personality change** and **mental slowness**/basal motor symptoms (**extrapyramidal, bipyramidal**, and **pseudobulbar**) preponderate over **instrumental difficulties**, *and* the predominant brain syndrome is not global

9   not evaluated/not possible to evaluate
0   no evidence of a frontosubcortical brain syndrome
I   evidence of a frontosubcortical brain syndrome

49. Frontoparietal brain syndrome refers to a condition in which **personality change** and **instrumental difficulties** preponderate over **mental slowness**/basal motor symptoms (**extrapyramidal, bipyramidal**, and **pseudobulbar**), *and the* predominant brain syndrome is not global

9   not evaluated/not possible to evaluate
0   no evidence of a frontoparietal brain syndrome
I   evidence of a frontoparietal brain syndrome

50. Other complex brain syndrome (e.g. the frontoparietosubcortical brain syndrome)

9   not evaluated/not possible to evaluate
0   no
I   yes
     (What syndrome?) _____

	9	0	1	2	3
PRIMARY VARIABLES					
1. Reduced wakefulness	☐	☐	☐	☐	☐
2. Concentration difficulties	☐	☐	☐	☐	☐
3. Hallucinatory behaviour	☐	☐	☐	☐	☐
4. Paranoid symptoms	☐	☐	☐	☐	☐
5. Restless movements	☐	☐	☐	☐	☐
6. Depressed mood	☐	☐	☐	☐	☐
7. Elevated mood	☐	☐	☐	☐	☐
8. Apathy	☐	☐	☐	☐	☐
9. Disinhibition	☐	☐	☐	☐	☐
10. Vulnerability to stress	☐	☐	☐	☐	☐
11. Perseveration	☐	☐	☐	☐	☐
12. Mental slowness	☐	☐	☐	☐	☐
13. Memory disturbance	☐	☐	☐	☐	☐
14. Disorientation	☐	☐	☐	☐	☐
15. Reduced capacity for abstract thinking	☐	☐	☐	☐	☐
16. Visuospatial disturbance	☐	☐	☐	☐	☐
17. Poverty of language	☐	☐	☐	☐	☐
18. Sensory aphasia	☐	☐	☐	☐	☐
19. Visual agnosia	☐	☐	☐	☐	☐
20. Apraxia	☐	☐	☐	☐	☐
21. Dysarthria	☐	☐	☐	☐	☐
22. Dysphagia	☐	☐	☐	☐	☐
23. Positive masseter reflex	☐	☐	☐		
24. Tremor	☐	☐	☐	☐	☐
25. Rigidity	☐	☐	☐	☐	☐
26. Paratonia	☐	☐	☐	☐	☐
27. Hypokinesia	☐	☐	☐	☐	☐
28. Marche à petit pas	☐	☐	☐	☐	☐
29. Increased reflexes	☐	☐	☐	☐	☐
30. Babinski's phenomenon	☐	☐	☐	☐	
31. Ataxia	☐	☐	☐	☐	☐
32. Body agnosia	☐	☐	☐	☐	☐
33. Myoclonus	☐	☐	☐	☐	☐
34. Focal neurologic symptoms	☐	☐	☐		
35. Other emotional, cognitive, or neurologic symptoms	☐	☐	☐		
COMPOUND VARIABLES					
36. General symptoms of dementia	☐	☐	☐	☐	☐
37. Delirium	☐	☐	☐	☐	☐
38. Personality change ('frontal-lobe symptoms')	☐	☐	☐	☐	☐
39. Instrumental difficulties ('parietal-lobe symptoms')	☐	☐	☐	☐	☐
40. Dementia	☐	☐	☐	☐	☐
41. Extrapyramidal symptoms	☐	☐	☐	☐	☐
42. Bipyramidal symptoms	☐	☐	☐	☐	☐
43. Pseudobulbar symptoms	☐	☐	☐	☐	☐
COMPLEX VARIABLES					
44. Global (nonregional) brain syndrome	☐	☐	☐		
45. Frontal brain syndrome	☐	☐	☐		
46. Subcortical brain syndrome	☐	☐	☐		
47. Parietal brain syndrome	☐	☐	☐		
48. Frontosubcortical brain syndrome	☐	☐	☐		
49. Frontoparietal brain syndrome	☐	☐	☐		
50. Other complex brain syndrome	☐	☐	☐		

Chapter 2b

Neuropsychiatric assessments

These are traditionally considered to consist of psychiatric symptoms and behavioural disturbances (also known as non-cognitive features to distinguish them from cognitive deficits such as amnesia, aphasia, apraxia and agnosia). Compared with the assessment of cognitive impairment, these non-cognitive features have only relatively recently been subject to quantitative assessment. There are a large number of scales which purport to assess a wide range of features, including many neuropsychiatric problems found in the more severe stages of the illness. Often, the scales measure symptoms and signs which have more in common with lay descriptions of behaviour such as agitation, uncooperativeness and obstreperousness. They are often assessed in common with deficits in Activities of Daily Living, because of the high association between the two. Many of the scales represent a laudable attempt to assess the degree of disturbance present and use this as a measure for the amount of time carers need to spend with an individual. A significant advance has been the development of scales to measure more specific symptom profiles in patients. Measures of aggression have been devised, as have scales dealing specifically with agitation. A number of instruments have recently been published that provide a global measure of psychiatric symptoms, and as such are akin to the quantified assessments of cognitive function produced 20 years ago.

The BEHAVE-AD (behavioral symptoms in Alzheimer's disease: phenomenology and treatment) scale (page 125) was one of the first to be published, and has the advantage of being sensitive to change, making it suitable to measure the effects of drugs. A cluster of other scales include the Manchester and Oxford Universities Scale for the Psychopathological Assessment of Dementia (MOUSEPAD; page 133) derived from the Present Behavioural Examination (PBE; page 137), the Neuropsychiatric Inventory (NPI; page 128), the Columbia University Scale for Psychopathology in Alzheimer's Disease (CUSPAD; page 130) and the Consortium to Establish a Registry for Alzheimer's Disease (CERAD) Behavioral Rating Scale (page 138). These have relatively little to choose between them, and each has its own proponents and detractors. Reliability and validity data are available for them all, and all have been published in peer-reviewed journals. The NPI is an efficient scale and has been used by pharmaceutical companies assessing the effects drugs have on these features. Many include questions of depression, and so overlap with those scales described in Chapter 1 is to be found.

Specific measures of aggression can be found (e.g. the Rating Scale for Aggressive Behaviour in the Elderly (RAGE; page 142), an observational scale for the assessment of inpatients, the Overt Aggression Scale (OAS; page 144), which measures the severity and frequency of all types of aggression, and the Ryden Aggression Scale (page 154), which is all-encompassing). Agitation is best assessed by the Cohen-Mansfield Agitation Inventory (CMAI; page 159) which has a short and a long form plus a direct observational scale, something also found in the Pittsburgh Agitation Scale (PAS; page 163). A much shorter version of the scale exists (Brief Agitation Rating Scale (BARS; page 158)). Measures for irritability and apathy also exist. This leaves a host of other tools which assess a wide range of behavioural disturbances in patients and which the reader has to familiarize him or herself with to decide which is the most appropriate for use. These include: the BEAM-D (page 169), the Comprehensive Psychopathological Rating Scale (CPRS; page 255), the Dysfunctional Behaviour Rating Instrument (DBRI; page 165) (validated on community patients), the Dementia Behavior Disturbance Scale (page 162), the Nurses' Observation Scale for Geriatric Patients (NOSGER; page 288) and the Neurobehavioral Rating Scale (NRS; page 146) (which includes cognitive tests). The Clinical Rating Scale for Symptoms of Psychosis in Alzheimer's Disease (SPAD; page 171) measures specifically psychotic features.

The choice of scale depends on the question to be answered. If a rating of a specific behaviour is required (e.g. to measure the effects of an intervention such as a behaviour programme or drug), then one of the specific scales should be chosen. If the rater wishes to have a more general measure of the dependency of a ward or section of a nursing home to compare them with another group, then a more global measure is appropriate which may also include an assessment of cognition and activities of daily living.

Personality Inventory

Reference: **Brooks DN, McKinlay W (1983) Personality and behavioural change after severe blunt head injury – a relative's view.** *Journal of Neurology, Neurosurgery, and Psychiatry 46: 336–44*

Time taken 20 minutes (reviewer's estimate)

Rating on a visual analogue scale by relatives

Main indications

Assessment of personality changes after severe head injury; also used to assess personality in dementia.

Commentary

The original study using the Personality Inventory describes the scale ratings on 55 severely head-injured adults at 3, 6 and 12 months post-injury. No reliability or validity data were presented. Petry et al (1988) describe 30 control subjects pre- and post-retirement together with patients suffering from dementia of the Alzheimer type, and examined their changing score after the onset of dementia. No significant changes were found in the control group, but there were highly significant changes on 12 of the 18 items – patients became more passive, more coarse and less spontaneous. In this study, ratings were made on a –2 to +2, five-point rating scale with 0 indicating no change. Petry et al (1989) carried out a follow-up of the 30 original patients, describing four response pattern: change at onset with little subsequent change,

ongoing change, no change and regression of previously disturbed behaviour. Cummings et al (1990) described personality changes in patients with dementia of the Alzheimer type and multi-infarct dementia, and found that while personality alterations were universal, patients with Alzheimer's disease had greater alterations in maturity and had less personal control compared with patients with vascular dementia, who had more apathy and remained more affectionate and easy-going. A few correlations were found between the severity of dementia and the magnitude of behavioural change.

Additional references

Cummings JL, Petry S, Dian L et al (1990) Organic personality disorder in dementia syndromes: an inventory approach. *Journal of Neuropsychiatry* **2**: 261–7.

Petry S, Cummings JL, Hill MA et al (1988) Personality alterations in dementia of Alzheimer type. *Archives of Neurology* **45**: 1187–90.

Petry S, Cummings JL, Hill MA et al (1989) Personality alterations in dementia of Alzheimer type: a three-year follow-up study. *Journal of Geriatric Psychiatry and Neurology* **2**: 184–8.

Personality Inventory

	+2	+1	0	–1	–2	
Talkative	___	___	___	___	___	Quiet
Even-tempered	___	___	___	___	___	Quick-tempered
Relies on others	___	___	___	___	___	Does things himself
Affectionate	___	___	___	___	___	Cold
Fond of company	___	___	___	___	___	Dislikes company
Irritable	___	___	___	___	___	Easy-going
Unhappy	___	___	___	___	___	Happy
Excitable	___	___	___	___	___	Calm
Energetic	___	___	___	___	___	Lifeless
Down to earth	___	___	___	___	___	Out of touch
Rash	___	___	___	___	___	Cautious
Listless	___	___	___	___	___	Enthusiastic
Mature	___	___	___	___	___	Childish
Sensitive	___	___	___	___	___	Insensitive
Cruel	___	___	___	___	___	Kind
Generous	___	___	___	___	___	Mean
Unreasonable	___	___	___	___	___	Reasonable
Stable	___	___	___	___	___	Changeable

Source: Brooks DN *et al.* *J Neurol Neurosurg Psychiatry* 1983, **46**: 336–44, with permission from the BMJ Publishing Group.

BEHAVE-AD

Reference: **Reisberg B, Borenstein J, Salob SP, Ferris SH, Franssen E, Georgotas A (1987) Behavioral symptoms in Alzheimer's disease: phenomenology and treatment.** *Journal of Clinical Psychiatry* **48 (suppl 5): 9–15**

Time taken 20 minutes

Rating by clinician

Main indications

The BEHAVE-AD was designed particularly to be useful in prospective studies of behavioural symptoms and in pharmacological trials to look at behavioural symptoms in patients with Alzheimer's disease.

Commentary

The BEHAVE-AD is the original behaviour rating scale in Alzheimer's disease, the items having been lifted originally from a chart review of 57 outpatients with Alzheimer's disease. The areas covered were the main domains of symptomatology: paranoid and delusional ideation, hallucinations, activity disturbances, aggressiveness, diurnal rhythm disturbances, affective disturbances, and anxieties/phobias. A global rating of the trouble the various behaviours are to the caregiver is also noted. Reference is to the 2 weeks prior to the interview, which is directed to an informed carer.

Sclan et al (1996) determined inter-rater reliability of the scale transculturally, including patients from France. Inter-rater reliability was excellent, with agreement coefficients ranging from 0.65 to 0.91. Similar consistency was found in the French version. Measures were carried out on 140 patients with probable Alzheimer's disease, with the finding that the BEHAVE-AD scores were most severe in the moderate and moderately severe stages of the illness. Patterson et al (1990) reported similar very good reliability ratings (kappa value 0.62–1.00 on 20 of the 25 items with percentage agreement of between 82 and 100%). Reisberg et al (1989) demonstrated the variability of the different symptoms at the different stages of the disease measured with the Global Deterioration Scale (GDS; page 217).

Additional references

Patterson M, Schnell A, Martin R et al (1990) Assessment of behavioral and affective symptoms in Alzheimer's disease. *Journal of Geriatric Psychiatry and Neurology* **3**: 21–30.

Reisberg B, Franssen E, Sclan S et al (1989) Stage specific incidence of potentially remediable behavioral symptoms in aging and Alzheimer's disease; a study of 120 patients using the BEHAVE-AD. *Bulletin of Clinical Neuroscience* **54**: 95–112.

Sclan S, Saillon A, Franssen E et al (1996) The behavior pathology in Alzheimer's disease rating scale (BEHAVE-AD): reliability and analysis of symptom category scores. *International Journal of Geriatric Psychiatry* **11**: 819–30.

Address for correspondence

Barry Reisberg
Aging and Dementia Research Program
Department of Psychiatry
NYU Medical Center
550 First Avenue
NY 10016
USA

e-mail: barry.reisberg@med.nyu.edu

Part 1: Symptomatology

Assessment Interval: Specify: ———— wks.

Total Score: ————

a. Paranoid and Delusional Ideation

1. 'People are Stealing Things' Delusion
0 = Not present.
1 = Delusion that people are hiding objects.
2 = Delusion that people are coming into the home and hiding objects or stealing objects.
3 = Talking and listening to people coming into the home.

2. 'One's House is Not One's Home' Delusion
0 = Not present.
1 = Conviction that the place in which one is residing is not one's home (e.g. packing to go home; complaints, while at home, of 'take me home').
2 = Attempt to leave domiciliary to go home.
3 = Violence in response to attempts to forcibly restrict exit.

3. 'Spouse (or Other Caregiver) is an Imposter' Delusion
0 = Not present.
1 = Conviction that spouse (or other caregiver) is an imposter.
2 = Anger toward spouse (or other caregiver) for being an imposter.
3 = Violence towards spouse (or other caregiver) for being an imposter.

4. 'Delusion of Abandonment' (e.g. to an Institution).
0 = Not present.
1 = Suspicion of caregiver plotting abandonment or institutionalization (e.g. on telephone).
2 = Accusation of a conspiracy to abandon or institutionalize.
3 = Accusation of impending or immediate desertion or institutionalization.

5. 'Delusion of Infidelity'
0 = Not present.
1 = Conviction that spouse and/or children and/or other caregivers are unfaithful.
2 = Anger toward spouse, relative, or other caregiver for infidelity.
3 = Violence toward spouse, relative, or other caregiver for supposed infidelity.

6. 'Suspiciousness/Paranoia' (other than above)
0 = Not present.
1 = Suspicious (e.g. hiding objects that he/she later may be unable to locate).
2 = Paranoid (i.e. fixed conviction with respect to suspicions and/or anger as a result of suspicions).
3 = Violence as a result of suspicions.
Unspecified?
Describe

7. Delusions (other than above)
0 = Not present.
1 = Delusional.
2 = Verbal or emotional manifestations as a result of delusions.
3 = Physical actions or violence as a result of delusions.
Unspecified?
Describe

b. Hallucinations

8. Visual Hallucinations
0 = Not present.
1 = Vague: not clearly defined.
2 = Clearly defined hallucinations of objects or persons (e.g. sees other people at the table).
3 = Verbal or physical actions or emotional responses to the hallucinations.

9. Auditory Hallucinations
0 = Not present.
1 = Vague: not clearly defined.
2 = Clearly defined hallucinations of words or phrases.
3 = Verbal or physical actions or emotional response to the hallucinations.

10. Olfactory Hallucinations
0 = Not present.
1 = Vague: not clearly defined.
2 = Clearly defined
3 = Verbal or physical actions or emotional responses to the hallucinations.

11. Haptic Hallucinations
0 = Not present.
1 = Vague: not clearly defined.
2 = Clearly defined.
3 = Verbal or physical actions or emotional responses to the hallucinations.

12. Other Hallucinations
0 = Not present.
1 = Vague: not clearly defined.
2 = Clearly defined
3 = Verbal or physical actions or emotional responses to the hallucinations.
Unspecified?
Describe

c. Activity Disturbances

13. Wandering: Away From Home or Caregiver
0 = Not present.
1 = Somewhat, but not sufficient to necessitate restraint.
2 = Sufficient to require restraint.
3 = Verbal or physical actions or emotional responses to attempts to prevent wandering.

14. Purposeless Activity (Cognitive Abulia)
0 = Not present.
1 = Repetitive, purposeless activity (e.g. opening and closing pocketbook, packing and unpacking clothing, repeatedly putting on and removing clothing, opening and closing drawers, insistent repeating of demands or questions).
2 = Pacing or other purposeless activity sufficient to require restraint.
3 = Abrasions or physical harm resulting from purposeless activity.

15. Inappropriate Activity
0 = Not present.
1 = Inappropriate activities (e.g. storing and hiding objects in inappropriate places, such as throwing clothing in wastebasket or putting empty plates in the oven; inappropriate sexual behavior, such as inappropriate exposure).
2 = Present and sufficient to require restraint.
3 = Present, sufficient to require restraint, and accompanied by anger or violence when restraint is used.

cont.

d. Aggressiveness
16. Verbal Outbursts
0 = Not present.

1 = Present (including unaccustomed use of foul or abusive language).

2 = Present and accompanied by anger.

3 = Present, accompanied by anger, and clearly directed at other persons.

17. Physical Threats and/or Violence
0 = Not present.

1 = Threatening behavior.

2 = Physical violence.

3 = Physical violence accompanied by vehemence.

18. Agitation (other than above)
0 = Not present.

1 = Present.

2 = Present with emotional component.

3 = Present with emotional and physical component.

Unspecified?

Describe

e. Diurnal Rhythm Disturbances
19. Day/Night Disturbance
0 = Not present.

1 = Repetitive wakenings during night.

2 = 50% to 75% of former sleep cycle at night.

3 = Complete disturbance of diurnal rhythm (i.e. less than 50% of former sleep cycle at night).

f. Affective Disturbance
20. Tearfulness
0 = Not present.

1 = Present.

2 = Present and accompanied by clear affective component.

3 = Present and accompanied by affective and physical component (e.g. 'wrings hands' or other gestures).

21. Depressed Mood: Other
0 = Not present.

1 = Present (e.g. occasional statement 'I wish I were dead', without clear affective concomitants).

2 = Present with clear concomitants (e.g. thoughts of death).

3 = Present with emotional and physical component (e.g. suicide gestures).

Unspecified?

Describe

g. Anxieties and Phobias
22. Anxiety Regarding Upcoming Events (Godot Syndrome)
0 = Not present.

1 = Present: Repeated queries and/or other activities regarding upcoming appointments and/or events.

2 = Present and disturbing to caregivers.

3 = Present and intolerable to caregivers.

23. Other Anxieties
0 = Not present.

1 = Present.

2 = Present and disturbing to caregivers.

3 = Present and intolerable to caregivers.

Unspecified?

Describe

24. Fear of being Left Alone
0 = Not present.

1 = Present: Vocalized fear of being alone.

2 = Vocalized and sufficient to require specific action on part of caregiver.

3 = Volcalized and sufficient to require patient to be accompanied at all times.

25. Other Phobias
0 = Not present.

1 = Present.

2 = Present and of sufficient magnitude to require specific action on part of caregiver.

3 = Present and sufficient to prevent patient activities.

Unspecified?

Describe

Part 2: Global Rating
With respect to the above symptoms, they are of sufficient magnitude as to be:

0 = Not at all troubling to the caregiver or dangerous to the patient.

1 = Mildly troubling to the caregiver or dangerous to the patient.

2 = Moderately troubling to the caregiver or dangerous to the patient.

3 = Severely troubling or intolerable to the caregiver or dangerous to the patient.

Source: Reisberg B, Borenstein J, Salob SP, Ferris SH, Franssen E, Georgotas A, Behavioral symptoms in Alzheimer's disease: phenomenology and treatment, *Journal of Clinical Psychiatry*, Vol. 48 (Suppl 5), pp. 9–15, 1987. Copyright © 1986 Barry Reisberg. Reprinted by permission.

Neuropsychiatric Inventory (NPI)

Reference: **Cummings JL, Mega M, Gray K, Rosenberg-Thompson S, Carusi DA, Gornbein J (1994) The Neuropsychiatric Inventory: comprehensive assessment of psychopathology in dementia.** *Neurology* **44: 2308–14**

Time taken 10 minutes

Rating based on interview carried out with carer

Main indications

The Neuropsychiatric Inventory (NPI) evaluates a wider range of psychopathology than comparable instruments, and may help distinguish between different causes of dementia; it also records severity and frequency separately.

Commentary

The NPI is a relatively brief interview assessing 10 behavioural disturbances: delusions; hallucinations; dysphoria; anxiety; agitation/aggression; euphoria; disinhibition; irritability/lability; apathy; and aberrant motor behaviour. It uses a screening strategy to cut down the length of time the instrument takes to administer, but it obviously takes longer if replies are positive. It is scored from 1 to 144. Severity and frequency are independently assessed. The authors reported on 40 caregivers, and content and concurrent validity and inter-rater and test/retest reliability were assessed. Some 45 assessments were used for the inter-rater reliability and 20 for test/retest reliability. Concurrent validity was found to be satisfactory using a panel of appropriated experts; concurrent reliability was determined by comparing the NPI subscale with subscales of the BEHAVE-AD (page 125) and the Hamilton Depression Rating Scale (page 6). Highly significant correlations were found. A high level of internal consistency (0.88) was found using a Cronbach's coefficient. Inter-rater reliability revealed agreement in over 90 ratings, and test/retest reliability (a second interview within 3 weeks) was very highly significant. A training pack and further information is available from the author.

Address for correspondence

Dr JL Cummings
UCLA School of Medicine
Department of Neurology
710 Westwood Plaza RNRC 2-238
Los Angeles
CA 90095-1769
USA

e-mail: cummings@ucla.edu

Neuropsychiatric Inventory (NPI)

Description of the NPI

The NPI consists of 12 behavioral areas

Delusions	Apathy
Hallucinations	Disinhibition
Agitation	Irritability
Depression	Aberrant motor behavior
Anxiety	Night-time behaviors
Euphoria	Appetite and eating disorders

Frequency is rated as
1. Occasionally – less than once per week
2. Often – about once per week
3. Frequently – several times a week but less than every day
4. Very frequently – daily or essentially continuously present

Severity is rated as
1. Mild – produce little distress in the patient
2. Moderate – more disturbing to the patient but can be redirected by the caregiver
3. Severe – very disturbing to the patient and difficult to redirect

Distress is scored as
0 – no distress
1 – minimal
2 – mild
3 – moderate
4 – moderately severe
5 – very severe or extreme

For each domain there are 4 scores. Frequency, severity, total (frequency × severity) and caregiver distress. The total possible score is 144 (i.e. A maximum of 4 in the frequency rating × 3 in the severity rating × 12 remaining domains)
This relates to changes, usually over the 4 weeks prior to completion.

Source: Cummings JL, Mega M, Gray K, Rosenberg-Thompson S, Carusi DA, Gornbein J (1994) The Neuropsychiatric Inventory: comprehensive assessment of psychopathology in dementia. *Neurology* **44**: 2308–14.

Neuropsychiatric Inventory with Caregiver Distress Scale

Reference: **Kaufer DI, Cummings JL, Christine D, Bray T, Castellon S, Masterman D, MacMillan A, Ketchel P, DeKosky ST (1998) Assessing the impact of neuropsychiatric symptoms in Alzheimer's disease: the Neuropsychiatric Inventory Caregiver Distress Scale.** *Journal of the American Geriatrics Society* **46: 210–15**

Time taken 10–15 minutes

Rating by the clinician in an interview with the carer

Main indications

The Neuropsychiatric Inventory (NPI) is described on page 128. The NPI with Caregiver Distress Scale has an additional question on each domain specifically addressing the level of distress caused to carers by each specific symptom.

Commentary

When each domain is completed and the caregiver has completed the frequency and severity rating, an additional question may be addressed to the caregiver to look at distress associated with that particular domain. The caregiver is asked how much, if any, emotional/psychological distress the behaviour he/she has just discussed causes him or her. The distress is rated from 0 (no distress) up to 5 (very severe or extreme).

Address for correspondence

Dr JL Cummings
UCLA School of Medicine
Department of Neurology
710 Westwood Plaza RNRC 2-238
Los Angeles
CA 90095-1769
USA

e-mail: cummings@ucla.edu

Columbia University Scale for Psychopathology in Alzheimer's Disease (CUSPAD)

Reference: **Devanand DP, Miller L, Richards M, Marder K, Bell K, Mayeux R, Stern Y (1992) Columbia University Scale for Psychopathology in Alzheimer's Disease.** *Archives of Neurology* **49: 371–6**

Time taken 10–15 minutes

Rating most items on a categorical measure of presence or absence in the last month. Interview carried out with carer

Main indications

As a screening instrument for psychopathology in Alzheimer's disease.

Commentary

The Columbia University Scale for Psychopathology in Alzheimer's Disease (CUSPAD) uses operational definitions based on existing definitions of symptomatology. An important development is the differentiation of the delusion as being either fixed (i.e. not amenable to correction) or otherwise. A measure of whether the feature is persistent (more than three times a week) or transient is also made. If the symptom is present, depression items are scored on a five-point scale. The study consisted of reliability on 20 patients between a psychiatrist and lay interviewer. Further interviews were carried out with 91 patients with Alzheimer's disease to form the basis of a follow-up study. Inter-rater reliability was high, varying from 0.80 to 1.0 in the conjoint interviews and 0.30 to 0.73 in the independent interviews. The distinction between paranoid ideation and paranoid delusions was underscored by the striking difference in prevalence between a broad and narrow definition of the symptom (narrow corresponding to a true delusion, broad to the wider concept). The strength of the scale is its proven reliability by lay interviewers and its further definition of psychotic symptoms.

Address for correspondence

DP Devanand
New York State Psychiatric Institute
722 West 168 Street
New York
NY 10032
USA

Columbia University Scale for Psychopathology in Alzheimer's Disease (CUSPAD)

1. DELUSIONS (past month)

For all **delusions** ask:

(a) Was this the case some of the time or most of the time?

Score –		
	Persistent	0
	Transient	1
	N/A	2

(b) Will the patient accept the truth if corrected?

Score –		
	No	0
	Yes	1
	N/A	2

General

In the past month, has the patient talked about any strange ideas or unusual beliefs?

No	0
Yes	1

If 'Yes', can you describe them for me? _____

_____

_____

Paranoid Delusions (past month)

(a) Has the patient felt that others are stealing things from him/her?

No	0
Yes	1

(b) Has the patient suspected that his/her wife/husband is unfaithful? (circle N/A if patient is single or widowed)

No	0
Yes	1
N/A	2

(c) Has the patient had any other unfounded suspicions?

No	0
Yes	1

If 'Yes', can you describe them? _____

_____

_____

Delusions of Abandonment (past month)

Has the patient suspected or accused the caregiver of plotting to leave him/her?

No	0
Yes	1

Somatic Delusions (past month)

Has the patient has any false beliefs that he/she has cancer or another physical illness?

No	0
Yes	1

Misidentification syndromes (past month)

(a) Has the patient stated that people are in the house/home when nobody is there?

No	0
Yes	1

(b) Has the patient looked into the mirror and said it is someone else?

No	0
Yes	1

(c) Has the patient misidentified people, for example, said that the spouse/caregiver is an impostor?

No	0
Yes	1

(d) Has the patient said that his/her house or home is not his/her home?

No	0
Yes	1

(e) Has the patient believed that the characters on television are real or in the room? (Circle N/A if the patient has no access to a television)

No	0
Yes	1
N/A	2

Other Delusions (past month)

Has the patient had any other false beliefs or other strange ideas that I have not asked you about?

No	0
Yes	1

If 'Yes', can you describe them? _____

_____

_____

2. HALLUCINATIONS (past month)

(a) Has the patient heard voices or sounds when no one is there? (Auditory)

No	0
Yes: Vague	1
Clear	2

(b) Has the patient seen visions? (Visual)

No	0
Yes: Vague	1
Clear	2

(c) Has the patient reported unusual smells like burning rubber, gas or rotten eggs? (Olfactory)

No	0
Yes: Vague	1
Clear	2

(d) Has the patient felt that things are crawling under his/her skin?

No	0
Yes: Vague	1
Clear	2

(e) Has the patient reported any other hallucinations?

No	0
Yes: Vague	1
Clear	2

Scale continued overleaf

3.   ILLUSIONS (past month)

Has the patient reported that one thing is something else, for example, saying that a pillow looks like a person or a light bulb looks like a fire starting?

No	0
Yes: Vague	I
Clear	2

If 'Yes', can you describe them? _____

_____

_____

4.   BEHAVIORAL DISTURBANCES (past month)

(a)   Has the patient wandered away from home or from the caregiver?

No	0
Yes	I

(b)   Has the patient made verbal outburts?

No	0
Yes	I

(c)   Has the patient used physical threats and/or violence?

No	0
Threatening behavior	I
Physical violence	2

(d)   Has the patient shown agitation or restlessness?

No	0
Yes	I

(e)   Has the patient been more confused at night or during evening, compared to the day?

No	0
Yes	I

5. DEPRESSION (past month)

If the answer to items (a) to (c) below is 'Yes', circle the appropriate level of severity. If the answer is 'No', circle 'N/A'.

(a)   Has the patient been sad, depressed, blue or down in the dumps?

No	0
Yes	I

If 'Yes', how do you know they are sad, e.g. do they cry or complain they feel sad?

Write down details: _____

_____

_____

Was he/she depressed?:	N/A	0
occasionally		I
some of the time		2
most of the time		3
all of the time		4

(b)   Has the patient had difficulty sleeping?

	No	0
	Yes	I

If 'Yes', is there:	N/A	0
slight difficulty		I
at least 2 hours sleep at night		2
less than 2 hours sleep at night		3
excessive sleep/sleepiness		4

(c)   Has the patient's appetite changed?

	No	0
	Yes	I

If 'Yes', circle one:	N/A	0
slightly decreased		I
no appetite – food is tasteless		2
need persuasion to eat at all		3
excessive appetite		4

Symptomatology is absolute not relative.

Manchester and Oxford Universities Scale for the Psychopathological Assessment of Dementia (MOUSEPAD)

Reference: **Allen NHP, Gordon S, Hope T, Burns A (1996) Manchester and Oxford Universities Scale for Psychopathological Assessment of Dementia (MOUSEPAD).** *British Journal of Psychiatry* **169: 293–307**

Time taken 15–30 minutes

Rating by experienced clinician, most items on a 3-point severity scale. Interview with carers

Main indications

The measurement of psychiatric symptoms and behavioural changes in patients with dementia.

Commentary

There have been a number of different scales assessing non-cognitive features of dementia, and this is one of them. The Manchester and Oxford Universities Scale for the Psychopathological Assessment of Dementia (MOUSEPAD) is based on the longer Present Behavioural Examination (PBE; Hope and Fairburn, 1992), but was developed as being a shorter instrument and one with an equal emphasis on psychiatric symptomatology as much as behavioural changes. The 59-item instrument was developed from questions in the PBE as well as questions derived from empirical studies of the phenomenology of Alzheimer's disease (Burns et al, 1990). The paper presents reliability, sensitivity and validity. Thirty patients were interviewed four times over 6 weeks. The MOUSEPAD has the ability to measure the presence of phenomena in the last month as well as since the onset of dementia defined as the presence of the first change, whether this be memory loss, personality change or otherwise. Test/retest reliability in the main symptoms areas was generally above 0.6. Inter-rater reliability was of a similar magnitude. The range of kappa values for test/retest reliability was 0.4–0.93, 0.56–1.0 for inter-rater reliability and 0.43–0.67 for validity. It should be noted that the scale contains no items for depression, and the Cornell Scale for Depression in Dementia (page 9), is suggested as the additional instrument (Alexopoulos et al, 1988). Validity was compared with the PBE itself and, while ratings varied, generally there was excellent agreement. A global rating of change suggested that the MOUSEPAD is sensitive to change but that the degree of change observed was slight. Separate ratings of severity and frequency are made.

Additional references

Alexopoulos G, Abrahams R, Young R et al (1988) Cornell Scale for Depression in Dementia. *Biological Psychiatry* **23**: 271–84.

Burns A, Jacoby R, Levy R (1990) Psychiatric phenomena in Alzheimer's disease. I. Disorders of thought content. *British Journal of Psychiatry* **157**: 72–6.

Hope RA, Fairburn CG (1992) The Present Behavioural Examination (BPE): the development of an interview to measure current behavioural abnormalities. *Psychological Medicine* **22**: 223–30.

Address for correspondence

Harry Allen
Consultant Psychiatrist
York House
Manchester Royal Infirmary
Oxford Road
Manchester M13 9WL
UK

e-mail: hallen@psych/cmht.nwest.nhs.uk

Manchester and Oxford Universities Scale for the Psychopathological Assessment of Dementia (MOUSEPAD)

Descriptive psychopathology of dementia

Name _____

Date

No.

Informant

First, establish the duration of the dementia syndrome in months: How long ago was the first symptom you noticed?
(Cases referred to are 'she'/'her' purely for convenience)

Delusions
(These beliefs should be held firmly, be false, *last for more than seven days* and occur in the absence of acute physical illness.)

	Yes/no	Severity	Months from onset	Duration in months	In last month? Y/N	Convince otherwise
Has she ever said:						
she is being watched or spied upon?	–	–	–	–	–	–
her food or drink is being poisoned?	–	–	–	–	–	–
she is being followed?	–	–	–	–	–	–
her possessions are being hidden?	–	–	–	–	–	–
her possessions are being stolen?	–	–	–	–	–	–
her house is not her own home?	–	–	–	–	–	–
her spouse is having an affair?	–	–	–	–	–	–
she is involved in an amorous affair?	–	–	–	–	–	–
she is about to be abandoned by her family?	–	–	–	–	–	–
someone else is in the house?	–	–	–	–	–	–

Hallucinations
(These experiences can be considered present if the patient has spontaneously complained of the phenomenon or if there is evidence that she has been seen interacting with an apparently false perception. They must have occurred in the absence of acute illness and have lasted for **more than seven days**. NB. Do not rate here patients talking to mirror image, to photographs or to television – these should be rated under misidentifications.)

Has she heard voices or other sounds where there have been none apparent?

	Yes/no	Severity	Months from onset	Duration in months	In last month? Y/N
If so, have they been:					
voices?					
from known persons	–	–	–	–	–
from unknown persons	–	–	–	–	–
does she appear to understand the voices? Yes/No	–	–	–	–	–
music	–	–	–	–	–
animals	–	–	–	–	–
other noises	–	–	–	–	–

Has she seen things where there have been none apparent?

	Yes/no	Severity	Months from onset	Duration in months	In last month? Y/N
If so, have they been:					
people					
known persons	–	–	–	–	–
unknown persons	–	–	–	–	–
dwarf-like figures	–	–	–	–	–
children	–	–	–	–	–
animals	–	–	–	–	–
other					
Has the patient reported strange smells when none have been apparent?	–	–	–	–	–
Has the patient reported strange sensations in her body?	–	–	–	–	–
Has the patient reported an unusual taste in her food or drink	–	–	–	–	–

cont.

Misidentifications
(These experiences must have **lasted for at least seven days** and have occurred in the absence of acute physical illness.)

Has she acted unusually when seeing herself in the mirror?

	Yes/no	Severity	Months from onset	Duration in months	In last month? Y/N
If so, has she:					
claimed that her image is not her own self?	–	–	–	–	–
spent time conversing with her own image?	–	–	–	–	–
Has she ever apparently believed:					
that a close relative or carer is not who they claim to be?	–	–	–	–	–
that they have been replaced by an imposter?	–	–	–	–	–
that TV images or photographs are real events?	–	–	–	–	–
that she is infested with small animals?	–	–	–	–	–

Reduplications
(These experiences must have **lasted for at least seven days** and have occurred in the absence of acute physical illness.)

Has she ever said that things have been reduplicated?:
(e.g. that there are two of anyone or anything in existence)

If so what?	Yes/no	Severity	Months from onset	Duration in months	In last month? Y/N
Spouses or carers	–	–	–	–	–
Houses or other inanimate objects	–	–	–	–	–
Animate objects (pets etc.)	–	–	–	–	–

Behavioural changes in dementia
Note any physical problems which might significantly alter ratings (e.g. arthritis might affect her walking around). If physical problem makes rating inappropriate rate 8 and explain.

	Yes/no	Severity	Months from onset	Duration in months	In last month? Y/N
Walking					
Does she walk around more often than she used to just before the memory problems started?					
If yes then rate:					
1: mild: sits most days for more than 15 minutes at a time, awake					
2: severe: will not sit, most days, for as long as 15 minutes at a time, awake	–	–	–	–	–
Does she follow you (or anyone else) around?					
0: follows others around less than 30 minutes each day					
1: follows others around, most days, for more than 30 minutes but less than 2 hours					
2: follows others around for more than 2 hours, most days	–	–	–	–	–
Does she wander out of the house or home (beyond the garden)?					
0: absent or occasional only (less than 1 hour on a typical day)					
1: for less than 3 hours most days					
2: for more than 3 hours most days	–	–	–	–	–
Does she wander at night? (i.e. after she has gone to bed)					
Has she wandered away from home and had to be brought back home?	–	–	–	–	–

Scale continued overleaf

Manchester and Oxford Universities Scale for the Psychopathological Assessment of Dementia (MOUSEPAD)

Eating

Has her weight changed since onset of problems? No/clearly gained/clearly lost

	Yes/no	Severity	Months from onset	Duration in months	In last month? Y/N
Does she eat more than just before the onset of problems than she used to? 1: eats a little more 2: eats half as much again, or more	–	–	–	–	–
Does she eat more quickly than just before the onset of problems than she used to? 1: eats a little more quickly 2: eats much more quickly	–	–	–	–	–
Have you ever had to limit how much she eats because otherwise she would try to eat too much? 1: on a few occasions only 2: need to control intake much of the time	–	–	–	–	–
Does she eat more sweet things than she used to? (More of a sweet tooth)	Yes/No				

	Yes/no	Severity	Months from onset	Duration in months	In last month? Y/N
Sleep					
Is she restless/wakeful during the night?	–	–	–	–	–
Does she confuse night and day?	–	–	–	–	–
Does she 'doze' during the day, more than she did before the onset of her problems?	–	–	–	–	–
Sexual behaviour					
Does she talk inappropriately about sex?	–	–	–	–	–
Does she act in a sexually disinhibited manner?	–	–	–	–	–

Aggression

	Yes/No				
Has she been physically or verbally aggressive since onset of memory problems (**more** aggressive than before onset of dementia)?	Yes/No				
If yes, under what circumstances?					
While she was being cared for (e.g. washing, dressing)?	Yes/No				
Unprovoked or impatient?	Yes/No				
In response to hallucinations or mistaken ideas you were going to harm her?	Yes/No				
Is the aggression:					
physical – against other people	–	–	–	–	–
– against objects	–	–	–	–	–
verbal	–	–	–	–	–
Does she have outbursts of					
laughing	–	–	–	–	–
crying	–	–	–	–	–

Other types of behaviour in the last month

	Yes/No
Does she move objects and hide them, or put them in strange places?	–
Does she mislay things?	–

Rate symptoms, hallucinations, misidentifications and behavioural changes as follows (can be current or occurred in the past):
0 = Absent; 1 = Mild (< 1 × week); 2 = Moderate (1 day/week or more but < 4/7 days); 3 = Severe – present at least 4 × week; 8 = Not applicable/not asked; 9 = Interviewee does not know; Must explain why 8 or 9 given in any question.

Present Behavioural Examination (PBE)

Reference: **Hope T, Fairburn CG (1992) The present behavioural examination (PBE): the development of an interview to measure current behaviour abnormalities.** *Psychological Medicine* **22: 223–30**

Time taken up to 1 hour

Rating by trained observer

Main indications

Assessment of current behaviour of people with dementia.

Commentary

This is an extremely detailed assessment of the behaviour of people with dementia, equating to the Present State Examination for psychiatric patients and representing the gold standard in such scales. It is a lengthy interview assessing a number of different domains (number of questions in brackets): mental health (15); walking (28); eating (30); diurnal rhythm (19); aggressive behaviour (44); sexual behaviour (5); continence (26); individual behavioural abnormality (20). There are 121 main questions in total, with a further 66 subsidiary questions if a corresponding main question is answered positively. Some 115 of 121 main questions are on a discontinuous scale (i.e. between a two- and seven-point severity rating scale), with the remaining six on an unlimited ordinal scale. Inter-rater and test/retest reliability is presented, inter-rater reliability ranging from between 0.65 and 1.0 and between 0.16 and 0.74 for test/retest reliability. Some 96% of items were rated the same by each rater in the inter-rater reliability study and 83% in the test/retest reliability study.

Address for correspondence

Tony Hope
Reader in Medicine
Warneford Hospital
Oxford OX3 7JX
UK

e-mail: admin@ethox.ox.ac.uk

CERAD Behavioral Rating Scale

Reference: **Tariot PN, Mack JL, Patterson MB, Edland SD, Weiner MF, Fillenbaum G, Blazina L, Teri L, Rubin E, Mortimer JA, Stern Y and the Behavioral Pathology Committee of the Consortium to Establish a Registry for Alzheimer's Disease (1995) The behavioral rating scale for dementia of the Consortium to Establish a Registry for Alzheimer's Disease.** *American Journal of Psychiatry* 152: 1349–57

Time taken 20–30 minutes (reviewer's estimate)

Rating by a trained examiner who meets a predetermined certification standard

Main indications

Rating of psychopathology in patients with probable Alzheimer's disease.

Commentary

This rating scale comes out of the large CERAD (Consortium to Establish a Registry for Alzheimer's Disease) initiative. The scale has 46 questions, most rated on a five-point severity scale but some with a categoric yes/no response. The items were gleaned from existing scales and designed to be administered to a knowledgeable informant. Items were rated by frequency in view of the difficulty of making judgements of severity. Rating is limited to the previous month, although notes can be made of signs and symptoms occurring before that. The original sample consisted of 303 subjects attending 16 Alzheimer centres within the USA. Eight factors were revealed: depressive features; psychotic features; defective self-regulation; irritability/agitation; vegetative features; apathy; aggression; and affective lability. Inter-rater reliability ranges between 91 and 100% with a kappa value ranging from 0.77 to 1.0, the vast majority being over 0.9. A further study (Patterson et al, 1997) followed 64 health controls and 261 patients with Alzheimer's disease over 12 months to assess changes in behaviour over time. Test/retest reliability over 1 month was good, with correlation coefficients between 0.7 and 0.89 for patients with Alzheimer's disease (categorized in terms of scores on the Mini-Mental State Examination (MMSE; page 36)). There was relatively little change in total behaviour rating scores over 12 months, although there was a decrease in the total score in the normal control group and an increase in patients with Alzheimer's disease whose MMSE score was between 16 and 20. It was suggested that additive scores of correlated items would be a better measure of change in behaviour over time rather than a simple summation of total scores in view of the variability of behaviour over time.

Additional references

Patterson MB, Mack JL (1997) CERAD Behavior Rating Scale for Dementia (BRSD). *Alzheimer Disease and Associated Disorders* 11 (Suppl 2): S90–1.

Patterson MB, Mack JL, Mackell JA et al (1997) A longitudinal study of behavioral pathology across five levels of dementia severity in Alzheimer's disease: the CERAD behavior rating scale for dementia. *Alzheimer Disease and Associated Disorders* 11 (Suppl 2): S40–4.

Address for correspondence

Pierre N Tariot
Psychiatry Unit
Monroe Community Hospital
435 East Henrietta Road
Rochester
NY 14620
USA

CERAD Behavioral Rating Scale

Code

1. Has {S} **said** that {S} feels anxious, worried, tense, or fearful? (For example, has {S} expressed worry or fear about being left alone? Has {S} said {S} is anxious or afraid or certain situations?) If so, describe.　A

2. Has {S} shown **physical signs** of anxiety, worry, tension, or fear? (For example, is {S} easily startled? Does {S} appear nervous? Does {S} have a tense or worried facial expression?) If so, describe.　A

3. Has {S} appeared sad or blue or depressed?　A
4. Has {S} expressed feelings of hopelessness or pessimism?　A
5. Has {S} cried within the past month?　A
6. Has {S} said that {S} feels guilty? (For example, has {S} blamed {S's} self for things {S} did in the past?) If yes, describe nature and extent of guilt.　A
7. Has {S} expressed feelings of poor self-esteem? For example, has {S} said that {S} feels like a failure or that {S} feels worthless? This item is intended to reflect global loss of self-esteem rather than simply a concern over loss of, for example, a particular ability.　A
8. Has {S} said {S} feels life is not worth living? Or has {S} expressed a wish to die or done something that suggested {S} was considering suicide? If yes, specify what subject said or did.　A

If yes or a rating of 8, ask: Has {S} ever made a suicide attempt?
Include any suicidal gestures in rating this probe.

0 No
I Yes
9 NA

9. Have there been times when {S} doesn't enjoy the things {S} does as much as {S} used to before {S's} dementia began? This item refers to any specific loss of enjoyment so long as {S} actually engages in the activity in question. {S} need not be an active participant in this activity; {S} need only be present.　B

10. Do you find {S} sometimes can't seem to **get started** on things {S} used to do before {S's} dementia began, even though {S} is **capable** of doing them? (For example, do you find {S} won't start a task or pastime on {S's} own, but with a little encouragement {S} goes ahead and carries it out?) This item refers to any failure to initiate activities, so long as the activities are those which S is still capable of carrying out when given the opportunity.　B

11. Has {S} seemed tired or lacking in energy?　A

12. Was {S's} sleeping pattern in the past month different from the way it was before {S's} dementia began? (For example, does {S} sleep more or less than {S} used to? Does {S} sleep at a different time of day than {S} used to?) If yes, describe change.　B

13. Has {S} had difficulty falling asleep or remaining asleep? If yes, describe.　A

14. Has {S's} appetite during the past month changed from the way it was before {S's} dementia began? (For example, at meal times does {S's} desire to eat seem different?) 'Appetite' refers to S's response to food when it is presented in the usual manner.
If yes, circle either increased or decreased appetite, according to informant's judgment.　B

I Increased
2 Decreased

15. In the past month, has {S} gained or lost weight without intending to?　B
If yes, circle amount gained or lost.
Gained:

I Up to 5 lbs.
2 More than 5 lbs.

Lost:

I Up to 5 lbs.
2 More than 5 lbs.

16. Has {S} had physical complaints that seemed out of proportion to {S's} actual physical problems?　A
17. In the past month, has {S's} sexual interest been different from the way it was before {S's} dementia began? If yes, describe.　B
18. Has {S} shown sudden changes in {S's} emotions? (For example, does {S} go from laughter to tears quickly?)　A
19. Have there been times when {S} was agitated or upset? This item refers to **observable** signs of emotional distress, such as verbal comments, facial expressions, or gestures. It is the **emotional components that distinguishes this item from item 24.**　A
20. Have there been times when {S} was easily irritated or annoyed?　A
21. Has {S} been uncooperative? (For example, does {S} refuse to accept appropriate help? Does {S} insist on doing things {S's} own way?)　A
22. Has {S} been threatening or verbally abusive toward others?　A
23. Has {S} been physically aggressive toward people or things? (For example, has {S} shoved or physically attacked people or thrown or broken objects?)　A
24. Has {S} seemed restless or overactive? (For example, does {S} fidget or pace? Does {S} finger things or seem unable to sit still?) When the overactive behavior is associated with emotional agitation that is rated in item 19, it should **not** be rated here also.　A

Scale continued overleaf

25.	Has {S} done things that seem to have no clear purpose or a confused purpose? (For example, does {S} open and close drawers? Does {S} put things in inappropriate places? Does {S} hoard things or rummage through things?) If S's behavior shows a high level of motor activity rather than confusion or lack of purpose, it should be rated under item 24.	A
26.	Has there been a particular time of day during which {S} seemed more confused than at other times?	B
		1 Daytime
	If yes, circle time of day	2 Evening (6:00 pm to bedtime)
		3 Night
27.	Has {S} wandered or tried to wander for no apparent reason? 'Wandering' includes wandering away from one's residence or caregiver, as well as within the residence. If yes, describe incidents.	A
28.	Has tried to leave home or get away from whoever was taking care of {S} **with** an apparent purpose or destination in mind? If yes, describe incidents.	A
29.	Has {S} done socially inappropriate things? (For example, does {S} make vulgar remarks? Does {S} talk excessively to strangers? Has {S} sexually exposed {S's} self or done other things such as making gestures of touching people inappropriately? This item is intended to reflect a loss of propriety, not simply confusion. If inappropriate behavior can be rated under a more specific item, such as abusive behavior (item 22) or aggressive behavior (item 23), it should not be rated here.	A
30.	Does {S} tend to say the same things repeatedly? This item refers to repetitive statements, including questions, phrases, demands, etc.	A
31.	Does {S} withdraw from social situations? (For example, does {S} avoid groups of people or prefer to be alone? Does {S} avoid participating in activities with others?)	A
32.	Does {S} seek out more visual or physical contact with {S's} caregivers than before {S's} dementia began? (For example, has {S} seemed 'clingy'? Does {S} follow you about and seem to want to be in the same room with you?)	B
33.	Has {S} misidentified people? (For example, has {S} confused one familiar person with another, or has {S} thought that a familiar person was a stranger?) 'Misidentification' means an actual belief that one person was another, not simply a misnaming or failure to remember who someone is, and it refers to someone actually seen by {S}.	A
34.	Has {S} looked at {S's} -self in a mirror and not recognized {S's} -self?	A
35.	Has {S} misidentified things? Has {S} thought common things were someting else? (For example, has {S} said that a pillow was a person or that a light bulb was a fire?) If yes, describe.	A
36.	Has {S} done or said anything that suggests {S} believes people are harming, threatening, or taking advantage of {S} in some way? (For example, with no good reason has {S} thought things have been given away or stolen; has {S} thought {S} was mischarged or over charged for purchase; has {S} seemed suspicious or wary?)	A
		0 Yes
	If yes, ask: If you try to correct {S}, will {S} accept the truth?	1 No
		9 N/A
37.	Has {S} done or said anything that suggests {S} thinks {S's} spouse is unfaithful?	A
		0 Yes
	If yes, ask: If you try to correct {S}, will {S} accept the truth?	1 No
		9 N/A
38.	Has {S} done or said anything that suggests {S} thinks {S's} spouse or caregiver is plotting to abandon {S}?	A
		0 Yes
	If yes, ask: If you try to correct {S}, will {S} accept the truth?	1 No
		9 N/A
39.	Has {S} done or said anything that suggests {S} thinks {S's} spouse or caregiver is an imposter?	A
		0 Yes
	If yes, ask: If you try to correct {S}, will {S} accept the truth?	1 No
		9 N/A
40.	Has {S} done or said anything that suggests {S} thinks that characters on television are real? (For example, has {S} talked to them, acted as if they could hear or see {S}, or said that they were friends or neighbors?)	A
		0 Yes
	If yes, ask: If you try to correct {S}, will {S} accept the truth?	1 No
		9 N/A
41.	Has {S} done or said anything that suggests {S} believes that there are people in or around the house beyond those who are actually there?	A
		0 Yes
	If yes, ask: If you try to correct {S}, will {S} accept the truth?	1 No
		9 N/A

cont.

42. Has {S} done or said anything that suggests {S} believes that a dead person is still alive, even though {S} used to know they were dead? Do not rate memory problems. If {S} simply cannot remember whether a particular person has died, it should not be rated as a mistaken belief.

        A
        0 Yes

If yes, ask: If you try to correct {S}, will {S} accept the truth?

        1 No
        9 N/A

43. Has {S} done or said anything that suggests {S} thinks where {S} lives is not really {S's} home, even though {S} used to consider it home?

        A
        0 Yes

If yes, ask: If you try to correct {S}, will {S} accept the truth?

        1 No
        9 N/A

44. Has {S} heard voices or sounds when there was no sound? If yes, describe.
        A
If yes, rate for clarity.
        Vague 0   Clear 1

45. Has {S} seen things or people that were not there? If yes, describe.
        A
If yes, rate for clarity.
        Vague 0   Clear 1

46. Before we stop, I want to be sure we've covered all of {S's} problems, except, of course, for those related to memory loss. Has {S} done anything else in the past month that seemed strange or created difficulties? Has {S} said anything that suggests {S} has some unusual ideas or beliefs that I haven't asked you about? If response concerns purely cognitive symptoms, do not rate. If response contains behaviors that can be rated under other items, do so. Any behavior that is rated here should be described. Indicate the most frequently occurring problem and rate it.

        A

S = subject.

Code A:
0 = Not occurred since illness began
1 = 1–2 days in past month
2 = 3–8 days in past month (up to 2 × week)
3 = 9–15 days in past month
4 = 16 days or more in past month
8 = Occurred since illness began, but not in past month
9 = Unable to rate

Code B:
0 = Not occurred since illness began
1 = Yes, has occurred in past month
8 = Occurred since illness began, but not in past month
9 = Unable to rate

American Journal of Psychiatry, Vol. 152, pp. 1349–1357, 1995. Copyright 1995, The American Psychiatric Association. Reprinted by permission.

Rating Scale for Aggressive Behaviour in the Elderly (RAGE)

Reference: Patel V, Hope RA (1992) A rating scale for aggressive behaviour in the elderly – the RAGE. *Psychological Medicine* 22: 211–21

Time taken less than 5 minutes

Rating by trained interviewer

Main indications

Designed to be of value in studies involving the treatment and correlates of aggressive behaviour in psychogeriatric inpatients.

Commentary

The authors of the Rating Scale for Aggressive Behaviour in the Elderly (RAGE) note the wide availability of global rating scales, but while *useful* they are not reliable in assessing specific problems such as aggressive behaviour. The RAGE scale was specifically designed to be filled in by ward-based nursing staff. Aggression was defined as 'an overt act involving the delivery of noxious stimuli to (but not necessarily aimed at) another organism, object or self which is clearly not accidental'. The original set of items was generated following interviews with carers of 40 patients with dementia and the observation period was defined as the past few days (chosen to balance the risk of missing the behaviour if the period is too short and decreased sensitivity if the period is too long). On the basis of feedback from professionals, the scale was revised and underwent inter-rater reliability, test/retest reliability and validation using direct observation. Inter-rater reliability was 0.94 with 86% agreement. Test/retest reliability over 6 hours, 7 and 14 days was excellent. Sensitivity was evaluated by validating the scale scores against descriptions by the nursing staff for changes in behaviour. Other analyses incude intraclass correlation, split half reliability, correlation of individual items and principal components analysis.

Address for correspondence

Tony Hope
Reader in Medicine
Warneford Hospital
Oxford OX3 7JX
UK

e-mail:admin@ethox.ox.ac.uk

Rating Scale for Aggressive Behaviour in the Elderly (RAGE)

Has the patient in the past 3 days . . .

1.	Been demanding or argumentative?	0	1	2	3
2.	Shouted, yelled, or screamed?	0	1	2	3
3.	Sworn or used abusive language?	0	1	2	3
4.	Disobeyed ward rules, e.g. deliberately passed urine outside the commode?	0	1	2	3
5.	Been uncooperative or resisted help, e.g. whilst being given a bath or medication?	0	1	2	3
6.	Been generally in a bad mood, irritable or quick to fly off the handle?	0	1	2	3
7.	Been critical, sarcastic or derogatory, e.g. saying someone is stupid or incompetent?	0	1	2	3
8.	Been inpatient or got angry if something does not suit him/her?	0	1	2	3
9.	Threatened to harm or made statements to scare others?	0	1	2	3
10.	Indulged in antisocial acts, e.g. deliberately stealing food or tripping someone?	0	1	2	3
11.	Pushed or shoved others?	0	1	2	3
12.	Destroyed property or thrown things around angrily, e.g. towels, medicines?	0	1	2	3
13.	Been angry with him/herself?	0	1	2	3
14.	Attempted to kick anyone?	0	1	2	3
15.	Attempted to hit others?	0	1	2	3
16.	Attempted to bite, scratch, spit at, or pinch others?	0	1	2	3
17.	Used an object (such as a towel or a walking stick) to lash out or hurt someone?	0	1	2	3

In the past 3 days, has the patient inflicted any injury . . .

18.	On him/herself?	0	1	2	3
19.	On others?	0	1	2	3

    0   no
    1   mild e.g. a scratch
    2   moderate e.g. a bruise
    3   severe e.g. a fracture

20. Has the patient in the past 3 days been required to be placed under sedation or in isolation or in physical restraints, in order to control his/her aggressiveness?
    0   no; 1   yes

21. Taking all factors into consideration, do you consider the patient's behaviour in the last 3 days to have been aggressive?
    0   not at all
    1   mildly
    2   moderately
    3   severely

Total score:

Any additional comments:

Rating on frequency basis over last 3 days
0 = Never
1 = At least once in past 3 days
2 = At least once every day in past 3 days
3 = More than once every day in past 3 days

Source: Patel V, Hope RA (1992) A rating scale for aggressive behaviour in the elderly – the RAGE. *Psychological Medicine* **22**: 211–21. Reprinted by kind permission of Cambridge University Press.

Overt Aggression Scale (OAS)

Reference: **Yudofsky SC, Silver JM, Jackson W, Endicott J, Williams D (1986) The Overt Aggression Scale for the objective rating of verbal and physical aggression.** *American Journal of Psychiatry* **143: 35–9**

Time taken 5 minutes (reviewer's estimate)

Rating by nurses and nursing aides

Main indications

The scale is designed as an objective rating of verbal and physical aggression specifically to quantify the severity of the aggression and to distinguish those with chronic hostility from those with episodic outbursts.

Commentary

The Overt Aggression Scale (OAS) is divided into four categories: verbal aggression; physical aggression against objects; physical aggression against self; and physical aggression against other people. It is primarily designed to be used in psychiatric settings, and records the severity of the aggression, the timing and duration of the incident and the intervention. Correlation coefficients were greater than 0.5 in 95% of ratings and greater than 0.75 in 52%. The total aggression score had a correlation coefficient of 0.87. Buss and Durkee (1959) describe a hostility scale which forms the basis for many aggression ratings.

Additional reference

Buss A, Durkee A (1957) An inventory for assessing different kinds of hostility. *Journal of Consulting Psychology* **21**: 343–9.

Address for correspondence

Stuart C Yudofsky
Baylor College of Medicine
Houston Medical Center Building
One Baylor Plaza
Houston, TX 77030
USA

e-mail: stuarty@bcm.tmc.edu
www.bcm.tmc

Overt Aggression Scale (OAS)

AGGRESSIVE BEHAVIOR (check all that apply)

Verbal Aggression

__ Makes loud noise, shouts angrily.
__ Yells mild personal insults, e.g. 'You're stupid!'
__ Curses viciously, uses foul language in anger, makes moderate threats to others or self.
__ Makes clear threats of violence toward others or self ('I'm going to kill you') or requests to help control self.

Physical Aggression Against Objects

__ Slams door, scatters clothing, makes a mess.
__ Throws objects down, kicks furniture without breaking it, marks the wall.
__ Breaks objects, smashes windows.
__ Sets fires, throws objects dangerously.

Physical Aggression Against Self

__ Picks or scratches skin, hits self, pulls hair (with no or minor injury only).
__ Bangs head, hits fist into objects, throws self onto floor or into objects (hurst self without serious injury).
__ Small cuts or bruises, minor burns.
__ Mutilates self, causes deep cuts, bites that bleed, internal injury, fracture, loss of consciousness, loss of teeth.

Physical Aggression Against Other People

__ Makes threatening gesture, swings at people, grabs at clothes.
__ Strikes, kicks, pushes, pulls hair (without injury to them).
__ Attacks others, causing mild-moderate physical injury (bruises, sprain, welts).
__ Attacks others, causing severe physical injury (broken bones, deep lacerations, internal injury).

Time incident began: __ __:__ __ a.m. / p.m.

Duration of incident: __ __:__ __ (hours:minutes)

INTERVENTION (check all that apply)

__ None.
__ Talking to patient.
__ Closer observation.
__ Holding patient.

__ Immediate medication given by mouth.
__ Immediate medication given by injection.
__ Isolation without seclusion (time out).
__ Seclusion.

__ Use of restraints.
__ Injury requires immediate medical treatment for patient.
__ Injury requires immediate treatment for other person.

COMMENTS

Neurobehavioral Rating Scale (NRS)

Reference: **Sultzer DL, Levin HS, Mahler ME, High WM, Cummings JL (1992) Assessment of cognitive, psychiatric, and behavioral disturbances in patients with dementia: the Neurobehavioral Rating Scale.** *Journal of the American Geriatrics Society* **40: 549–55**

Time taken 30–40 minutes

Rating by observer

Main indications

Characterizes the cognitive, psychiatric and behavioural disturbance in patients with dementia.

Commentary

The Neurobehavioural Rating Scale (NRS) is a comprehensive instrument assessing a very wide range of changes, containing most of the items of the Brief Psychiatric Rating Scale (BPRS; page 272). The original validation study was performed on 83 patients with dementia (61 with Alzheimer's Disease and 22 with multi-infarct dementia). High correlations were found between the scale and depressive symptoms on the Hamilton Depression Rating Scale (page 6). Inter-rater reliability had been previously reported in patients with head injury. Principal components analysis revealed six factors: cognition/insight, agitation/disinhibition, behavioural retardation, anxiety/depression, verbal output disturbance and psychosis.

Additional references

Corrigan JD, Dickerson J, Fisher E et al (1990) The Neurobehavioral Rating Scale: replication in an acute inpatient rehabilitation setting. *Brain Injury* **4**: 215–22.

Hilton G, Sisson R, Freeman E (1990) The Neurobehavioral Rating Scale: an inter-rater reliability study in the HIV seropositive population. *Journal of Neuroscience Nursing* **22**: 36–42.

Levin HS, High WM, Goethe KE et al (1987) The Neurobehavioral Rating Scale: assessment of the behavioral sequelae of head injury by the clinician. *Journal of Neurology, Neurosurgery and Psychiatry* **50**: 183–93.

Address for correspondence

DL Sultzer
Behavioral Neurosciences Section
B-111
West LA VA Medical Center
11301 Wilshire Blvd
Los Angeles
CA 90073
USA

Neurobehavioral Rating Scale (NRS)

___ 1. Inattention/Reduced Alertness
        Decreased alertness; unable to sustain attention; easily distracted.
___ 2. Somatic Concern
        Volunteers complaints or elaborates excessively about somatic symptoms.
___ 3. Disorientation
        Confusion for person, place, or time.
___ 4. Anxiety
        Worry, apprehension, or overconcern.
___ 5. Expressive Deficit
        Aphasia, with nonfluent features.
___ 6. Emotional Withdrawal
        Lack of spontaneous interaction; poor relatedness during interview.
___ 7. Conceptual Disorganization
        Thought process is loose, disorganized, or tangential.
___ 8. Disinhibition
        Socially inappropriate comments or actions.
___ 9. Guilt Feelings
        Self-blame or remose for past behavior.
___ 10. Memory Deficit
        Difficulty learning new information.
___ 11. Agitation
        Excessive motor activity (e.g. restlessness, kicking, arm flailing, roaming).
___ 12. Inaccurate Insight
        Poor insight; exaggerated self-opinion; overrates level of ability.
___ 13. Depressed Mood
        Sadness, hopelessness, despondency, or pessimism.
___ 14. Hostility/Uncooperativeness
        Animosity, belligerence, or oppositional behavior.
___ 15. Decreased Initiative/Motivation
        Fails to initiate or persist in tasks; reluctant to accept new challenges.
___ 16. Suspiciousness
        Mistrust.
___ 17. Fatigability
        Rapidly tires on tasks or complex activities; lethargic.
___ 18. Hallucinations
        Sensory perceptions without corresponding external stimuli.
___ 19. Motor Retardation
        Slowed movements or speech; not primary weakness.
___ 20. Unusual Thought Content
        Odd, strange, or bizarre thoughts; delusions.
___ 21. Blunted Affect
        Reduced emotional tone; reduced range or intensity of affect.
___ 22. Excitement
        Increased emotional tone; elevated mood; euphoria.
___ 23. Poor Planning
        Unrealistic goals; poorly formulated plans for the future.
___ 24. Mood Lability
        Rapid changes in mood that are disproportionate to the situation.
___ 25. Tension
        Postural and facial expression of anxiety; autonomic hyperactivity.
___ 26. Comprehension Deficit
        Difficulty understanding verbal or written instructions.
___ 27. Speech Articulation Defect
        Misarticulation or slurring of words that affects intelligibility.
___ 28. Fluent Aphasia
        Aphasia, with fluent features.

Reproduced from Sultzer DL, Levin HS, Mahler ME, High WM, Cummings JL (1992) Assessment of cognitive, psychiatric, and behavioral disturbances in patients with dementia: the Neurobehavioral Rating Scale. *Journal of the American Geriatrics Society,* Vol. 40, no. 6, pp. 549–55.

Caretaker Obstreperous-Behavior Rating Assessment (COBRA) Scale

Reference: **Drachman DA, Swearer JA, O'Donnell BF, Mitchell AL, Maloon A (1992) The Caretaker Obstreperous-Behavior Rating Assessment (COBRA) Scale.** *Journal of the American Geriatrics Society* **40: 463–70**

Time taken 20 minutes (author's estimate)

Rating by observer

Main indications

For the assessment of 'obstreperous' behaviours in dementia (defined as difficult and troublesome behaviours).

Commentary

The Caretaker Obstreperous-Behavior Rating Assessment (COBRA) Scale is divided into four main areas: aggressive/assaultive, disordered ideas/personality, mechanical/motor and vegetative, with a total of 30 items. It measures both frequency and severity. A summary score is produced. The scale was validated on 67 patients with dementia. Inter-rater reliability (on seven patients) was between 0.73 and 0.99 for eight of the twelve summary measures and between 0.30 and 0.63 for four. Test/retest reliability correlaton coefficients were significant at $p < 0.01$. Validity was assessed with comparison to cognitive measures and global ratings of dementia.

Address for correspondence

DA Drachman
Department of Neurology
University of Massachusetts Medical Center
55 Lake Avenue North
Worcester
MA 01655
USA

Caretaker Obstreperous-Behavior Rating Assessment (COBRA) Scale

Illustrative examples of the operational definitions used in the COBRA Scale for each of the behavioral categories

Behavioral category	Target behavior	Operational definition
Aggressive/assaultive	Physical attack	Effort or actual physical injury to other, e.g. hit, kick, bite, scratch, etc. If the attack did not end in contact, it was because the patient was physically restrained.
Ideas/personality	Bradyphrenia	Responds slowly to questions and only after a long delay.
Mechanical/motor	Wandering	Aimlessly walks without guidance, frequently away from where he/she should be.
Vegetative	Change in sexuality Hypersexuality Hyposexuality	Increased and aggressive interest in sexual activities; Loss of interest in all sexual activities.

These are **Target Behaviors**
8 OBs = Aggressive/Assaultive
9 OBs = Disordered ideas/Personality
7 OBs = Mechanical/Motor
6 OBs plus subdivisions = Vegetative

Videos provided for each OB to facilitate recognition/description by caretaker.

Frequency and severity scales – an intensity assessment for each target OB.

Frequency
0 = Behavior **not** occurred within past 3 months.
1 =
2 =
3 =
4 = Behavior occurred daily or more often.

Severity – rate disruptiveness of behavior
0 = No appreciable disruptive effect.
1 =
2 =
3 =
4 = Significant danger.
Ceiling scores to differentiate maximum possible effects.

COBRA Scale summary scores

I. Total number of OBs in each category

Behavior	Number present
1. Aggressive/Assaultive	_____
2. Ideas/Personality	_____
3. Mechanical/Motor	_____
4. Vegetative	_____

II. Highest severity score in each category

Behavior	Highest Severity Score
5. Aggressive/Assaultive	_____
6. Ideas/Personality	_____
7. Mechanical/Motor	_____
8. Vegetative	_____

III. Most severe OBs – all categories
    9. Highest severity score for any OB   _____
    10. How many OBs had scores >3?   _____

IV. Most frequent OBs – all categories
    11. Highest frequency score for any OB   _____
    12. How many OBs had scores >3?   _____

Determines behavioral categories, number of different OBs, severity of disruption of OBs and frequency of OB occurrence

Reproduced from Drachman DA, Swearer JA, O'Donnell BF, Mitchell AL, Maloon A (1992) The Caretaker Obstreperous-Behavior Rating Assessment (COBRA) Scale. *Journal of the American Geriatrics Society,* Vol. 40, no. 5, pp. 463–70.

Nurses' Observation Scale for Inpatient Evaluation (NOSIE)

Reference: **Honigfeld G, Klett CJ (1965) Nurses' Observation Scale for Inpatient Evaluation: a new scale for measuring improvement in chronic schizophrenia.** *Journal of Clinical Psychology* **21: 65–71**

Time taken 20 minutes

Rating by nursing staff

Main indications

To assess change in psychopathology in patients with schizophrenia.

Commentary

The Nurses' Observation Scale for Inpatient Evaluation (NOSIE) was designed as a sufficiently sensitive scale to measure change resulting from therapy in older people with schizophrenia but could also be applied in clinical research to any elderly patient or for use in drug trials. The 100 initial items had been drawn from existing scales, and two scales were described: a rating scale of 80 items and a directly derived 30-item scale using only the items derived from a factor analysis which were most sensitive to therapeutic effects. The NOSIE-80 was derived from the initial 100 items by dropping 20 with insufficient inter-rater reliability.

Scoring is based on a three-day observation of the patient on a five-scale frequency score. Seven factors are identified in the NOSIE-80: social competence, social interests, personal neatness, cooperation, irritability, manifest psychosis and psychotic depression. The NOSIE-30 has six factors – cooperation and psychotic depression are absent, with the addition of retardation. Inter-rater reliability was found to be satisfactory.

Additional reference

Honigfeld G, Gillis RD, Klett CJ (1966) NOSIE-30: a treatment-sensitive ward behavior scale. *Psychological Reports* **19**: 180–2.

Nurses' Observation Scale for Inpatient Evaluation (NOSIE)

Instructions: For each of the 30 items below you are to rate this patient's behavior during the last **three days only**. Indicate your choice by placing a circle around the correct number before each item.

0 Never
1 Sometimes
2 Often
3 Usually
4 Always

1.	Is sloppy	0	1	2	3	4
2.	Is impatient	0	1	2	3	4
3.	Cries	0	1	2	3	4
4.	Shows interest in activities around him	0	1	2	3	4
5.	Sits, unless directed into activity	0	1	2	3	4
6.	Gets angry or annoyed easily	0	1	2	3	4
7.	Hears things that are not there	0	1	2	3	4
8.	Keeps his clothes neat	0	1	2	3	4
9.	Tries to be friendly with others	0	1	2	3	4
10.	Becomes easily upset if something doesn't suit him	0	1	2	3	4
11.	Refuses to do the ordinary things expected of him	0	1	2	3	4
12.	Is irritable and grouchy	0	1	2	3	4
13.	Has trouble remembering	0	1	2	3	4
14.	Refuses to speak	0	1	2	3	4
15.	Laughs or smiles at funny comments or events	0	1	2	3	4
16.	Is messy in his eating habits	0	1	2	3	4
17.	Starts up a conversation with others	0	1	2	3	4
18.	Says he feels blue or depressed	0	1	2	3	4
19.	Talks about his interests	0	1	2	3	4
20.	Sees things that are not there	0	1	2	3	4
21.	Has to be reminded what to do	0	1	2	3	4
22.	Sleeps, unless directed into activity	0	1	2	3	4
23.	Says that he is not good	0	1	2	3	4
24.	Has to be told to follow hospital routine	0	1	2	3	4
25.	Has difficulty completing even simple tasks on his own	0	1	2	3	4
26.	Talks, mutters, or mumbles to himself	0	1	2	3	4
27.	Is slow moving and sluggish	0	1	2	3	4
28.	Giggles or smiles to himself without any apparent reason	0	1	2	3	4
29.	Quick to fly off the handle	0	1	2	3	4
30.	Keeps himself clean	0	1	2	3	4

Source: Guy (W), Ed.: ECDEU Assessment Manual for Psychopharmacology. Ed. revised. Rockville, Maryland, US Department of Health, Education and Welfare, 1976.
Reproduced from Honigfeld G, Klett C (1965) Nurses' Observational Scale for Inpatient Evaluation (NOSIE): a new scale for measuring improvement in chronic schizophrenia. *Journal of Clinical Psychology* **21**: 65–71. Copyright © 1965, John Wiley & Sons, Inc. Reprinted with permission.

Disruptive Behavior Rating Scales (DBRS)

Reference: **Mungas D, Weiler P, Franzi C, Henry R (1989) Assessment of disruptive behavior associated with dementia: the Disruptive Behavior Rating Scales.** *Journal of Geriatric Psychiatry and Neurology* **2: 196–202**

Time taken 10 minutes (reviewer's estimate)

Rating by nurses or carers looking after a patient

Main indications

Assessment of disruptive behaviour in patients with dementia.

Commentary

The Disruptive Behavior Rating Scales (DBRS) rate the severity of four categories of disruptive behaviour: physical aggression, verbal aggression, agitation and wandering. The behaviours were defined to minimize clinical judgement in making the ratings, which are made on a five-point severity scale. The scale was designed to assess a narrower range of behaviour than similar scales but to do so in a more detailed manner. A checklist is completed daily and the DBRS ratings made on a weekly basis. Inter-rater reliability gave values of greater than 0.83. Validity was measured against nursing assessment, and principal components analysis was used to measure convergent and discriminant validity showing four main factors: wandering, agitation and aggression.

Address for correspondence

D Mungas
Alzheimer's Disease and Diagnostic Treatment Center
UC Davis Medical Center
2000 Stockton Blvd
Sacramento
CA 95817
USA

Disruptive Behavior Rating Scales (DBRS)

Definition of behaviors
Physical aggression
Overt behavior with clear aggressive intent that is directed at either persons or objects.
Accidental behavior that otherwise fits this definition should not be rated as physical aggression.

Verbal aggression
Verbal behavior with clear aggressive intent directed at persons or objects.

Agitation
Overt behavior that indicates restlessness, hyperactivity, or subjective distress.
Verbal or physical aggressive behavior not directed at a specific target should be rated as agitation.

Wandering
Leaving authorized premises in a manner that clearly indicates that the individual does not have a rational plan for or awareness of where he/she is going.
Total disruptive behavior: an average of measures one through four.

Name: _____

Week beginning: _____

		Day						
Behavior		1	2	3	4	5	6	7
1.	Hitting							
2.	Kicking							
3.	Biting							
4.	Spitting							
5.	Throwing things							
6.	Using weapons							
7.	Other physical aggression							
8.	Yelling/screaming							
9.	Swearing							
10.	Threatening physical harm							
11.	Criticizing							
12.	Scolding							
13.	Other verbal aggression							
14.	Pacing							
15.	Hand wringing							
16.	Unable to sit/lie still							
17.	Rapid speech							
18.	Increased psychomotor activity							
19.	Repeated expressions of distress							
20.	Other signs of agitation							
21.	Wandering							

Rating:
0 = insufficient data
1 = does not occur
2 = occurs but no intervention results
3 = occurs and intervention required
4 = occurs and has major effect, e.g. injury, or results in major intervention
5 = occurs and has severe effect or extreme intervention

Reprinted with kind permission of the *Journal of Geriatric Psychiatry and Neurology*, **2**: 196–202, Mungas D, Weiler P, Franzi C, Henry R (1989) Assessment of disruptive behavior associated with dementia: the Disruptive Behavior Rating Scales.

Ryden Aggression Scale

Reference: **Ryden MB (1988) Aggressive behavior in persons with dementia who live in the community.** *Alzheimer Disease and Associated Disorders* **2: 342–55**

Time taken 20 minutes

Rating by informant

Main indications

To measure aggressive behaviour in community-based persons with dementia.

Commentary

The Ryden Aggression Scale is based on Lanza's model of aggression, and looks at three subscales to measure physical, verbal and sexually aggressive behaviour. The inventory consists of 25 items, each of which is a specific observable aggressive behaviour. It was initially used in a pilot study on 183 community-living patients with dementia. Overall inter-rater consistency was 0.88 with test/retest reliability of 0.86.

Additional reference

Lanza M (1983) Origins of aggression. *Journal of Psychosocial Nursing and Mental Health Services* **12:** 11–16.

Ryden Aggression Scale

DIRECTIONS: This rating scale is to be completed by the persons who are most knowledgeable about the individual's behavior.

Below is a list of specific behaviors. To the right of each behavior is a statement about frequency. For each behavior, circle the statement that best describes how often the person demonstrates this behavior.

Ratings are to be based on information you have as to how the person has acted in the past, but you need not have actually observed each of the behaviors reported.

EXAMPLE: If the person doubled up his/her fist without hitting once or twice every week, you would complete the item as shown below.

MAKING THREATENING GESTURES	Never	Less than once a year	1–11 times a year	1–3 times a month	(1–6 times a week)	1 or more times daily

EXAMPLE: If the person has never bit anyone, you would complete the item as shown below.

BITING	(Never)	Less than once a year	1–11 times a year	1–3 times a month	1–6 times a week	1 or more times daily

Be sure to respond to every item by circling the response that best describes how often the person demonstrates that particular behavior. Do not leave any items unanswered.

PHYSICALLY AGGRESSIVE BEHAVIOR

BEHAVIOR	(0)	(1)	(2)	(3)	(4)	(5)
1. PUSHING/SHOVING	Never	Less than once a year	1–11 times a year	1–3 times a month	1–6 times a week	1 or more times daily
2. SLAPPING	Never	Less than once a year	1–11 times a year	1–3 times a month	1–6 times a week	1 or more times daily
3. HITTING/PUNCHING	Never	Less than once a year	1–11 times a year	1–3 times a month	1–6 times a week	1 or more times daily
4. PINCHING/ SQUEEZING	Never	Less than once a year	1–11 times a year	1–3 times a month	1–6 times a week	1 or more times daily
5. PULLING HAIR	Never	Less than once a year	1–11 times a year	1–3 times a month	1–6 times a week	1 or more times daily
6. SCRATCHING	Never	Less than once a year	1–11 times a year	1–3 times a month	1–6 times a week	1 or more times daily
7. BITING	Never	Less than once a year	1–11 times a year	1–3 times a month	1–6 times a week	1 or more times daily
8. SPITTING	Never	Less than once a year	1–11 times a year	1–3 times a month	1–6 times a week	1 or more times daily
9. ELBOWING	Never	Less than once a year	1–11 times a year	1–3 times a month	1–6 times a week	1 or more times daily
10. KICKING	Never	Less than once a year	1–11 times a year	1–3 times a month	1–6 times a week	1 or more times daily
11. TACKLING	Never	Less than once a year	1–11 times a year	1–3 times a month	1–6 times a week	1 or more times daily
12. MAKING THREATENING GESTURES	Never	Less than once a year	1–11 times a year	1–3 times a month	1–6 times a week	1 or more times daily
13. THROWING AN OBJECT	Never	Less than once a year	1–11 times a year	1–3 times a month	1–6 times a week	1 or more times daily
14. STRIKING A PERSON WITH AN OBJECT	Never	Less than once a year	1–11 times a year	1–3 times a month	1–6 times a week	1 or more times daily
15. BRANDISHING A WEAPON	Never	Less than once a year	1–11 times a year	1–3 times a month	1–6 times a week	1 or more times daily
17. DAMAGING PROPERTY	Never	Less than once a year	1–11 times a year	1–3 times a month	1–6 times a week	1 or more times daily

If the person has shown other physically aggressive behavior that was not listed above, please describe the behavior.

HOW OFTEN DOES IT OCCUR?	Never	Less than once a year	1–11 times a year	1–3 times a month	1–6 times a week	1 or more times daily

Scale continued overleaf

Ryden Aggression Scale – *continued*

VERBALLY AGGRESSIVE BEHAVIOR	(0)	(1)	(2)	(3)	(4)	(5)
18. NAME CALLING	Never	Less than once a year	1–11 times a year	1–3 times a month	1–6 times a week	1 or more times daily
19. MAKING VERBAL THREATS	Never	Less than once a year	1–11 times a year	1–3 times a month	1–6 times a week	1 or more times daily
20. CURSING, DIRECTED AT A PERSON	Never	Less than once a year	1–11 times a year	1–3 times a month	1–6 times a week	1 or more times daily
21. HOSTILE, ACCUSATORY LANGUAGE DIRECTED AT A PERSON	Never	Less than once a year	1–11 times a year	1–3 times a month	1–6 times a week	1 or more times daily

If the person has shown other verbally aggressive behavior that was not listed above, please describe the behavior.

HOW OFTEN DOES IT OCCUR?	Never	Less than once a year	1–11 times a year	1–3 times a month	1–6 times a week	1 or more times daily

SEXUALLY AGGRESSIVE BEHAVIOR

Many of the following behaviors are ways in which we customarily show love and affection for each other. Such behaviors are considered to be sexually aggressive ONLY IF THEY ARE AGAINST THE EXPRESSED WILL AND/OR DESPITE THE RESISTANCE OF THE OTHER PERSON.

If the person has not acted sexually toward anyone against their will and/or despite their resistance, then circle 'Never' opposite each behavior. If the person has ever done any of the listed behaviors in a sexually aggressive way, then circle the item opposite each behavior that indicates how often this happened.

	(0)	(1)	(2)	(3)	(4)	(5)
22. KISSING	Never	Less than once a year	1–11 times a year	1–3 times a month	1–6 times a week	1 or more times daily
23. HUGGING	Never	Less than once a year	1–11 times a year	1–3 times a month	1–6 times a week	1 or more times daily
24. TOUCHING BODY PARTS	Never	Less than once a year	1–11 times a year	1–3 times a month	1–6 times a week	1 or more times daily
25. INTERCOURSE	Never	Less than once a year	1–11 times a year	1–3 times a month	1–6 times a week	1 or more times daily
26. MAKING OBSCENE GESTURES	Never	Less than once a year	1–11 times a year	1–3 times a month	1–6 times a week	1 or more times daily

If the person has shown other sexually aggressive behavior that was not listed above, please describe the behavior.

HOW OFTEN DOES IT OCCUR	Never	Less than once a year	1–11 times a year	1–3 times a month	1–6 times a week	1 or more times daily

Source: Ryden MB (1988) Aggressive behavior in persons with dementia who live in the community. *Alzheimer Disease and Associated Disorders* **2**: 342–55. Reproduced with permission from Lippincott-Raven Publishers.

Agitated Behavior Mapping Instrument (ABMI)

References: **Cohen-Mansfield J, Watson V, Meade W, Gordon M, Leatherman J, Emor C (1989) Does sundowning occur in residents of an Alzheimer unit?** *International Journal of Geriatric Psychiatry* **4: 294–8**

Cohen-Mansfield J, Marx MS, Rosenthal AS (1989) A description of agitation in a nursing home. *Journal of Gerontology* **44: M77–M84**

Time taken see below

Rating by trained observers (rating from the manual and appropriate training are essential – contact Jiska Cohen-Mansfield at address below for further details)

Main indications

For the observation of behavioural disturbance in residents of nursing facilities.

Commentary

The Agitated Behavior Mapping Instrument (ABMI) is a way of quantifying agitated behaviour by direct observation. It is based on the Cohen-Mansfield Agitation Inventory (CMAI, Cohen-Mansfield, 1986). Twenty-five specific agitated behaviours are assessed encompassing the following categories: verbal non-aggressive, physical non-aggressive, verbal aggressive and physical aggressive behaviours. A training programme familiarizes observers with behaviour mapping techniques in general and continues throughout the course of any study. Observers are instructed to remain at an unobtrusive distance from the resident and, in this study, observe residents for 3 minutes during each hour of a

24-hour day stratified randomly over a period of 2 months. Eight residents were observed over a 1-hour period and a rating made if a particular behaviour remained constant during the 3-minute observation periods. Numerical values were assigned in accordance with this.

Additional references

Cohen-Mansfield J (1986) Agitated behaviors in the elderly. II. Preliminary results in the cognitively deteriorated. *Journal of the American Geriatrics Society* 34: 722–7.

Cohen-Mansfield J, Billig N (1986) Agitated behaviors in the elderly. I. A conceptual review. *Journal of the American Geriatrics Society* 34: 711–21.

Address for correspondence

Jiska Cohen-Mansfield
Director of Research
Hebrew Home
Greater Washington
6121 Montrose Road
Rockville, MD 20852
USA
e-mail: cohenmaj@gunet.georgetown.edu

The Cohen-Mansfield Agitation Inventory (CMAI) – Short Form

1. Cursing or verbal aggression
2. Hitting (including self), Kicking, Pushing, Biting, Scratching, Aggressive spitting (include at meals)
3. Grabbing onto people, Throwing things, Tearing things or destroying property
4. Other aggressive behaviors or self-abuse including: Intentional falling, Making verbal or physical sexual advances, Eating/drinking/chewing inappropriate substances, Hurt self or other
5. Pace, aimless wandering, Trying to get to a different place (e.g. out of the room, building)
6. General restlessness, Performing repetitious mannerisms, tapping, strange movements
7. Inappropriate dress or disrobing
8. Handling things inappropriately
9. Constant request for attention or help
10. Repetitive sentences, calls, questions or words
11. Complaining, Negativism, Refusal to follow directions
12. Strange noises (weird laughter or crying)
13. Hiding things, Hoarding things
14. Screaming

Rating:

1 = Never; 2 = < 1 × per week; 3 = Once or several times/week; 4 = Once or several times a day; 5 = A few times an hour or continuous for ½ hour or more; If more than one occurred per group then summate occurrences.

NB This is the short form CMAI. Other forms exist, e.g. Community Form CMAI, Disruptiveness Relatives CMAI

Brief Agitation Rating Scale (BARS)

Reference: Finkel SI, Lyons JS, Anderson RL (1993) A Brief Agitation Rating Scale (BARS) for nursing home elderly. *Journal of the American Geriatrics Society* 41: 50–2

Time taken 5 minutes (reviewer's estimate)

Rating by caregiver

Main indications

A brief scale to assess agitation in nursing home residents based on the Cohen-Mansfield Agitation Inventory (CMAI; page 159).

Commentary

The Brief Agitation Rating Scale (BARS) was developed after the CMAI was administered to 232 nursing home residents by inteviewers trained by a psychiatrist. The BARS was developed following a three-stage process. First, correlations of individual items against total score were rated, with those having a high correlation selected for possible inclusion. Secondly, inter-rater reliability was assessed. Thirdly, items were selected to be representative of the original CMAI scale. Cronbach's alpha showed reliability of 0.74–0.82, depending on the time of day when the scale was completed. Inter-rater reliability as assessed by intraclass correlation was 0.73. Validity was assessed using the BEHAVE-AD (page 125) and the Behavioural Syndrome Scale for Dementia (quoted in the paper). Correlations were generally high, although greater on those taken throughout the day than those in the evening or at night.

The following ten behaviours were rated in the BARS: hitting, grabbing, pushing, pacing or aimless wandering, performing repetitive mannerisms, restlessness, screaming, repetitive sentences or questions, strange noises and complaining.

Additional reference

Devanand DP, Brockington CD, Moody BJ et al (1992). Behavioral syndromes in Alzheimer's disease. *International Psychogeriatrics* **4**: 161–84.

Address for correspondence

SI Finkel
Department of Psychiatry and Behavioral Sciences
446 E Ontario #830
Chicago
IL 60611
USA

e-mail: sfinkel104@aol.com

Cohen-Mansfield Agitation Inventory (CMAI) – Long Form

References: **Cohen-Mansfield J (1986) Agitated behaviors in the elderly. II. Preliminary results in the cognitively deteriorated.** *Journal of the American Geriatrics Society* 34: 722–7

Cohen-Mansfield J, Marx MS, Rosenthal AS (1989) A description of agitation in a nursing home. *Journal of Gerontology* 44: M77–M84

Time taken 10–15 minutes

Rating by carers (rating from the manual and appropriate training are essential – contact Jiska Cohen-Mansfield at address below for further details)

Main indications

To look at agitated behaviour in patients with cognitive impairment.

Commentary

A seven-point rating scale assessing the frequency with which patients manifest up to 29 agitated behaviours.

Address for correspondence

Jiska Cohen-Mansfield
Director of Research
Hebrew Home
Greater Washington
6121 Montrose Road
Rockville
MD 20852
USA

www.medafile.com/zyweb/CMAI.htm

Cohen-Mansfield Agitation Inventory (CMAI) – Long Form

1. Pace, aimless wandering
2. Inappropriate dress or disrobing
3. Spitting (include at meals)
4. Cursing or verbal aggression
5. Constant unwarranted request for attention or help
6. Repetitive sentence or questions
7. Hitting (including self)
8. Kicking
9. Grabbing onto people
10. Pushing
11. Throwing things
12. Strange noises (weird laughter or crying)
13. Screaming
14. Biting
15. Scratching
16. Trying to get to a different place (e.g. out of the room, building)
17. Intentional falling
18. Complaining
19. Negativism
20. Eating/drinking inappropriate substances
21. Hurt self or other (cigarette, hot water, etc.)
22. Handling things inappropriately
23. Hiding things
24. Hoarding things
25. Tearing things or destroying property
26. Performing repetitive mannerisms
27. Making verbal sexual advances
28. Making physical sexual advances
29. General restlessness

As manifest during last fornight
Rating:
1 = Never
2 = < 1 × week
3 = 1–2 × per week
4 = Several times a week
5 = Once or twice per day
6 = Several times per day
7 = Several times an hour

Observed Agitation in Patients with DAT (SOAPD)

Reference: **Hurley AC, Volicer L, Camberg L, Ashley J, Woods P, Odenheimer G, Ooi WL, McIntyre K, Mahoney E (1999) Measurement of Observed Agitation in Patients with Dementia of the Alzheimer Type.** *Journal of Mental Health and Aging* **5: 117–33**

Time taken 5 minutes

Main indications

Assessment of agitation in dementia.

Commentary

The authors describe the Scale for the Observation of Agitation in Patients with DAT (dementia of the Alzheimer Type, SOAPD). Agitation was defined as those observed patient behaviours which communicate to others that the patient is experiencing an unpleasant state of excitement and which remain after interventions to reduce internal and external stimuli by managing resistiveness, alleviating aversive physical signs and decreasing sources of accumulated stress have been carried out. Items for the SOAPD were derived from existing inventories following eight steps: content domain identification; concept clarification and specification; content validity determination; initial tool development with items, definitions, demarcat-

ing characteristics and administration procedures; initial development of rater training materials; assessment and refinement of initial tool with corresponding training procedures; rater training and evaluation; and development of the scoring system. In the original paper, 57 subjects with Alzheimer's disease in nine long-term care sites during 2136 5-minute observation periods were examined to assess the reliability and validity of the SOAPD. The 26 observers' kappa values ranged from 0.55 to 0.90, with an alpha coefficient of 0.70. Both the duration and the intensity of the experience are scored on a 0–3-point scale

Address for correspondence

Dr Ann C Hurley (182B)
Center for Excellence in Nursing Practice
Brigham and Women's Hospital
The School of Nursing
Bouve College of Health Sciences
Northeastern University
Boston Mass
USA

Demarcating Characteristics SOAPD

1. Total Body Movements. From One Place – The whole body is moving in a repetitive way. There is a sense of urgency, speed, hyperactivity, restlessness, or purposelessness. Includes: (a) disturbed pacing and disturbed walking: repetitively walking back and forth, following a pattern or walking in a hyperactive way regardless of a pattern. (b) Moving while confined to a chair: attempting to move or scoot a chair, geriatric chair, or wheelchair either back and forth or down the hall.

2. Up/Down Movements. A person's body actions are carried out in more than one place and with more speed and/or intensity than is used for purposeful or goal-directed activity. Includes: (a) getting up–sitting down–getting up repetitively, (b) repeated attempts to get out of a chair or to climb out of bed, (c) sitting up in bed–lying back down–sitting up repetitively, (d) rolling from one side of the bed to the other repetitively.

3. Repetitive Body Motions in Place. This category means making repeated movements (not directed outwardly – includes self and clothes) that have a restless or fidgeting quality. A restless quality gives the appearance of being jittery, tense, nervous, uneasy, or unsettled. A fidgeting quality means body movements that look like one is squirming or 'itchy-twitchy'. A key to the category is that the movement is done repetitively. Includes: (a) rubbing: the thighs, hands, feet or rubbing body part against a surface, (b) picking: at clothes (as if to remove lint that is not there), (c) clapping, (d) hand wringing, (e) scratching, (f) squeezing, (g) tapping: continued movement of feet or fingers on a surface, (h) rocking in place, (i) marching in place, (j) clothing actions: taking off or putting on shoes or clothing. The action may result in the person wearing more or less clothing than others in the same environment, or being in undergarments in a nonprivate setting.

4. Outward Motions. Body actions of the extremities that are directed outwardly. Generally, this category includes repetitive behaviors which involve contact with a surface, object, or person and include: (a) hitting, (b) pinching, (c) pushing, (d) shoving, (e) punching, (f) threatening gestures [making a motion which would be universally considered to cause alarm or signal that a harmful behavior may follow. Includes: shaking a clenched fist, or pointing a finger at someone, (g) banging or pounding [such as banging on a table, door, or other object], (h) kicking, (i) elbowing or jabbing, (j) slapping, (k) throwing [under circumstances where it is not appropriate to throw an object, e.g. throwing food and other objects on the floor], (l) messing [playing or randomly spreading substances such as food/feces/soap, etc.], (m) shaking [moving an object back and forth], (n) flipping objects [randomly and purposelessly flipping papers or the pages of books or magazines], (o) tapping, scratching, rubbing an external surface.

5. High-Pitched or Loud Noise. Words or other sounds that are made in a louder than usual volume or in which the sound has a high-pitched quality or tone. A guide for this category is whether or not the sound is louder or higher pitched than conversational level. Includes: (a) calling out, (b) shouting or yelling, (c) crying out [an inarticulate sound of distress with a shrill tone], (d) screaming [sounds with a high-pitched or wailing tone].

6. Repetitive Vocalization. Words or sounds that are made over and over again. It can also include repeated requests for information or other assistance, and running streams of talk or self-talk in which only some words are repeated. Includes: (a) repeated requests for information [using a few words over and over in a questioning tone, e.g. 'where am I? Can I go home now?'], (b) repeated words, (c) whining [repeating words or sounds in a moaning, groaning, or sing-song way], (d) muttering [using a low-volume sound which may include garbled speech or words with a grumbling tone], (e) mumbling [using a low-volume complaining tone, babbling], (f) rapid speech [speaking at a rate faster than the speed of conversational speech], (g) crying, (h) self-talk.

7. Negative Words. Words that express negativity or a tone that is argumentative or demanding. Includes: (a) name calling [using a negative name for an individual], (b) swearing, cursing, profane language, (c) hostile, threatening language [words that connote a belligerent or menacing theme, e.g. 'Get away from me,' or 'Don't come near me'], (d) abusive or obscene language [using insulting or lewd words], (e) argumentative [using quarrelsome speech with a heated tone of voice, e.g. 'I don't have to ...'], (f) demanding [calling urgently, e.g. 'I want to eat now'].

Source: Hurley AC *et al. J Mental Health Aging* 1999; **5:** 131–3. Reproduced by permission from Springer Publishing Co., Inc., New York 10012. © 1999.

Dementia Behavior Disturbance Scale

Reference: **Baumgarten M, Becker R, Gauthier S (1990) Validity and reliability of the Dementia Behavior Disturbance Scale.** *Journal of the American Geriatrics Society* **38: 221–6**

Time taken 10–15 minutes (reviewer's estimate)

Rating in an interview with the patient's primary caregiver, or as a self-administered scale by the carer

Main indications

Measurement of behavioural disturbances in dementia.

Commentary

The Dementia Behavior Disturbance Scale is a 28-item scale developed to avoid some of the problems with earlier scales, for example the confusion of collecting information about cognitive and non-cognitive features in the same instrument. A need for assessment outside the clinical setting was also considered. Two samples were assessed: community-residing patients assessed at a geriatric assessment unit and patients taking part in a drug trial. Test/retest reliability (2 weeks later) was 0.71, internal consistency was 0.84 and construct validity was described in terms of positive correlations with the Behavioural and Mood Disturbance Scale (BMDS; page 340).

Address for correspondence

M Baumgarten
Community Health Department
St Justine Hospital
3175 Cote St Catherine
Montreal
Quebec H3T 1C5
Canada

Dementia Behavior Disturbance Scale

Asks same question repeatedly
Loses, misplaces, or hides things
Lack of interest in daily activities
Wakes up at night for no obvious reason
Makes unwarranted accusations
Sleeps excessively during the day
Paces up and down
Repeats the same action over and over
Is verbally abusive, curses
Dresses inappropriately
Cries or laughs inappropriately
Refuses to be helped with personal care
Hoards things for no obvious reason
Moves arms or legs in a restless or agitated way

Empties drawers or closets
Wanders in the house at night
Gets lost outside
Refuses to eat
Overeats
Is incontinent of urine
Wanders aimlessly outside or in the house during the day
Makes physical attacks (hits, bites, scratches, kicks, spits)
Screams for no reason
Makes inappropriate sexual advances
Exposes private body parts
Destroys property or clothing
Is incontinent of stool
Throws food

Patient's primary caregiver is respondent. There are five possible responses corresponding to behaviour frequency in preceding week:

0 = Never
4 = All the time

Thus, higher scores indicate more disturbance.

Reproduced from Baumgarten M, Becker R, Gauthier S (1990) Validity and reliability of the Dementia Behavior Disturbance Scale. *Journal of the American Geriatrics Society*, Vol. 38, no. 3, pp. 221–6.

Pittsburgh Agitation Scale (PAS)

Reference: **Rosen J, Burgio L, Kollar M, Cain M, Allison M, Fogleman M, Michael M, Zubenko GS (1994) The Pittsburg Agitation Scale: a user-friendly instrument for rating agitation in dementia patients.** *American Journal of Geriatric Psychiatry* **2: 52–9**

Time taken less than 1 minute

Rating by direct observation for between 1 and 8 hours by clinical staff

Main indications

To assess agitation in patients with dementia.

Commentary

The Pittsburgh Agitation Scale (PAS) provides a quantification of the severity of disruptive behaviour within four general behaviour groups: aberrant vocalizations; motor agitation; aggressiveness; resisting care on a scale ranging from 0 to 4. The score reflects the most disruptive or severe behaviour within each behaviour group, and thus an improvement in the PAS score may reflect a decline in a severely disruptive behaviour but other symptoms of agitation may exist. The score is useful when taken in the context that levels of agitation can vary within environments, and should the patient change environments the scores may alter. Inter-rater reliability exceeded 0.80 – validity was assessed by the number of interventions needed.

Address for correspondence

Jules Rosen
Western Psychiatric Institute and Clinic
3811 O'Hara Street
Pittsburgh
PA 15213
USA

Pittsburgh Agitation Scale (PAS)

Hours of sleep this rating period

Circle only the highest intensity score for each behavior group that you observed during this rating period. Use the anchor points as a guide to choose a suitable level of severity. (Not all anchor points need be present. Choose the more severe level when in doubt.)

Behavior groups

Aberrant vocalization

(repetitive requests or complaints, nonverbal vocalizations, e.g. moaning, screaming)

Intensity during rating period

0. Not present
1. Low volume, not disruptive in milieu, including crying
2. Louder than conversational, mildly disruptive, redirectable
3. Loud, disruptive, difficult to redirect
4. Extremely loud screaming or yelling, highly disruptive, unable to redirect

Motor agitation

(pacing, wandering, moving in chair, picking at objects, disrobing, banging on chair, taking others' possessions. Rate 'intrusiveness' by normal social standards, not by effect on other patients in milieu. If 'intrusive' or 'disruptive' due to noise, rate under 'Vocalization'.)

0. Not present
1. Pacing or moving about in chair at normal rate (appears to be seeking comfort, looking for spouse, purposeless movements)
2. Increased rate of movements, mildly intrusive, easily redirectable
3. Rapid movements, moderately intrusive or disruptive, difficult to redirect
4. Intense movements, extremely intrusive or disruptive, not redirectable verbally

Aggressiveness

(score '0' if aggressive only when resisting care)

0. Not present
1. Verbal threats
2. Threatening gestures; no attempt to strike
3. Physical toward property
4. Physical toward self or others

Resisting care

(circle associated activity)
Washing
Dressing
Eating
Meds
Other

0. Not present
1. Procrastination or avoidance
2. Verbal/gesture of refusal
3. Pushing away to avoid task
4. Striking out at caregiver

Were any of the following used during this rating period because of behavior problems?
(Circle interventions used.)

Seclusion
PRN Meds (specify)
Restraint
Other interventions

Reproduced from Rosen J, Burgio L, Kollar M, Cain M, Allison M, Fogleman M, Michael M, Zubenko GS (1994) The Pittsburg Agitation Scale: a user-friendly instrument for rating agitation in dementia patients. *American Journal of Geriatric Psychiatry* **2**: 52–9, with permission.

Dysfunctional Behaviour Rating Instrument (DBRI)

Reference: **Molloy DW, McIlroy WE, Guyatt GH, Lever JA (1991) Validity and reliability of the Dysfunctional Behaviour Rating Instrument.** *Acta Psychiatrica Scandinavica* 84: 103–6

Time taken 10–15 minutes (reviewer's estimate)

Rating by nurse observer

Main indications

Rating of behaviour in community-living elderly people.

Commentary

The Dysfunctional Behaviour Rating Instrument (DBRI) was developed as a short, simple, comprehensive instrument to be completed by the caregiver which measures the frequency of, and caregiver's responses to, a range of behaviours found in elderly people with cognitive impairment. The specific goal was to assess the effect of behavioural disturbances on carers of patients suffering from dementia. Some 240 consecutive referrals were assessed in addition to the DBRI, the Mini-Mental State Examination (MMSE; page 36) and the Lawton and Brody Instrumental Activities of Daily Living Scale (IADL; page 186). The scale consists of 25 questions rated on a six-point scale. Inter-rater reliability was assessed using a subgroup of 35 subjects and caregivers who were assessed three times at three week intervals. Construct validity of the DBRI was assessed by comparing it with the BPC, the Standardized MMSE (page 40) and the IADL Scale. The intraclass correlation coefficient for intra-observer reliability of DBRI was 0.75. Validity was shown by early significant correlation between the DBRI items and the BPC items. Significant negative correlations were found between the MMSE and the DBRI.

Additional reference

Molloy DW, Bédard M, Guyatt GH, Lever J (1996) Dysfunctional Behavior Rating Instrument. *International Psychogeriatrics* **8** (suppl 3): 333–41.

Address for correspondence

DW Molloy
Henderson General Hospital
711 Concession Street
Hamilton
Ontario L8V 1C3
Canada

Dysfunctional Behaviour Rating Instrument (DBRI)

1. Ask same questions over and over
2. Repeats stories over and over
3. Refused to cooperate
4. Became angry
5. Was withdrawn (did not speak or do anything unless he/she was asked)
6. Was demanding
7. Was afraid to be left alone
8. Was aggressive
9. Was hiding things
10. Was suspicious
11. Had temper outbusts
12. Had delusions, i.e. thought that:
    Spouse was 'not my wife/husband'
    Home was 'not my home'
    There were 'people in the house'
    That 'people were stealing things'
    Other:
13. Hallucinations:
    Saw things that were not there
    Heard things or people that were not there
    Other:
14. Was agitated, e.g. pacing
15. Was crying
16. Was frustrated
17. Wandered, got lost in house, property or elsewhere
18. Was up at night
19. Wanted to leave
20. Kept changing mind
21. Embarrassing behaviour in public
22. Are there any other behaviours not mentioned above that [patient's name] had?

If yes, how often does this occur?
Rating: 0 = never; 1 = about every 2 weeks; 2 = about 1 × week; 3 = > 1 × week; 4 = at least 1 × day; 5 = > 5 × a day;
Then – how much of a problem is this?
Rating: 0 = No problem; 1 = Very little problem; 2 = Little problem; 3 = Somewhat of a problem; 4 = Moderate problem; 5 = Great deal of a problem

---

Irritability, Aggression and Apathy Scale

Reference: **Burns A, Folstein S, Brandt J, Folstein M (1990) Clinical assessment of irritability, aggression and apathy in Huntington and Alzheimer's Disease.** *Journal of Nervous and Mental Disease* **178: 20–6**

Time taken 10 minutes

Rating by semi-structured interview with informant

Main indications

The scale is designed to measure non-cognitive features of irritability and apathy in dementia.

Commentary

The Irritability, Aggression and Apathy scale incorporated the Yudofsky Aggression Scale in conjunction with questions relating to irritability and pathy. It was validated on 31 patients with Alzheimer's disease and 26 with Huntington's disease. Inter-rater reliability was over 0.85, scores correlated with those on the Psychogeriatric Dependency Rating Scales (PGDRS; page 243) and were significantly greater than controls.

Additional references

Yudofsky SC, Silver JM, Jackson W et al (1986) The Overt Aggression Scale for the objective rating of verbal and physical aggression. *American Journal of Psychiatry* **143** 35–39.

Address for correspondence

Professor Alistair Burns
University of Manchester
School of Psychiatry and Behavioural Sciences
Education and Research Centre
Wythenshawe Hospital
Manchester M23 9LT
UK

e-mail: a_burns@man.ac.uk

Irritability, Aggression and Apathy Scale

Please answer the following questions about your ＿＿＿ according to how he/she is not, compared with how he/she was before his/her health problems began. (It may be necessary to emphasize that the questionnaire relates to behaviour since the onset of illness and not in the very recent past. An open-ended question such as 'what effect has your ＿＿＿ illness had on him/her' may be used.)

Irritability

1. How irritable would you say he/she was?   Score

    1   2   3   4   5

    not at all   extremely   ＿＿＿
    irritable   irritable

		Never (score = 1)	Sometimes (score = 2)	Always (score = 3)
2.	Does he/she sulk after he/she is angry?	＿＿＿	＿＿＿	＿＿＿
3.	Does he/she 'pout' if he/she does not get his/her own way?	＿＿＿	＿＿＿	＿＿＿
4.	Does he/she get into arguments?	＿＿＿	＿＿＿	＿＿＿
5.	Does he/she raise his/her voice in anger?	＿＿＿		＿＿＿
			Total score	＿＿＿

(maximum = 17)

Apathy

1. Has his/her interest in everyday events changed?   Score

    1   2   3   4   5

    much more   just the   much less
    interested   same   interested   ＿＿＿

2. How long does he/she stay lying in bed or sitting in a chair doing nothing during the day?

    1   2   3   4   5

    no more than   all the
    anyone else   time   ＿＿＿

3. How active is he/she in day to day activities?

    1   2   3   4   5

    very active   normal   very inactive   ＿＿＿

4. How busy does he/she keep him/herself?

    1   2   3   4   5

    same   less so   prefers doing   prefers   if left
    hobbies   but still   nothing but   watching TV   alone does
    as   has   does with   or watches   nothing
    usual   hobbies   prompting   others doing
                                                                      things   ＿＿＿

5. Does the patient seem withdrawn from things?

    1   2   3   4   5

    not at   a little   more than   much more   yes,
    all   more than   usual   than   definitely
                          usual   usual   ＿＿＿

                                                                      Total score   ＿＿＿
                                                                      (maximum = 25)

Reproduced from Burns A, Folstein S, Brandt J, Folstein M (1990) Clinical assessment of irritability, aggression and apathy in Huntington and Alzheimer's Disease. *Journal of Nervous and Mental Disease*, Vol. 178, no. 1, pp. 20–6.

Apathy Scale for Parkinson's Disease

Reference: **Starkstein SE, Mayberg HS, Preziosi TJ, Andrezejewski P, Leiguarda R, Robinson RG (1992) Reliability, validity and clinical correlates of apathy in Parkinson's disease.** *Journal of Neuropsychiatry and Neurosciences* **4: 134–9**

Time taken 5–10 minutes (reviewer's estimate)

Rating by clinician during interview with patient

Main indications

Assessment of apathy in patients with Parkinson's disease.

Commentary

This scale is an abridged version of a larger scale (Marin, 1990). The scale consists of 14 items rated on a three-point scale. The total score possible is 42; the higher the score the greater the apathy. Inter-rater and test/retest reliability (Spearman correlation) was above 0.80 and internal consistency, as demonstrated by Cronbach's alpha, was 0.76. Validity was assessed by asking a clinician to rate apathy independently, and whilst there did not seem to be an association between apathy and depression, apathy was associated with deficits of verbal memory and time-dependent tasks. A number of neuropsychological tests confirmed the validity of the scale and there seems no reason why the scale (properly validated) could not be used to assess apathy in other conditions.

Additional reference

Marin R (1990) Differential diagnosis and classification of apathy. *American Journal of Psychiatry* **147**: 22–30.

Address for correspondence

Dr S Starkstein
School of Psychiatry and Clinical Neurosciences
University of Western Australia
Queen Elizabeth II Medical Centre (SCGH)
Nedlands, Perth, WA 6009
Australia

e-mail: quistar@infovia.com.au

Apathy Scale for Parkinson's Disease

1. Are you interested in learning new things?
2. Does anything interest you?
3. Are you concerned about your condition?
4. Do you put much effort into things?
5. Are you always looking for something to do?
6. Do you have plans and goals for the future?
7. Do you have motivation?
8. Do you have the energy for daily activities?
9. Does someone have to tell you what to do each day?
10. Are you indifferent to things?
11. Are you unconcerned with many things?
12. Do you need a push to get started on things?
13. Are you neither happy nor sad, just in between?
14. Would you consider yourself apathetic?

Scoring:

Questions 1–8:   3 points = not at all; 2 points = slightly; 1 point = some; 0 point = a lot

Questions 9–14:   3 points = a lot; 2 points = some; 1 point = slightly; 0 point = not at all

Scores range from 0 to 42
Higher scores indicate more severe apathy

Reproduced from Starkstein SE, Mayberg HS, Preziosi TJ, Andrezejewski P, Leiguarda R, Robinson RG (1992) Reliability, validity and clinical correlates of apathy in Parkinson's disease. *Journal of Neuropsychiatry and Neurosciences* **4**: 134–9, with permission.

BEAM-D

Reference: **Sinha D, Zemlan FP, Nelson S, Bienenfeld D, Thienhaus O, Ramaswamy G, Hamilton S (1992) A new scale for assessing behavioral agitation in dementia.** *Psychiatry Research* **41: 73–88**

Time taken 20 minutes (reviewer's estimate)

Rating by trained raters

Main indications

To assess the effects of treatment on behavioural problems of inpatients with dementia.

Commentary

Approximately 45 patients with a diagnosis of primary degenerative dementia were assessed. The BEAM-D scale consists of 16 items – target behaviour and inferred states.

Inter-rater reliabilities ranged from 0.70 to 1.0, with individual kappa statistics varying from 0.56 to 1.0.
Concurrent validity was assessed using the Brief Psychiatric Rating Scale (BPRS; page 272) and the Sandoz Clinical Assessment – Geriatric (SCAG; page 253).

Address for correspondence

FP Zemlan
Alzheimer's Research Center
University of Cincinnati
College of Medicine
Cincinnati
OH 45267–0559
USA

BEAM-D

Target behaviors

1. Hostility/aggression
Verbal and nonverbal expressions of anger and resentment
0 = No information; not assessed; unable to assess.
1 = Patient has neither expressed nor manifested any hostile/aggressive behavior.
2 = Patient has openly expressed verbally aggressive/hostile behavior – at least one to two separate instances.
3 = Patient has been overtly aggressive at least one to two separate instances; physically assaultive behavior may be manifested.
4 = Patient has been overtly aggressive – at least three or more separate instances; physically assaultive behavior may be manifested.

2. Destruction of property (belonging to self or others)
Extent to which the patient willfully damages, or causes destruction of property.
0 = No information; not assessed; unable to assess.
1 = Patient has not damaged personal or others' property.
2 = At least one or two separate instances.
3 = At least three or four separate instances.
4 = Continuously engaged in destructive activities.

3. Disruption of others' activities
Extent to which the patient disrupts the activities of others.
0 = No information; not assessed; unable to assess.
1 = Patient has not interrupted the activities of others at any time.
2 = 3 or fewer instances.
3 = 4 or more instances.
4 = Continuously disruptive to others.

4. Uncooperativeness
Extent to which the patient is responsive and receptive to the feelings and needs of others.
0 = No information; not assessed; unable to assess.
1 = Rarely exhibits inconsiderate, discourteous behavior.
2 = Generally unconcerned about the needs and feelings of others.
3 = Inconsiderate of and unconcerned about the needs and feelings of others; neither cooperativeness nor courtesy; patient's presence is still tolerated by others.
4 = Consistently inconsiderate of and unconcerned about the needs and feelings of others; patient's presence is infrequently tolerated by others.

5. Noncompliance
0 = No information; not assessed; unable to assess.
1 = Patient has been responsive to requests made of him/her.
2 = Several occasions been noncompliant.
3 = Frequently noncompliant with requests.
4 = Consistently noncompliant with requests.

6. Attention-seeking behavior
0 = No information; not assessed; unable to assess.
1 = Patient has not exhibited attention-seeking behavior.
2 = Occasionally exhibited attention-seeking behavior.
3 = Frequently exhibited attention-seeking behavior.
4 = Continuously exhibited attention-seeking behavior. This occurs several times per day.

7. Sexually inappropriate behavior
0 = No information; not assessed; unable to assess.
1 = No sexually inappropriate behavior observed.
2 = Patient observed to touch, kiss, hug others in socially inappropriate settings.
3 = Patient occasionally exposes himself/herself.
4 = Patient frequently (tries to) expose(s) self and masturbate(s).

8. Wandering
0 = No information; not assessed; unable to assess.
1 = Patient has not wandered from designated area.
2 = Patient has on at least 1 to 2 instances wandered from designated area.
3 = Patient has on at least 3 to 4 instances wandered from designated area.
4 = Patient has wandered on several (numerous) occasions. Patient may be restrained for this behavior.

9. Hoarding behavior
0 = No information; not assessed; unable to assess.
1 = Patient has not shown any hoarding behavior.
2 = Patient has occasionally collected/hidden objects.
3 = Patient has regularly collected/hidden objects.
4 = Patient has constantly engaged in hoarding behavior.

Inferred states
1. Depression
2. Delusions
3. Hallucinations
4. Anxiety
5. Appropriateness/stability of affect
6. Increased/decreased appetite
7. Sleep

Insomnia – Early
0 = No information; not assessed; unable to assess.
1 = No difficulty falling asleep.
2 = Complains of occasional difficulty falling asleep – i.e. more than ½ hour.
3 = Complains of nightly difficulty falling asleep.

Insomnia – Middle
0 = No information; not assessed; unable to assess.
1 = No difficulty.
2 = Patient complains of being restless and disturbed during the night.
3 = Waking during the night – any getting out of bed rated 2 (except for purposes of voiding).

Insomnia – Late
0 = No information; not assessed; unable to assess.
1 = No difficulty.
2 = Waking in early hours of the morning but goes back to sleep.
3 = Unable to fall asleep again if he gets out of bed.

Rating:
Scales 1–9:
0 = No information, not able/not assessed; 1 = None; 2 = Mild; 3 = Moderate; 4 = Severe

Reprinted from *Psychiatry Research*, 41, Sinha D et al, A new scale for assessing behavioural agitation in dementia, 73–88, © 1992, with permission from Elsevier Science.

Clinical Rating Scale for Symptoms of Psychosis in Alzheimer's Disease (SPAD)

Reference: **Reisberg B, Ferris SH (1985) A clinical rating scale for symptoms of psychosis in Alzheimer's disease.** *Psychopharmacology Bulletin* 21: 101–4

Time taken 10 minutes (reviewer's estimate)

Rating by clinician on the basis of a caregiver report

Main indications

Assessment of psychotic features in patients with Alzheimer's disease.

Commentary

The Clinical Rating Scale for Symptoms of Psychosis in Alzheimer's Disease (SPAD) represents the precursor of the BEHAVE-AD (page 125). It consists of nine questions regarding psychiatric symptoms and rated on a three-point scale of frequency. The stimulus for development appears to have been the lack of measures to assess changes in behavioural disturbances in dementia, only one example of which had been found in the literature (Barnes et al, 1982).

Additional reference

Barnes R, Veith R, Okimoto J et al (1982) Efficacy of antipsychotic medications in behaviorally disturbed dementia patients. *American Journal of Psychiatry* **139**: 1170–4.

Address for correspondence

Barry Reisberg
Department of Psychiatry
Ageing and Dementia Research Center
NYU Medical Center
550 First Avenue
New York 10016
USA

e-mail: barry.reisberg@med.nyu.edu

Clinical Rating Scale for Symptoms of Psychosis in Alzheimer's Disease (SPAD)

	Score *Symptomatology*	*Not present* *0*	*Mild* *1*	*Moderate* *2*	*Severe* *3*
I.	'People are stealing things'	☐ Not present	☐ Delusion that people are hiding objects	☐ Delusion that people are coming into the home and hiding or stealing objects	☐ Talking and listening to people coming into the home
II.	'One's house is not one's home'	☐ Not present	☐ Conviction that the place in which one is residing is not one's home (e.g. packing to go home)	☐ Attempt to leave domiciliary to go home	☐ Violence in response to attempts to forcibly restrict exit
III.	'Spouse (or other caregiver) is an imposter'	☐ Not present	☐ Conviction that spouse (or other caregiver) is an imposter	☐ Anger toward spouse (or other caregiver) for being an imposter	☐ Violence toward spouse (or other caregiver) for being an imposter
IV.	'Delusion of abandonment' (e.g. to an institution)	☐ Not present	☐ Suspicion of caregiver plotting abandonment or institutionalization (e.g. on telephone)	☐ Accusation of a conspiracy to abandon or institutionalize	☐ Accusation of impending or immediate desertion or institutionalization
V.	Cognitive abulia (purposeless activity)	☐ Not present	☐ Repetitive purposeless activity (e.g. packing and unpacking clothing; repeatedly putting on and removing clothing; insistent repeating of demands or questions)	☐ Pacing	☐ Abrading
VI.	Day/night disturbance	☐ Not present	☐ Repetitive wakenings during night	☐ 50 to 75% of former sleep cycle at night	☐ Complete disturbance of diurnal rhythm (i.e. less than 50% of former sleep cycle at night)
VII.	Visual hallucinatory experiences	☐ Not present	☐ Occasional (less than 5 in preceding 6-month period) episodes noted	☐ Frequent (more than 5 in preceding 6-month period), definite (clearly defined hallucinations of objects or persons noted) episodes	☐ Daily (or more frequent) hallucinatory experiences (minimum of 3 consecutive days)
VIII.	Auditory hallucinatory experiences	☐ Not present	☐ Occasional (less than 5 in preceding 6-month period) episodes noted	☐ Frequent (more than 5 in preceding 6-month period), definite (clearly defined hallucinations of words or phrases noted) episodes	☐ Daily (or more frequent) hallucinatory experiences (minimum of 3 consecutive days)
IX.	Other behavioral symptoms which may respond to neuroleptics (specify all that apply and total severity rating)	☐	☐	☐	☐

*General criteria for scoring:
(a)   To be scored by clinician on the basis of primary caregivers' experiences;
(b)   Information may be obtained from more than one primary caregiver with respect to the presence of each symptom;
(c)   Score '0' if a symptom is not present;
      Score '1' if symptom is present and judged to be mild by the primary caregiver;
      Score '2' if symptom is present and judged to be of moderate severity by the primary caregiver;
      Score '3' if symptom is present and judged to be severe by the primary caregiver.

Georagsobber Vatieschaal voor de Intramurale Psychogeriatrie (GIP)

Reference: **Verstraten PFJ (1988) The GIP: an observational ward behavior scale.** *Psychopharmacology Bulletin* **24: 717–19**

Time taken 10 minutes (reviewer's estimate)

Rating by ward staff

Main indications

Assessment of behaviour in psychogeriatric inpatients.

Commentary

The Georagsobber Vatieschaal voor de Intramurale Psychogeriatrie (GIP) reports four separate behaviour subtypes: social; cognitive; psychomotor; and affective. This has been expanded to a total of 14 selected scales, and in total the GIP contains 82 items with an average of about six items in each scale. Patients are rated on each item on a 4-point scale indicating the frequency of the behaviour stated in that item during the last two weeks. The scale was validated on 567 patients from psychogeriatric hospital wards, nursing home residents and day care visitors. Inter-rater reliability (correlation coefficiency) ranged from 0.53 to 0.90. Interval consistency was greater than 0.75.

Address for correspondence

Peter FJ Verstraten
Stationsstraat 36
5451 AN Mill
The Netherlands

Georagsobber Vatieschaal voor de Intramurale Psychogeriatrie (GIP)

- social behavior types:
  1. nonsocial behavior;
  2. apathetic behavior;
  3. distorted consciousness;
  4. loss of decorum; and
  5. rebellious behavior

- cognitive behavior types:
  6. incoherent behavior
  7. distorted memory; and
  8. disoriented behavior;

- psychomotor behavior types:
  9. senseless repetitive behavior; and
  10. restless behavior;

- emotional or affective behavior types:
  11. suspicious behavior;
  12. melancholic or sorrowful behavior;
  13. dependent behavior; and
  14. anxious behavior.

Rated on a 4-point scale: never – always/often/continuously

Reproduced from Verstraten PFJ (1988) The GIP: an observational ward behavior scale. *Psychopharmacology Bulletin* **24**: 717–19.

Nursing Home Behavior Problem Scale (NHBPS)

Reference: **Ray WA, Taylor JOA, Lichtenstein MJ and Meador KG (1992) The Nursing Home Behavior Problem Scale.** *Journal of Gerontology* 47: M9–16.

Time taken 3–5 minutes

Rating by nurse or nursing assistant who knows the patient

Main indications

The measurement of specific behaviour problems in the nursing home setting which are so disruptive as to lead to the use of medications or physical restraint.

Commentary

The Nursing Home Behavior Problem Scale (NHBPS) is a 29 item scale based on existing scales, omitting some passive behaviours and including others which specifically call for the prescription of medication. The study reported on 500 residents in 2 nursing home populations. Six subscales were described – uncooperative/aggressive, irrational/restless, sleep problems, annoying behaviour, inappropriate behaviour and dangerous behaviour. Validation was with the Nurses' Observation Scale for Inpatient Evaluation (NOSIE; page 150) and the Cohen-Mansfield Agitation Inventory (CMAI; page 159). Correlations with these scales were –0.747 and +0.911 respectively. Inter-rater reliability for the subscales ranged from 0.467 for dangerous behaviour to 0.768 for sleep problems.

Address for correspondence

Wayne A Ray
Department of Preventive Medicine and
Department of Psychiatry
Vanderbilt University School of Medicine
Nashville, TN
USA

Nursing Home Behavior Problem Scale (NHBPS)

DIRECTIONS
Please rate this resident's behavior during the last 3 days only.
Indicate your choice by circling a number for each item, using this key:

0 = Never 1 = Sometimes 2 = Often 3 = Usually 4 = Always

Resists care
Becomes upset or loses temper easily
Enters others' rooms inappropriately
Awakens during the night
Talks. mutters, or mumbles to herself
Tries to hurt herself
Refuses care
Fights or is physically aggressive: hits, slaps, kicks, bites, spits, pushes, pulls
Fidgets. Is unable to sit still, restless
Has difficulty falling asleep
Goes to the bathroom in inappropriate places (not incontinence)

Says things that do not make sense
Damages or destroys things on purpose
Screams, yells, or moans loudly
Argues, threatens, or curses
Tries to get in or out of wheelchair, bed, or chair unsafely
Asks or complains about her health, even though it is unjustified
Has inappropriate sexual behavior
Sees or hears things that are not there
Disturbs others during the night
Wanders, tries to escape or go to off-limits places
Accuses others of things that are not true
Asks for attention or help, even though it is not needed
Is uncooperative
Paces: walks or moves in wheelchair aimlessly back and forth
Tries to escape physical restraints
Complains or whines
Does something over and over, even though it doesn't make sense
Tries to do things that are dangerous

The California Dementia Behavior Questionnaire Caregiver and Clinical Assessment of Behavioral Disturbances

Reference: **Victoroff J, NielsonK, Mungas D (1997) Caregiver and Clinical Assessment of Behavioral Disturbances: the California Dementia Behavior Questionnaire.** *International Psychogeriatrics* **9: 155–74**

Time taken estimated 20–30 minutes

Rater caregiver completed with minimal prompts

Main indications

A comprehensive caregiver–rater questionnaire for non-cognitive behavioural disturbances in dementia.

Commentary

A three-part instrument consisting of:

(a) A 62-item questionnaire rating behaviours by frequency on a four-step Likart-type scale of degree of frequency for each behaviour
(b) A 19-item section rating mood and emotion on a three-step scale of severity

(c) A six-item section for caregiver ratings of their own stress and depressive symptoms.

Caregivers showed good test/retest reliability for ratings of all types of patient behavioural disturbance. Caregiver inter-rater reliability was highest for depression and lowest for psychosis. The correlation between caregiver reports and professional assessments was highest for agitation, intermediate for psychosis and lowest for depression.

Address for correspondence

Jeff Victoroff MD
Department of Neurology
University of Southern California School of Medicine
Rancho Los Amigos Medical Center
7601 E Imperial Highway
Dwoney
CA 90242
USA

Harmful Behaviours Scale

References: **Draper B, Brodaty H, Low Lee-Fay, Richards U, Paton H, Lie D (2002) Self-destructive behaviours in nursing home residents.** *Journal of the American Geriatrics Society* **50: 354–8**

Draper B, Brodaty H, Low Lee-Fay (2002) Types of nursing home residents with self-destructive behaviours: analysis of the Harmful Behaviours Scales. *International Journal of Geriatric Psychiatry* **17: 670–5**

Time taken 10–15 minutes (reviewer's estimate)

Main indications

To evaluate self-destructive behaviour in nursing home residents.

Commentary

The Harmful Behaviours Scale assess direct and indirect self-destructive behaviours in nursing home residents. In the original study, 61% of 610 residents in 11 nursing homes in Australia had indirect harmful behaviours occurring at least once a week with direct behaviours occurring in 14% of subjects over the same interval. The HBS was significantly correlated with the BEHAVE-AD and was associated with a score on the Hamilton 'suicide' item. Younger patients, those with a diagnosis of dementia, and those who are more functionally impaired had higher scores.

Draper et al (2002) carried out a latent class analysis of the scale and identified groups of residents – aggressive resistant (35%), food refusal (27%), behaviourally disturbed (5%) and asymptomatic (33%).

Address for correspondence

Dr B Draper
Academic Department for Old Age Psychiatry
Prince of Wales Hospital
Randwick, 2031
NSW
Australia
b.draper@unsw.edu.au

The Challenging Behaviour Scale (CBS)

Reference: **Moniz-Cook E, Woods R, Gardiner E, Silver M, Agar S (2001) The Challenging Behaviour Scale (CBS): development of a scale for staff caring for older people in residential and nursing homes.** *British Journal of Clinical Psychology* **40: 309–22**

Time taken 5–7 minutes (if you know the patient)

Rating by staff on interview

Main indications

The scale was developed to measure challenging behaviour in residential nursing home settings.

Commentary

The scale is a staff report of behaviour that they consider to be challenging. Challenging behaviours that are measured using this scale are physical aggression (pushing, grabbing, hitting, kicking, spitting), verbal aggression and noise-making (swearing, shouting, screaming), wandering, urinating in public, stripping, inappropriate sexual behaviour and deviant behaviour in keeping with dementia (perseveration, delusions, hallucinations and underactive talking).

The CBS should be completed by a member of staff, usually a key worker who is familiar with the resident.

There are four measures on the scale, three of which are rated by the staff, and the fourth is a calculated score.

First the staff indicate whether the resident has displayed such behaviour in the past 8 weeks. If the behaviour is present, the frequency is rated on a scale of 1–4:1 indicating occasionally present, less than once per month, 4 indicating present on a daily basis. Severity of the behaviour on a scale of 1–4 is also measured, 1 being minimal management difficulty, 4 being extreme management difficulty. The fourth measure is the total level of challenge and is calculated as a sum of the products of frequency and difficulty reading for each behavioural item on the scale. There are 35 items on the scale. The CBS has good internal consistency, test/retest and inter-rater reliability.

Address for correspondence

Esme Moniz-Cook
Senior Lecturer in Psychology
c/o Coltman Street Day Hospital
39–41 Coltman Street
Hull HU3 2SG
UK

Behavioural Activities in Demented Geriatric Patients

Reference: Ferm L (1974) Behavioural Activities in Demented Geriatric Patients. *Gerontology Clinics* 16: 185–94

Time taken 10 minutes (reviewer's estimate)

Main indications

The assessment of behavioural disturbances in older patients with dementia.

Commentary

Ferm (1974) described the application of the scale in 136 patients from long-stay old age psychiatry wards. The rationale of the original investigation was to explore the relationship between behavioural disturbances, the stage of dementia and psychometric tests. Subjects were evaluated on a six-point rating scale (scores 1–6) and short, precise instructions for screening evaluation were given for every variable. In the several areas of performance the scale values were defined as follows:

1. Completely independent and adequate performance
2. Uncertain performance
3. Partial performance, requiring control and slight help
4. Partial performance requiring control and considerable help
5. Little spontaneity, requiring virtually constant help
6. Complete care necessary.

In participation and hobbies, ascending scale values denoted a declining level of activity, score 1 showing great activity and score 6 a complete lack of activity. In evaluating sleep behaviour, the medication used was taken into account. Scale values 1–3 indicated good sleeping ability, score 1 indicating ability to sleep without sleep-inducing drugs, score 2 with temporary use of such drugs, and score 3 with constant use of average doses of usual sedatives, whereas the scale values 4–6 were used to indicate increasing disturbance of sleep in spite of increasing doses of drugs. In evaluating quietness, by contrast, medication was not taken into consideration, score 1 indicating constant quietness and score 6 constant disturbed behaviour, irrespective of the use of tranquillizers.

Forty-seven per cent of the group had severe dementia (described as 'grave'), 30% had moderate and 20% had mild dementia. Generally speaking, behavioural disturbances were more severe in people with more advanced disease. The authors were able to show that in the course of dementia independent hobbies are lost first, loss of ability to wash and dress second, orientation, recognition of others and communication disappeared after that, and the ability to walk and eat were the longest-preserved functions. Sleep and 'quietness' were independent of the degree of dementia.

Although this is a very early paper, the study does show the value of simply observing people with dementia. The study has been used recently in trials of memantine.

Additional reference

Winblad B, Poritis N (1999) Memantine in severe dementia: result of the 9M-Best Study (benefit and efficacy in severely demented patients during treatment with memantine). *International Journal of Geriatric Psychiatry* 14: 135–46.

Address for correspondence

Dr Liisa Ferm
Koskela Geriatric Hospital
Helsinki
Finland

Behavioural Activities in Demented Geriatric Patients

Field of behaviour	Scale of evaluation					
	1	2	3	4	5	6
Ability to move						
Ability to wash						
Ability to dress						
Ability to eat						
Control of the bladder						
Control of the bowels						
Ability to communicate						
Orientation in space						
Recognition of persons						
Participation						
Hobbies						
Sleep						
Quietness						

Behavior Rating Scale for Dementia (BRSD)

Reference: **Mack JL, Patterson MB, Tariot PN (1999) Behavior Rating Scale for Dementia: development of test scales and presentation of data for 555 individuals with Alzheimer's disease.** *Journal of Geriatric Psychiatry and Neurology* **12: 211–23**

Time taken approximately 25 minutes

Rating by carer/informant interview

Main indications

The Behavior Rating Scale for Dementia (BRSD) was designed to measure the extent and severity of behavioral pathology in people with dementia

Commentary

The scale consists of 48 items concerned with the presence or absence of specific behaviours. Information is obtained during an interview with a relative or informant. The BRSD items are scaled by frequency as 0–4, with 0 indicating only 1–2 days in the past month and 4 indicat-ing 16 or more days in the past month. Severity is rated on 11 items by the inclusion of a probe which is administered when the items receive a rating of 1–4.

Factor analysis of BRSD identifies six factors, and six subscales have been developed: depressive symptoms, inertia, vegetative symptoms, irritability/aggression, behavioural dysregulation and psychotic symptoms. The instructions for scoring are included in a BRSD manual.

Address for correspondence

Dr James L Mack
Department of Neurology
University Hospitals of Cleveland
1110 Euclid Avenue
Cleveland
OH 44106-5040
USA

Appendix: Behavior Rating Scale for Dementia (BRSD)

Item number 1996	Item number 1992	Item content	Subjects rated present (%)	Correlation with MMSE total*
1	1	Feelings of anxiety	36.4	0.09
2	2	Physical signs of anxiety	48.1	−0.14
3	3	Sad appearance	53.7	
4	4	Feelings of hopelessness	28.1	
5	5	Crying	38.0	
6	6	Feelings of guilt	7.4	
7	7	Poor self-esteem	25.2	
8	8	Feels life is not worth living	16.6	
9	10	Loss of enjoyment	52.6	
10	11	Loss of initiative	57.1	0.13
11	12	Tiredness	55.9	
12	14	Change in sleeping pattern	51.5	−0.18
13	15	Trouble falling asleep	27.2	−0.11
14	16	Change in appetite	33.7	
15	17	Change in weight	31.0	−0.10
16	13	Excessive physical complaints	11.0	
17	18	Change in sexual interest	30.3	−0.17
18	19	Sudden changes in emotion	13.3	−0.17
19	20	Agitation	65.6	
20	28	Irritability	55.1	
21	29	Uncooperativeness	44.9	−0.17
22	30	Verbal aggression	17.8	−0.13
23	31	Physical aggression	13.7	−0.22
24	21	Restlessness	46.8	−0.30
25	22	Purposeless behaviour	60.4	−0.10
26	24	Diurnal confusion	46.5	−0.11
27	26	Wandering	14.1	−0.23
28	27	Trying to leave home	9.7	−0.10
29	25	Socially inappropriate behaviour	20.0	−0.09
30	23	Repetitive behaviour	64.1	0.34
31	33	Social withdrawal	34.1	−0.09
32	34	Clingy, dependent behaviour	51.0	
33	43	Misidentification of people	23.1	−0.19
34	44	Doesn't recognize self in mirror	7.9	−0.24
35	45	Misidentification of things	12.8	−0.19
36	35	Feeling threatened, suspicious	20.2	
37	36	Belief that spouse is unfaithful	6.1	
38	37	Belief that one is being abandoned	7.9	−0.10
39	38	Beflief that spouse is imposter	4.9	
40	39	Belief that TV characters are real	12.6	−0.21
41	40	Belief that people are in house	23.2	−0.19
42	41	Belief that dead person is still alive	23.4	−0.19
43	42	Belief that house is not home	19.8	−0.16
44	46	Auditory hallucinations	11.5	−0.17
45	47	Visual hallucinations	15.5	−0.22
46	48	Nonspecific item	11.5	

*Pearson product-moment correlations with significance of $p < 0.05$ or better.

Source: Mack JL et al. J Geriatr Psychiatry Neurol 1999; **12**: 211–23. Reproduced by permission from BC Decker Inc.

Resistiveness to Care Scale (RTC-DAT)

Reference: **Mahoney EK, Hurley AC, Volicer L, Bell M, Gianotis P, Hartshorn M, Lane P, Lesperance R, MacDonald S, Novakoff L, Rheaume Y, Timms R, Warden V (1999) Development and testing of the Resistiveness to Care Scale.** *Research in Nursing and Health* **22: 27–38**

Time taken 5 minutes of observation

Rating by trained observer after 5 minutes' observation

Main indications

This scale measures resistive behaviour in individuals with Alzheimer's disease.

Commentary

The RTC-DAT has 13 items. Scoring procedures and methods are described for rating videos or conducting clinical observations of resistiveness to particular activities of daily living. The period of observation for any particular ADL is 5 minutes. The items are rated as present or absent.

Address for correspondence

Ellen K Mahoney
Boston College School of Nursing
Cushing Hall 116
140 Commonwealth Avenue
Chestnut Hill
MA 01267-3812
USA

Resistiveness to Care Scale

Behaviour

Push away
Gegenhalten
Grab person
Pull away
Turn away
Scream
Threaten
Say no
Cry
Clench
Adduct
Hit/kick
Grab object
Eigenvalue
Percent variance

The Agitated Behavior in Dementia Scale

Reference: Logsdon RG, Teri L, Weiner MF, Gibbons LE, Raskind M, Peskind E, Grundman M, Koss E, Thomas RG, Thal LJ and members of the Alzheimer's Disease Cooperative Study (1999) Assessment of agitation in Alzheimer's disease: the agitated behavior in dementia scale. *Journal of the American Geriatrics Society* 47: 1354–8

Time taken 15 minutes

Rating by caregiver

Main indications

A measure of agitation in an outpatient sample of patients with mild to moderate Alzheimer's disease.

Commentary

The ABID consists of a 16-item questionnaire designed specifically to evaluate the frequency of and the caregiver's reaction to common agitated behaviours in patients with dementia. It was designed to provide a sensitive objective assessment of observable behaviours, evaluating the frequency of occurrence of agitated behaviour during two 1-week intervals. Also provides an assessment of the caregiver's level of distress about each behaviour.

Caregivers rated each behaviour according to frequency of occurrence during each of the 2 weeks immediately before the assessment on a scale of 0–3: 0 = did not occur during the week; 1 = occurred once or twice during the week; 2 = occurred three to six times in the week; 3 = occurred daily or more often. Reliability of results showed internal consistency of 0.7 and test/retest reliability of 0.6–0.73. Validity was confirmed by correlations with related measures and lack of correlation with unrelated constructs.

Address for correspondence

Dr Rebecca G Logsdon
Box 357263
University of Washington
Seattle
WA 98195-7263
USA

e-mail: logsdon@u.washington.edu

Rating Anxiety in Dementia (RAID)

Reference **Shankar KK, Walker M, Frost D, Orrell MW (1999) The development of a valid and reliable scale for rating anxiety in dementia (RAID).** *Aging and Mental Health* **3: 39–49**

Time taken 5–10 minutes

Rating by experienced interviewer

Main indications

To measure anxiety in patients suffering from dementia.

Commentary

The instrument was developed based on the author's previous work in this field in an attempt to develop an instrument measuring anxiety symptoms in people suffering from dementia. The absence of any specific instrument to assess these symptoms, and using the corollary of the Cornell Scale for Depression in Dementia, was the stimulus for developing the instrument. The items were derived from general concepts of anxiety and rated according to the person's symptoms and signs of anxiety over the previous 2 weeks. Six subgroups were described: worry, apprehension, vigilance, motor tension, autonomic hyperactivity, phobias and panic attacks. Criterion validity and construct validity were assessed. The instrument was piloted on 51 inpatients and 32 day hospital patients who had a DSM-IV diagnosis of dementia. Anxiety scores were not related to sex, age, where the person lived or the type of dementia, but were associated with physical illness and the preservation of insight. Inter-rater reliability and test/retest reliability were moderate, with an overall agreement of over 80% for individual items. The scale correlated significantly with other anxiety scales and with independent ratings.

Address for correspondence

Dr Martin Orrell
Reader in Psychiatry of Ageing
University College London
Department of Psychiatry
Wolfson Building
48 Riding House Street
London W1N 8AA
UK

e-mail: m.orrell@ucl.ac.uk

Rating Anxiety in Dementia – RAID

Patient's Name: **DOB:**   **Hospital no:**

Rater's Name: **Occupation:**   **Date:**

Patient's status at evaluation:
1. Inpatient. 2. Outpatient. 3. Day hospital/day centre patient. 4. Other (specify) ....

Scoring system:
U. unable to evaluate. 0. absent. 1. mild or intermittent. 2. moderate. 2. severe
Rating should be based on symptoms and signs occurring during two weeks prior to the interview.
No score should be given if symptoms result from physical disability or illness.
Total score is the sum of items 1 to 18. A score of 11 or more suggests significant clinical anxiety.

Score

Worry	1.	Worry about physical health
	2.	Worry about cognitive performance (failing memory, getting lost when goes out, not able to follow conversation)
	3.	Worry over finances, family problems, physical health of relatives
	4.	Worry associated with false belief and/or perception
	5.	Worry over trifles (repeatedly calling for attention over trivial matters)
Apprehension and vigilance	6.	Frightened and anxious (keyed up and on the edge)
	7.	Sensitivity to noise (exaggerated startle response)
	8.	Sleep disturbance (trouble falling or staying asleep)
	9.	Irritability (more easily annoyed than usual, short tempered and angry outbursts)
Motor tension	10.	Trembling
	11.	Motor tension (complain of headache, other body aches and pains)
	12.	Restlessness (fidgeting, cannot sit still, pacing, wringing hands, picking clothes)
	13.	Fatiguability, tiredness
Autonomic hypersensitivity	14.	Palpitations (complains of heart racing or thumping)
	15.	Dry mouth (not due to medication), sinking feeling in the stomach
	16.	Hyperventilating, shortness of breath (even when not exerting)
	17.	Dizziness or light-headedness (complains as if going to faint)
	18.	Sweating, flushes or chills, tingling or numbness of fingers and toes

Phobias: (fears which are excessive, that do not make sense and tend to avoid – like afraid of crowds, going out alone, being in a small room, or being frightened by some kind of animals, heights, etc.) *Describe*

Panic attacks: (Feelings of anxiety of dread that are so strong that think they are going to die or have a heart attack and they simply have to do something to stop them, like immediately leaving the place, phoning relatives, etc.) *Describe*

Source: Shankar KK *et al. Aging Mental Health* 1999; **3:** 39–49. Reproduced by permission.

Chapter 2c

Activities of daily living

The main use of activities of daily living (ADL) scales is in people with dementia whose functioning is impaired secondarily to cognitive decline. Their use in other conditions is analogous to that in any cognitively impaired older person, with the exception that an individual who is severely depressed or psychotic may not function because of apathy or withdrawal. Activities of daily living can be categorized into two types: basic physical activities such as eating, toileting, washing, walking and dressing (sometimes referred to as physical self maintenance) and instrumental activities, which are more complex tasks including shopping, using the telephone, cooking, housekeeping, self medicating and use of transport. Measurement of function is an essential part of clinical practice and is one of the major outcomes used in the assessment of interventions in dementia. It is also one of the main determinants of people being admitted to long-term care. The development of these types of scales is underscored by the distinction between impairments, functional limitations and disability. Functional disability refers to dependence in basic daily activities taken in the context of a physical and social environment as opposed to problems with work or social interactions. It is the lack of ability to cope within a set environment which renders the person disabled rather than simply impaired.

Scales can be divided into those which are generic or disease-specific and those which are self report, informant or performance (i.e. observer) scales. Generic scales include the Barthel Index, which was originally used in the rehabilitation field and measures functional abilities in older people but has been adapted for and validated for use in people with dementia. It taps more functional items than other scales in that it includes items such as the ability to walk up and down stairs. Criticism of the use of these scales in specific conditions such as dementia revolves round their presumed insensitivity to functional loss resulting from physical impairments, rather than that resulting from and secondary to cognitive deficits. Measures on ADL scores vary between the sexes and between cultures, and so variation in a demented group would not be surprising. However, generic scales tend to have been tested on larger numbers of patients, often in a variety of settings, and reliability and validity are well documented.

Specific instruments used in dementia are mainly observer and performance tests, the latter being particularly labour-intensive, especially if carried out by a trained observer. Depending on the severity of dementia and the setting, it may be important to know which functions are intact in terms of basic daily living tasks or more complex instrumental tasks. The commonest used informant measures are the Blessed Dementia Scale (page 46), the Cleveland Scale for Activities of Daily Living (page 200) and the Functional Assessment Staging (FAST; page 235). The Blessed Dementia Scale has been validated against pathological diagnosis, and includes both ADL and Instrumental Activities of Daily Living (IADL) measures, but nothing on selection of clothing. It was originally validated on an inpatient population, the accompanying Blessed Information–Memory–Concentration Test (page 46) demonstrating this by including the question about identifying people (e.g. a cleaner or nurse on the ward), making it less applicable to someone living at home. The need for measures which span the whole range of cognitive impairments from mild (where IADLs are more affected) to severe (where both ADLs and IADLs are affected) is important, particularly in longitudinal studies over time where patient characteristics would be expected to change with deterioration in their clinical condition. The FAST is an advance in this area, allowing the extremes of cognitive function to be rated. Performance tests have been more recently developed which allow separate analysis of individual aspects of a task, e.g. initiation, sequencing, safety and recognition of completion (Structured Assessment of Individual Living Skills (SALES; page 212)). Attention to physical (gross and fine motor movements) is given priority in some measures (e.g. the Performance Test of Activities of Daily Living (PADL; page 210)), and cognitive aspects of the tests are important. The majority of these tests do correlate with measures of cognitive function, validating their use in tapping disabilities associated with progressive mental impairment. The development of scales specifically for dementia has involved breaking up task performance, allowing, for example, prompting (all that may be necessary to allow a cognitively impaired person to complete a task) and help with sequencing to be rated separately. Several of the new scales have been developed by nurses and occupational therapists.

Instrumental Activities of Daily Living Scale (IADL)

Reference: **Lawton MP, Brody EM (1969) Assessment of older people: self-maintaining and instrumental activities of daily living.** *The Gerontologist* **9: 179–86**

Time taken 5 minutes

Rating by trained interviewer

Main indications

To assess the functional ability of older people in relation to activities of daily living.

Commentary

Two scales are reported in the paper: the Physical Self-Maintenance Scale (PSMS), detailing more basic self-care tasks and based on an instrument described by Lowenthal (1964), and the Instrumental Activities of Daily Living (Barrabee et al, 1955; Phillips, 1968), concerning more complex daily tasks. Validity was assessed compared with a measure of general physical health, a mental status questionnaire and a behaviour and adjustment rating scale. Inter-rater reliability was found to be 0.87 and 0.91 on two separate substudies.

Additional references

Barrabee P, Barrabee E, Finesinger J (1955) A normative social adjustment scale. *American Journal of Psychiatry* 112: 252–9.

Khan RL, Goldfarb AI, Pollock M et al (1960) The relationship of mental and physical status in institutionalized aged persons. *American Journal of Psychiatry* 117: 120–4.

Lowenthal MF (1964) *Lives in distress.* New York: Basic Books.

Phillips LG (1968) *Human adaptation and its failures.* New York: Academic Press.

Instrumental Activities of Daily Living Scale (IADL)

A Ability to use telephone

1.	Operates telephone on own initiative – looks up and dials numbers, etc	1
2.	Dials a few well-known numbers	1
3.	Answers telephone but does not dial	1
4.	Does not use telephone at all	0

B Shopping

1.	Takes care of all shopping needs independently	1
2.	Shops independently for small purchases	0
3.	Needs to be accompanied on any shopping trip	0
4.	Completely unable to shop	0

C Food preparation

1.	Plans, prepares and serves adequate meals independently	1
2.	Prepares adequate meals if supplied with ingredients	0
3.	Heats, serves and prepares meals, or prepares meals but does not maintain adequate diet	0
4.	Needs to have meals prepared and served	0

D Housekeeping

1.	Maintains house alone or with occasional assistance (e.g. 'heavy work domestic help')	1
2.	Performs light daily tasks such as dish-washing, bedmaking	1
3.	Performs light daily tasks but cannot maintain acceptable level of cleanliness	1
4.	Needs help with all home maintenance tasks	1
5.	Does not participate in any housekeeping tasks	0

E Laundry

1.	Does personal laundry completely	1
2.	Launders small items – rinses stockings, etc	1
3.	All laundry must be done by others	0

F Mode of transportation

1.	Travels independently on public transportation or drives own car	1
2.	Arranges own travel via taxi, but does not otherwise use public transportation	1
3.	Travels on public transportation when accompanied by another	1
4.	Travel limited to taxi or automobile with assistance of another	0
5.	Does not travel at all	0

G Responsibility for own medications

1.	Is responsible for taking medication in correct dosages at correct time	1
2.	Takes responsibility if medication is prepared in advance in separate dosage	0
3.	Is not capable of dispensing own medication	0

H Ability to handle finances

1.	Manages financial matters independently (budgets, writes checks, pays rent, bills, goes to bank), collects and keeps track of income	1
2.	Manages day-to-day purchases, but needs help with banking, major purchases, etc.	1
3.	Incapable of handling money	0

Physical self-maintenance scale

A Toilet

1.	Cares for self at toilet completely, no incontinence	1
2.	Needs to be reminded, or needs help in cleaning self, or has rare (weekly at most) accidents	0
3.	Soiling or wetting while asleep more than once a week	0
4.	Soiling or wetting while awake more than once a week	0
5.	No control of bowels or bladder	0

B Feeding

1.	Eats without assistance	1
2.	Eats with minor assistance at meal times and/or with special preparation of food, or help in cleaning up after meals	0
3.	Feeds self with moderate assistance and is untidy	0
4.	Requires extensive assistance for all meals	0
5.	Does not feed self at all and resists efforts of others to feed him	0

C Dressing

1.	Dresses, undresses, and selects clothes from own wardrobe	1
2.	Dresses and undresses self, with minor assistance	0
3.	Needs moderate assistance in dressing or selection of clothes	0
4.	Needs major assistance in dressing, but cooperates with efforts of others to help	0
5.	Completely unable to dress self and resists efforts of others to help	0

D Grooming
(neatness, hair, nails, hands, face, clothing)

1.	Always neatly dressed, well-groomed, without assistance	1
2.	Grooms self adequately with occasional minor assistance, e.g. shaving	0
3.	Needs moderate and regular assistance or supervision in grooming	0
4.	Needs total grooming care, but can remain well-groomed after help from others	0
5.	Actively negates all efforts of others to maintain grooming	0

E Physical ambulation

1.	Goes about grounds or city	1
2.	Ambulates within residence or about one block distant	0
3.	Ambulates with assistance of (check one) a ( ) cane, d ( ) walker, e ( ) wheel chair.	0
	1 ——— Gets in and out without help	
	2 ——— Needs help in getting in and out	
4.	Sits unsupported in chair or wheelchair but cannot propel self without help	0
5.	Bedridden more than half the time	0

F Bathing

1.	Bathes self (tub, shower, sponge bath) without help	1
2.	Bathes self with help in getting in and out of tub	0
3.	Washes face and hands only, but cannot bathe rest of body	0
4.	Does not wash self but is cooperative with those who bathe him	0
5.	Does not wash self and resists efforts to keep him clean	0

Interview for Deterioration in Daily Living Activities in Dementia (IDDD)

Reference: **Teunisse S, Derix MMA (1991) Measuring functional disability in community dwelling dementia patients: development of a questionnaire. *Tijdschrift voor Gerontologie en Geriatrie* 22: 53–9**

Time taken 15 minutes (reviewer's estimate)

Rating by interview with main caregiver

Main indications

To assess activities of daily living in dementia.

Commentary

The scale covers 33 activities such as washing, dressing, and eating as well as more complex activities such as shopping, writing and answering the telephone, tasks performed equally by men and women (earlier scales of activities of daily living tended to rely more heavily on female-dominated and less complex tasks). Both the initiative to perform activities and the performance itself were evaluated. There was high internal consistency ($\alpha = 0.94$) and two groups of items were discriminated: those related to self-care activity and those to more complex tasks. Functioning of the patient is examined in a structured verbal interview with the carer. The scoring is rated on a three-point scale: 1 where help is almost never needed or there has been no change, 2 where help is sometimes needed or when help is needed more often than previously, and 3 when help is almost always needed or help is needed much more than previously. The scoring is carried out by referring to behaviour in the last month, comparing it with how it was before the onset of the dementia. After a negative response the questioner is asked to check that the behaviour is unchanged compared with what it was like previously, and

after a positive response questions are asked: 'Is the help really necessary?' 'What happens if you don't help?' and 'Do you have to help more often than before?'

The original paper rated functional disability along with cognitive impairment (measured by the CAMCOG), behavioural disturbances (measured by the GIP (page 173)) and carer burden (measured by an instrument related to the Zarit Burden Interview (page 327)). Inter-relationships were found in 30 mild to moderately impaired patients with dementia. Functional disability was strongly related to cognitive deterioration and behavioural disturbances, and moderately related to burden experienced by carers. Since 1991, the IDDD has been translated into several languages and a paper-and-pencil version has been used in the measurement of treatment effects.

Additional reference

Teunisse S, Derix MMA, van Crevel H (1991) Assessing the severity of dementia: patient and caregiver. *Archives of Neurology* **48**: 274–7.

Address for correspondence

S Teunisse
Psychology Department
William Guild Building
King's College
University of Aberdeen
Aberdeen AB24 2UB
UK

Interview for Deterioration in Daily Living Activities in Dementia (IDDD)

1.	Do you have to tell her that she should wash herself (take the initiative to wash herself; not only washing of hands or face, but also washing of whole body)?	1	2	3	8	9
2.	Do you have to assist her in washing (finding face cloth, soap; soaping and rinsing of the body)?	1	2	3	8	9
3.	Do you have to tell her that she should dry herself (take the initiative to dry herself, for example looking or fetching for the towel)?	1	2	3	8	9
4.	Do you have to assist her in drying (drying individual body-parts)?	1	2	3	8	9
5.	Do you have to tell her that she should dress herself (take the initiative to dress herself, for example walking to the wardrobe)?	1	2	3	8	9
6.	Do you have to assist her in dressing herself (putting on individual clothes in right order)?	1	2	3	8	9
7.	Do you have to assist her in doing up her shoes, using zippers or buttons?	1	2	3	8	9
8.	Do you have to tell her that she should brush her teeth or comb her hair?	1	2	3	8	9
9.	Do you have to assist her in brushing her teeth?	1	2	3	8	9
10.	Do you have to assist her in combing her hair?	1	2	3	8	9
11.	Do you have to tell her that she should eat (take the initiative to eat; in case eating is elicited by others, it should be asked if she would take the initiative spontaneously)?	1	2	3	8	9
12.	Do you have to assist her in preparing a slice of bread?	1	2	3	8	9
13.	Do you have to assist her in carving meat, potatoes?	1	2	3	8	9
14.	Do you have to assist her in drinking or eating?	1	2	3	8	9
15.	Do you have to tell her that she should use the lavatory (take the initiative to go to the lavatory when necessary)?	1	2	3	8	9
16.	Do you have to assist her in using the toilet (undressing herself, using toilet, using closet paper)?	1	2	3	8	9
17.	Do you have to assist her in finding her way in the house (finding different rooms)?	1	2	3	8	9
18.	Do you have to assist her in finding her way in familiar neighbourhood outside the house?	1	2	3	8	9
19.	Does she – as often as before – take the initiative shopping (take the initiative to figure out what is needed)?	1	2	3	8	9
20.	Do you have to assist her in shopping (finding her way in the shops; getting goods in needed quantity)?	1	2	3	8	9
21.	Do you – or the shop-assistant – have to tell her that she should pay?	1	2	3	8	9
22.	Do you – or the shop-assistant – have to assist her in paying (knowing how much she should pay and how much should be reimbursed)?	1	2	3	8	9
23.	Is she – as often as before – interested in newspaper, book or post?	1	2	3	8	9
24.	Do you have to assist her in reading (understanding written language)?	1	2	3	8	9
25.	Do you have to assist her in writing a letter or card, or completing a form (writing of more than one sentence)?	1	2	3	8	9
26.	Does she – as often as before – start a conversation with others?	1	2	3	8	9
27.	Do you have to assist her in expressing herself verbally?	1	2	3	8	9
28.	Does she – as often as before – pay attention to conversation by other people?	1	2	3	8	9
29.	Do you have to assist her in understanding spoken language?	1	2	3	8	9
30.	Does she – as often as before – take the initiative to use the phone (both answering the phone and calling someone)?	1	2	3	8	9
31.	Do you have to assist her in using the phone (both answering the phone and calling someone)?	1	2	3	8	9
32.	Do you have to assist her in finding things in the house?	1	2	3	8	9
33.	Do you have to tell her to put out gas or coffee machine?	1	2	3	8	9

Rating:
1 = (nearly) no help needed/no change in help needed
2 = sometimes help needed/help more often needed
3 = (nearly) always help needed/help much more often needed
8 = no evaluation possible
9 = not applicable

Barthel Index

Reference: Mahoney FI, Barthel DW (1965) Functional evaluation: the BARTHEL index. *Maryland State Medical Journal* 14: 61–5

Time taken 5 minutes

Rating by informant

Main indications

Assessment of physical disability in elderly people.

Commentary

The Barthel Index represents probably the oldest and most widely used scale to assess physical disability in elderly patients in general. It is often used in studies in psychiatry. Its reliability has been assessed thoroughly in four ways: by self-report, by a trained nurse, and by two independent skilled observers. Agreement was generally present in over 90% of situations. Validity, reliability, sensitivity and clinical utility are all excellent, and have been reviewed (Wade and Collin, 1988). Explicit guidelines for rating have been suggested for the scale (Novak et al, 1996), and Wade and Collins have suggested an amended scoring system of 20.

Additional references

Collin C, Wade DT, Davis S et al (1988) The Barthel ADL Index: a reliability study. *International Disability Studies* 10: 61–3.

Novak S, Johnson J, Greenwood R (1996) Barthel revisited: making guidelines work. *Clinical Rehabilitation* 10: 128–34.

Wade DT, Collin C (1988) The Barthel ADL Index: a standard measure of physical disability? *International Disability Studies* 10: 64–7.

www.strokecenter.org/trials/scales/barthel.pdf

Barthel Index

		With help	Independent
1.	Feeding (if food needs to be cut up = help)	5	10
2.	Moving from wheelchair to bed and return (includes sitting up in bed)	5–10	15
3.	Personal toilet (wash face, comb hair, shave, clean teeth)	0	5
4.	Getting on and off toilet (handling clothes, wipe, flush)	5	10
5.	Bathing self	0	5
6.	Walking on level surfaces	10	15
	(if unable to walk, propel wheelchair)	0	5
7.	Ascend and descend stairs	5	10
8.	Dressing (includes tying shoes, fastening fasteners)	5	10
9.	Controlling bowels	5	10
10.	Controlling bladder	5	10

A score of 100 indicates independence in activities of daily living.

Mahoney FI, Barthel DW. Functional Evaluation: The BARTHEL Index. *Maryland State Medical Journal* 1965; 14(2): 61–5. Used with permission.

Progressive Deterioration Scale (PDS)

Reference: DeJong R, Osterlund OW, Roy GW (1989) Measurement of quality-of-life changes in patients with Alzheimer's disease. *Clinical Therapeutics* 11: 545–54

Time taken 10–15 minutes (based on interview lasting 90 minutes)

Rating by a carer

Main indications

Assesses changes in the quality of life of patients with Alzheimer's disease.

Commentary

The need for measures to assess the effects of medication on quality of life prompted the development of the Progressive Deterioration Scale (PDS), which involved three steps: step 1 – interviews with caregivers detailing particular facets of the disease which affected quality of life; step 2 – testing and preparation of questionnaires using the factors which were found to discriminate between various stages of Alzheimer's disease as characterized by the Global Deterioration Scale (GDS; page 236) leading to a final version; and step 3 – validation of the final version on a differ-

ent group of patients and measures of reliability. The 27 items came from a number of different content areas.

Content areas for questionnaire items that differentiate Global Deterioration Scale stages in Alzheimer's disease:

- Extent to which patient can leave immediate neighbourhood.
- Ability to travel distances safely alone.
- Confusion in familiar settings.
- Use of familiar household implements.
- Participation/enjoyment of leisure/cultural activities.
- Extent to which patient does household chores.
- Involvement in family finances, budgeting, etc.
- Interest in doing household tasks.
- Travel on public transportation.
- Self-care and routine tasks.
- Social function/behaviour in social settings.

The scale achieved 95% accuracy in discriminating between normal controls and patients with Alzheimer's disease and an overall 80% accuracy in discriminating between controls and patients with early, middle and late Alzheimer's disease. Coefficients of reliability ranged from 0.92 to 0.95. Test/retest reliability was generally significant at 0.80.

Summary of content areas for the Progressive Deterioration Scale (PDS)

- Extent to which patient can leave immediate neighbourhood.
- Ability to safely travel distances alone.
- Confusion in familiar settings.
- Use of familiar household implements.
- Participation/enjoyment of leisure/cultural activities.
- Extent to which patient does household chores.
- Involvement in family finances, budgeting, etc.
- Interest in doing household tasks.
- Travel on public transportation.
- Self-care and routine tasks.
- Social function/behaviour in social settings.

Functional Activities Questionnaire (FAQ)

Reference: **Pfeffer RI, Kurosaki TT, Harrah CH, Chance JM, Filos S (1992) Measurement of functional activities in older adults in the community.** *Journal of Gerontology* **37: 323–9**

Time taken 10 minutes (reviewer's estimate)

Rating by clinician

Main indications

For the assessment of functional capacity in older people, with or without dementia.

Commentary

The rationale for the scale was to provide operational descriptions of various levels of function, independent of education, socioeconomic status and intelligence. The Functional Activities Questionnaire (FAQ) was validated on a study of 195 adults aged over 60 with normal or very mild dementia and, after a screening test for cognitive impairment and depression, they were rated on three cognitive scales: the Mini-Mental State Examination (MMSE; page 36), the Symbol Digit Test and Subtest B of the Raven's Progressive Colour Matrices. The FAQ is rated on a seven-point scale, 1 being normal and 7 being severely incapacitated and helpless. Comparisons were made with the Instrumental Activities of Daily Living Scale (IADL; page 186). Inter-rater reliability was excellent, with correlation = 0.97, and correlation with the IADL was 0.72. The scale showed high sensitivity and specificity (0.85 and 0.81, respectively) in distinguishing between demented and non-demented people.

Address for correspondence

RI Pfeffer
Department of Neurology
University of California at Irving Medical Center
101 City Drive South
Orange
CA 92668
USA

Functional Activities Questionnaire (FAQ)

Functional capacity level	Descriptive title	Description	Residual mental function estimate (%)
1	Normal	Fully independent with no restriction: No cognitive impairment. Either no assistance or advice is required in the 10 areas of daily activities, IADL, or activities of daily living (ADL), or this does not deviate from an established life-long pattern (e.g. utilization of an accountant or business advisor).	100
2	Questionably affected: uncertain status	Qualified independence: (a) participant or alternate informant report less skill or greater difficulty than formerly in 10 areas of daily activities or IADL, but independent of others. Only compensation, if any, is self-imposed (e.g. notes, reminder) or (b) study staff observe minor word-finding problems, minimal impairment of immediate recall of recent events, questionable problem with spatial orientation in unfamiliar surroundings, but normally oriented to person, place, and date (± 1 day).	90
3	Mildly affected	Definite but mild restriction in normal activities or independence: Another supervises or advises in two or more of 10 formerly mastered areas of daily activities, or one or more areas of IADL, but participant still carries out activity. Example: requires very explicit or written directions to drive out of neighborhood, guidance in balancing checkbook but still handles own money. Alternatively, significant difficulty with activity, but spouse tolerates performance they described as substandard. Probably could not be gainfully employed, but lives independently and normally with slight environmental modification or intervention, such as one to three visits per week from friend/relative or redistribution of spouse's responsibilities.	75
4	Moderately affected	Require assistance in IADL, but carry out a portion of this function (e.g. writes own checks or pays at supermarket but another balances check book, submits medical bills, drives them to appointments or accompanies on bus. More severely affected persons in this category need intermittent supervisor (two times weekly reminders) in ADL (e.g. coordinating items of apparel, missed areas in shaving or makeup) but perform the function. Requires active external intervention for 'normal' home life, but takes care of basic personal needs.	60
5	Moderately severely affected	Half or more of IADL (e.g. shopping, laundry, handling money, making appointments, transport, dispensing medication) are performed by other. Require three times weekly assistance with toilette, although may participate in dressing and feed themselves. Most are spontaneously ambulatory. Requires major readjustments of family routine, adult daycare, or variable degress of attendant assistance; they may be placed in nursing homes.	40
6	Severely affected	Requires major, daily assistance in ADL (dressing, feeding, using toilet) and total assistance with IADL. Any ambulation with assistance. Initiates almost no activity other than for feeding, toilet, comfort. Institutional care is usual.	25
7	Severely incapacitated: helpless	Totally dependent. Mute, wheelchair, or bedfast. Almost all are institutionalized and require a higher level of nursing care than available outside most acute/rehabilitation hospitals.	10

Daily Activities Questionnaire (DAQ)

Reference: Oakley F, Sunderland T, Hill JL, Phillips SL, Makahon R, Ebner JD (1991) The Daily Activities Questionnaire: a functional assessment for people with Alzheimer's disease. *Physical and Occupational Therapy in Geriatrics* 10: 67–81

Time taken 15 minutes (reviewer's estimate)

Rating from caregiver

Main indications

An objective clinical research measure of activities in daily living (ADLs) in people with Alzheimer's disease.

Commentary

The Daily Activities Questionnaire (DAQ) consists of 12 visual analogue scales (100 mm lines ranging from totally dependent to totally independent). The domains assessed are money management, cooking, shopping, recreation, home care, phone use, dressing, grooming,

bathing, walking, sleeping, feeding, toileting and a global measure. The paper described significant differences in 32 patients with Alzheimer's disease and 18 normal controls. Inter-rater reliability (intraclass correlation coefficients) were all significant, with the exception of the items on recreation, walking and toileting. There were significant correlations between the severity of illness and ADLs. Normal controls were able to fill in their own questionnaire.

Address for correspondence

Frances Oakley
Occupational Therapy Service
NIH
Bethesda MD 20892
USA

Examples of visual analogue scales and clinical questions from the Daily Activities Questionnaire (DAQ)

Dressing

| Totally dependent | | Totally independent |

Cooking

| Totally dependent | | Totally independent |

Money management

| Totally dependent | | Totally independent |

When dressing:

Dresses without assistance 0

May occasionally need some supervision or direction to dress . 1

Usually needs much supervision or direction to dress 2

Must be physically dressed by another 3

If 1, 2, or 3 describe assistance provided: ——————

——————————————————————————

Not applicable. Why? ——————————————————

Reproduced with permission from *Physical and Occupational Therapy in Geriatrics*, 1991, The Haworth Press.

Bristol Activities of Daily Living Scale

Reference: **Bucks RS, Ashworth DL, Wilcock GK, Siegfried K (1996) Assessment of activities of daily living in dementia: development of the Bristol Activities of Daily Living Scale.** *Age and Ageing* **25: 113–20**

Time taken 15 minutes (reviewer's estimate)

Rating by carer

Main indications

Assessment of activities of daily living in patients with dementia either in the community or on clinical research trial.

Commentary

The scale was designed specifically for use in patients with dementia, and consists of 20 daily living abilities. Face validity was measured by way of carer agreement that the items were important, construct validity was confirmed by principal components analysis, concurrent validity by assessment with observed performance and good test/retest reliability. Three phases in the design of the scale were described. Anyone designing a scale should read this to serve as a model of clarity.

Additional reference

Patterson MB, Mack JL, Neundorfer MM et al (1992) Assessment of functional ability in Alzheimer's disease: a review and preliminary report on the Cleveland Scale for Activities of Daily Living. *Alzheimer Disease and Associated Disorders* **6**: 145–63.

Address for correspondence

GK Wilcock
Department of Care of the Elderly
Frenchay Hospital
Bristol BS16 1LE
UK
e-mail: Gordon.wilcock@bris.ac.uk

Bristol Activities of Daily Living Scale

1. Food

a.	Selects and prepares food as required	[ ]
b.	Able to prepare food if ingredients set out	[ ]
c.	Can prepare food if prompted step by step	[ ]
d.	Unable to prepare food even with prompting and supervision	[ ]
e.	Not applicable	[ ]

2. Eating

a.	Eats appropriately using correct cutlery	[ ]
b.	Eats appropriately if food made manageable and/or uses spoon	[ ]
c.	Uses fingers to eat food	[ ]
d.	Needs to be fed	[ ]
e.	Not applicable	[ ]

3. Drink

a.	Selects and prepares drinks as required	[ ]
b.	Can prepare drinks if ingredients left available	[ ]
c.	Can prepare drinks if prompted step by step	[ ]
d.	Unable to make a drink even with prompting and supervision	[ ]
e.	Not applicable	[ ]

4. Drinking

a.	Drinks appropriately	[ ]
b.	Drinks appropriately with aids, beaker/straw etc.	[ ]
c.	Does not drink appropriately even with aids but attempts to	[ ]
d.	Has to have drinks administered (fed)	[ ]
e.	Not applicable	[ ]

5. Dressing

a.	Selects appropriate clothing and dresses self	[ ]
b.	Puts clothes on in wrong order and/or back to front and/or dirty clothing	[ ]
c.	Unable to dress self but moves limbs to assist	[ ]
d.	Unable to assist and requires total dressing	[ ]
e.	Not applicable	[ ]

6. Hygiene

a.	Washes regularly and independently	[ ]
b.	Can wash self if given soap, flannel, towel, etc.	[ ]
c.	Can wash self if prompted and supervised	[ ]
d.	Unable to wash self and needs full assistance	[ ]
e.	Not applicable	[ ]

cont.

7. Teeth

a. Cleans own teeth/dentures regularly and independently [ ]

b. Cleans teeth/dentures if given appropriate items [ ]

c. Requires some assistance, toothpaste on brush, brush to mouth, etc. [ ]

d. Full assistance given [ ]

e. Not applicable [ ]

8. Bath/shower

a. Bathes regularly and independently [ ]

b. Needs bath to be drawn/shower turned on but washes independently [ ]

c. Needs supervision and prompting to wash [ ]

d. Totally dependent, needs full assistance [ ]

e. Not applicable [ ]

9. Toilet/commode

a. Uses toilet appropriately when required [ ]

b. Needs to be taken to the toilet and given assistance [ ]

c. Incontinent of urine or faeces [ ]

d. Incontinent of urine and faeces [ ]

e. Not applicable [ ]

10. Transfers

a. Can get in/out of chair unaided [ ]

b. Can get into a chair but needs help to get out [ ]

c. Needs help getting in and out of a chair [ ]

d. Totally dependent on being put into and lifted from chair [ ]

e. Not applicable [ ]

11. Mobility

a. Walks independently [ ]

b. Walks with assistance, i.e. furniture, arm for support [ ]

c. Uses aids to mobilize, i.e. frame, sticks etc. [ ]

d. Unable to walk [ ]

e. Not applicable [ ]

12. Orientation – time

a. Fully orientated to time/day/date etc. [ ]

b. Unaware of time/day etc but seems unconcerned [ ]

c. Repeatedly asks the time/day/date [ ]

d. Mixes up night and day [ ]

e. Not applicable [ ]

13. Orientation – space

a. Fully orientated to surroundings [ ]

b. Orientated to familiar surroundings only [ ]

c. Gets lost in home, needs reminding where bathroom is, etc. [ ]

d. Does not recognize home as own and attempts to leave [ ]

e. Not applicable [ ]

14. Communication

a. Able to hold appropriate conversation [ ]

b. Shows understanding and attempts to respond verbally with gestures [ ]

c. Can make self understood but difficulty understanding others [ ]

d. Does not respond to or communicate with others [ ]

e. Not applicable [ ]

15. Telephone

a. Uses telephone appropriately, including obtaining correct number [ ]

b. Uses telephone if number given verbally/visually or predialled [ ]

c. Answers telephone but does not make calls [ ]

d. Unable/unwilling to use telephone at all [ ]

e. Not applicable [ ]

16. Housework/gardening

a. Able to do housework/gardening to previous standard [ ]

b. Able to do housework/gardening but not to previous standard [ ]

c. Limited participation even with a lot of supervision [ ]

d. Unwilling/unable to participate in previous activities [ ]

e. Not applicable [ ]

17. Shopping

a. Shops to previous standard [ ]

b. Only able to shop for 1 or 2 items with or without a list [ ]

c. Unable to shop alone, but participates when accompanied [ ]

d. Unable to participate in shopping even when accompanied [ ]

e. Not applicable [ ]

18. Finances

a. Responsible for own finances at previous level [ ]

b. Unable to write cheque but can sign name and recognizes money values [ ]

c. Can sign name but unable to recognize money values [ ]

d. Unable to sign name or recognize money values [ ]

e. Not applicable [ ]

19. Games/hobbies

a. Participates in pastimes/activities to previous standard [ ]

b. Participates but needs instruction/supervision [ ]

c. Reluctant to join in, very slow, needs coaxing [ ]

d. No longer able or willing to join in [ ]

e. Not applicable [ ]

20. Transport

a. Able to drive, cycle or use public transport independently [ ]

b. Unable to drive but uses public transport or bike etc [ ]

c. Unable to use public transport alone [ ]

d. Unable or unwilling to use transport even when accompanied [ ]

e. Not applicable [ ]

Rating:

Tick only 1 box per activity. Answer with respect to last 2 weeks

Score: a = 0, b = 1, c = 2, d = 3, e = 0

Reprinted from Bucks RS, Ashworth DL, Wilcock GK, Siegfried K (1996) Assessment of activities of daily living in dementia: development of the Bristol Activities of Daily Living Scale. *Age and Ageing*, **25**: 113–20. By kind permission of Oxford University Press.

Direct Assessment of Functional Status (DAFS)

Reference: **Loewenstein DA, Amigo E, Duara R, Guterman A, Hurwitz D, Berkowitz N, Wilkie F, Weinberg G, Black B, Gittelman B, Eisdorfer C (1989) A new scale for the assessment of functional status in Alzheimer's disease and related disorders.** *Journal of Gerontology* **44: 114–21**

Time taken 25 minutes (reviewer's estimate)

Rating by trained interviewer

Main indications

Direct assessment of functional capacities in Alzheimer's disease and other disorders.

Commentary

The Direct Assessment of Functional Status (DAFS) consists of a number of domains: time orientation; transportation; financial skills; shopping skills; eating skills;

and dressing/grooming skills. Inter-rater reliability revealed kappa values of over 0.9 for all the domains, and test/retest reliability was also excellent, with all kappa values 0.86 or above. Correlations were described between the scale and the Blessed Dementia Scale (page 46) which were highly significant.

Address for correspondence

David A Loewenstein
Wien Center for Alzheimer's Disease
Mount Sinai Medical Center
Miami Beach FL 33140
USA

Direct Assessment of Functional Status (DAFS)

I. Time Orientation (16 points)

	Correct (2 points)	Incorrect (0 points)
A. Telling Time (Use large model of a clock)		
3:00	____	____
8:00	____	____
10:30	____	____
12:15	____	____

	Correct (2 points)	Incorrect (0 points)
B. Orientation to Date		
What is the date?	____	____
What day is it today?	____	____
What month are we in?	____	____
What year are we in	____	____

II. Communication (14 points) (Using a pushbotton telephone) (If at any point the patient dials, picks up, or hangs up the phone, he/she is given credit for items tapping these specific subskills.)

	Correct (1 point)	Incorrect (0 points)
A. Using the Telephone		
Dial Operator (0)	____	____
Dial number from book	____	____
Dial number presented orally	____	____
Dial number written down	____	____
Pick up receiver	____	____
Ability to dial	____	____
Hang up phone	____	____
Correct sequence across all previous trials	____	____

	Correct (1 point)	Incorrect (0 points)
B. Preparing a Letter for Mailing		
Fold in half	____	____
Put in envelope	____	____
Seal envelope	____	____
Stamp envelope	____	____
Address (has to be exact duplicate of examiner's copy)	____	____
Return address (has to put correct address in upper lefthand corner)	____	____

III. Transportation (13 points)
(Patient has to correctly identify a driver's correct response to these road signs.)

	Correct (1 point)	Incorrect (0 points)
Stop	____	____
Yield	____	____
One way	____	____
No right turn	____	____
Green light	____	____
Yellow light	____	____
Red light	____	____
No "U' turn	____	____
Railroad crossing	____	____
Do not enter	____	____
Double yellow line	____	____
Passing line	____	____
Speed limit	____	____

cont.

At this point the examiner should instruct the patient that he/she will be going to a grocery store in 10 minutes and that the patient will be asked to pick out four grocery items from memory. Patient is given each grocery item, repeats it and again is asked to commit the list of four grocery items to memory.

IV. Financial (21 points) (Lay out one $10 bill, three $1 bills, one $5 bill, 3 quarters, 2 dimes, 1 nickel, 3 pennies.) Subskills include making change for grocery items.

	Correct (1 point)	Incorrect (0 points)
A. Identifying Currency		
Identify penny	___	___
Identify nickel	___	___
Identify dime	___	___
Identify quarter	___	___
Identify dollar bill	___	___
Identify $5 bill	___	___
Identify $10 bill	___	___

		Correct (1 point)	Incorrect (0 points)
B. Counting Change			
Lay out			
1–$10 bill	6 cents	___	___
1–$5 bill	102 cents (in change)	___	___
3–$1 bill	$6.73	___	___
3–quarters	$12.17	___	___
2–dimes		___	___
1–nickel		___	___
3–pennies		___	___

	Correct (1 point)	Incorrect (0 points)
C. Writing a Check		
Signature	___	___
Pay to order of	___	___
Written amount	___	___
Numeric amount	___	___
Date (location)	___	___
(Does not have to be correct)		

	Correct (1 point)	Incorrect (0 points)
D. Balancing a Checkbook		
Amount A ($500–$350) correct $150	___	___
Amount B ($323–$23.50) correct $299.50	___	___
Amount C ($21.75–$3.92) correct $17.83	___	___

V. Shopping (16 points) Patients told to look over the 20 grocery items and asked to select the four which were presented to him/her 10 minutes earlier.

	Correct (2 points)	Incorrect (0 points)
A. Memory for Grocery Items		
Orange juice	___	___
Soup	___	___
Cereal	___	___
Tuna fish	___	___

All of the items selected by the patient on the previous test are put back and the patient is given a written grocery list.

	Correct (2 points)	Incorrect (0 points)
B. Selecting Groceries Given a Written List		
Milk	___	___
Crackers	___	___
Eggs	___	___
Laundry detergent	___	___

	Correct (2 points)	Incorrect (0 points)
C.		
Correct change	___	___

Give the patient a $5 bill and say the bill is $2.49. Put the money out in front of them (currency from the Financial Subskills Test) and ask them to count out the change they should receive.

VI. Grooming (14 points)
The patient is taken to the bathroom and asked to:

	Correct (2 points)	Incorrect (0 points)
Take cap off toothpaste	___	___
Put toothpaste on brush	___	___
Turn on water	___	___
Brush teeth	___	___
Dampen wash cloth	___	___
Put soap on cloth	___	___
Clean face	___	___
Turn off water	___	___
Brush hair	___	___
Put on coat	___	___
Button	___	___
Tie	___	___
Zip	___	___

VII. Eating (10 points)
(Place eating utensils in front of patient.)

	Correct (2 points)	Incorrect (0 points)
Fork	___	___
Knife	___	___
Spoon	___	___
Pour water	___	___
Drink from glass	___	___

Activities of Daily Living (ADL) Index

Reference: **Sheikh K, Smith DS, Meade TW, Goldenberg E, Brennan PJ, Kinsella G (1979) Repeatability and validity of a modified Activities of Daily Living (ADL) Index in studies of chronic disability.** *International Rehabilitation Medicine* 1: 51–8

Time taken 10 minutes (reviewer's estimate)

Rating by observer

Main indications

Assessment of activities of daily living function in chronic disability – modified to be sufficiently repeatable and valid.

Commentary

This is a 17-item scale tested on a number of different groups of patients. Inter-rater reliability and test/retest reliability were assessed in hospital and home settings, the relationship between the score and the size of the cerebral lesion was determined, and the score was compared with the patient's own perception of disability. Inter-rater reliability was 0.986 (over 2000 paired observations). Test/retest reliability (340 observations) was excellent, and the other substudies confirmed the validity of the scale.

ADL Index (Activity items)

Transfer from floor to chair
Transfer from chair to bed
Walking indoors
Walking outdoors
Ascending a flight of stairs
Descending a flight of stairs
Dressing (overgarments)
Washing (simulated)
Bathing (simulated)

Using lavatory (simulated)
Continence (bladder and bowel control)
Grooming (brushing hair or shaving)
Brushing teeth (simulated)
Preparing for making tea
Making tea
Using taps (ordinary sink taps)
Feeding (simulated)

Score as follows:
1 = Performed without assistance (physical aids allowed)
2 = Performed greater part without assistance; some verbal or physical assistance required
3 = Complete inability to perform, even with assistance, or refusal to perform even if deemed able
Minimum score = 17, indicating no apparent handicap.
If totally unable to carry out any activity even with help then would score 51.

Source: *International Rehabilitation Medicine*, 1, 51–58, 1979. Reprinted by permission of Taylor & Francis.

Cleveland Scale for Activities of Daily Living (CSADL)

Reference: **Patterson MB, Mack JL, Neundorfer MM, Martin RJ, Smyth KA, Whitehouse PJ (1992) Assessment of functional ability in Alzheimer disease: a review and a preliminary report on the Cleveland Scale for Activities of Daily Living.** *Alzheimer Disease and Associated Disorders* **6: 145–63**

Time taken 25 minutes (reviewer's estimate)
Rating by primary caregiver by nurse, clinician or trained interviewer

Main indications

Assessment of activities of daily living (ADLs) in Alzheimer's disease.

Commentary

The Cleveland Scale for Activities of Daily Living (CSADL) was designed specifically to reflect changes in the nature and extent of the broad spectrum of functional difficulties seen in individuals with Alzheimer's disease. Some 113 patients diagnosed as having Alzheimer's disease were assessed with the scale, and it was compared with the Blessed Dementia Scale (page 46) and the Mini-Mental State Examination (MMSE; page 36). The scale consists of 66 items in 16 domains of everyday activities, including both physical and instrumental ADLs, and represented all the physical and instrumental activities included in the Older Americans Resources and Services (OARS), the Functional Assessment Questionnaire (Duke University, 1978) plus several items suggested by Pfeffer in the Functional Activities Questionnaire (FAQ; page 192), as well as other items assessing more complex activities such as hobbies, communication skills and social behaviour. Within each domain, activities are broken down into several components. In the paper, five basic ADL domains were examined: bearing, dressing, eating, toileting and hygiene. Descriptions were given of the proportion of rating according to dependency level. Rating of individual items and intercorrelations of the items within each domain. The usefulness of the CSADL and its improved sensitivity of the detection of basic ADL functions were discussed.

Additional reference

Duke University Center for the Study of Aging (1978) *Multidimensional function assessment: the OARS methodology.* 2nd edition. Durham, NC: Duke University.

Address for correspondence

MB Patterson
Department of Neurology
University Hospitals of Cleveland
2074 Abington Road
Cleveland
OH 44106
USA

Cleveland Scale for Activities of Daily Living (CSADL)

Bathing –	initiates bath		Medications	
	prepares bath			
	gets in/out		Eating –	eats at appropriate intervals
	cleans self			eats at appropriate time
				feeds self
Toileting –	controls urination			acceptable manners
	controls bowels			
	recognizes need		Meal preparation	
	eliminates at toilet		Mobility	
	rearranges clothes		Shopping	
			Travel	
Personal hygiene and appearance –	initiates grooming		Hobbies, personal interests, employment	
	washes hands/face		Housework/home maintenance	
	brushes teeth		Telephone	
	combs hair		Money management	
			Communication skills	
Dressing –	initiates dressing		Social behavior	
	selects clothes			
	puts on garments			
	fastens clothing			

Score as follows: 0 = Activities carried out effectively and fully independent. Normal; 1 = Generally independent, sometimes needs direction/assistance; 2 = Usually requires direction and/or assistance but independent in some situations/occasions; 3 = Completely dependent on others for direction/assistance

---

Cognitive Performance Test

Reference: **Burns T, Mortimer JA, Merchak P (1994) Cognitive performance test: a new approach to functional assessment in Alzheimer's disease.** *Journal of Geriatric Psychiatry and Neurology* **7: 46–54.**

Time taken 45 minutes

Rating by trained interviewer

Main indications

Assessment of functional capacity in dementia.

Commentary

The Cognitive Performance Test claims to be different from other similar tests in that, rather than focusing on the ability to perform specific tasks, the emphasis is on the degree to which deficits in information processing compromise activities. Seventy-seven patients with mild to moderate Alzheimer's disease were studied. Inter-rater reliability was 0.91 and test/retest reliability over 4 weeks was 0.89. Validity was assessed by comparison with the Mini-Mental State Examination (MMSE; page 36) and the Instrumental Activities of Daily Living Scale (IADL; page 186). Correlations with these scales were 0.67, 0.64 and 0.49 respectively. The scale strongly predicted the rate of institutionalization over a 4-year follow-up period.

The scale is rated on 6 ordinal levels, profoundly disabled (level 1) and normal functioning (level 6).

Address for correspondence

Theressa Burns
Veterans Affairs Medical Center
1 Veterans Drive
Minneapolis
MN 55417
USA

Cognitive Performance Test

Initial Directions for Tasks

Dress: This test has to do with getting dressed. I want you to get dressed as if you were going outside on a cold, rainy day. You can use any of the things here. There are men's and women's things. Get dressed over your own clothes for going outside on a cold, rainy day.

Shop: I'd like to see how you do with money when you're shopping. I want you to buy a belt. Here is a wallet with some money in it. Choose a belt that fits you and one that you can pay for with the money in the wallet; then pay me the exact amount for the belt.

Toast: This next test has to do with preparing food. Make one slice of toast, then put some butter and jam on it. The supplies are on this table.

Phone: This next test has to do with using the phone. I'd like you to use the phone to find out the cost of one gallon of white paint.

Wash: Here are the directions for the next test; listen carefully. I want you to clean your hands as if you had been working outside in the yard. Take what you need from this box and use whatever you need in this room.

Travel: I want to see how well you're able to get from one place to another. This is a map of the hallways in this area. See if you can find this particular set of stairs. We are standing here. Follow the map to these stairs and point them out to me.

Source: Burns T, Mortimer JA, Merchak P (1994) Cognitive Performance Test: a new approach to functional assessment in Alzheimer's disease, *Journal of Geriatric Psychiatry and Neurology* **7**: 46–54.

Present Functioning Questionnaire (PFQ) and Functional Rating Scale (FRS)

Reference: **Crockett D, Tuokko H, Koch W, Parks R (1989) The assessment of everyday functioning using the Present Functioning Questionnaire and the Functional Rating Scale in elderly samples.** *Clinical Gerontologist* **8: 3–25**

Time taken PFQ: 20 minutes (reviewer's estimate)
FRS: 15 minutes (reviewer's estimate)

Rating PFQ: informant-based
FRS: ideally a multidisciplinary assessment

Main indications

Estimation of everyday functioning in elderly patients.

Commentary

The Functional Rating Scale (FRS) assesses information in eight areas: memory; social/community/occupational; home/hobbies; personal care; language skills; problem solving; affect; and orientation. The Present Functioning Questionnaire (PFQ) collates reported problems in five areas: personality; everyday tasks; language skills; memory functioning; and self-care. Subjects were chosen who were either normal volunteers living in the community or referrals to an Alzheimer's disease clinic. A reliability study confirmed high internal consistency for the scales, with an ability to differentiate between groups of subjects.

Additional reference

Tuokko T, Crockett D, Beattie B et al (1986) The use of rating scales to assess psycho-social functioning in demented patients. Paper presented at the International Neuropsychological Society Annual Meeting. Denver, CO.

Address for correspondence

D Crockett
Division of Psychology
Department of Psychiatry
University of British Columbia
Vancouver BC
V6T 2A1
Canada

Present Functioning Questionnaire (PFQ)

Personality:
Being irritable or angry —
Being miserable or depressed —
Being tense or panicky —
Being apathetic —
Being agitated or hyperactive —
Being anxious or afraid —
Stating that 'things aren't real' —
Complaining of 'upsetting thoughts' —
Being aggressive —
Being suspicious —
Being insensitive to others' feelings —
Showing inappropriate smiles or laughter —
Showing decreased hobby involvement —
Talking to imaginery others —
Exhibiting inappropriate sexual activities —

Everyday tasks:
Problems performing household tasks —
Problems handling money —
Problems shopping —
Problems finding their way inside a house or building —
Problems finding their way around familiar streets —
Problems recognizing surroundings —
Problems recognizing the date or day of week —
Problems recognizing the time of day —
Awakening at night and thinking it is day —
Problems reading (except as caused by poor vision) —
Problems performing job —
Problems driving a car (if could before) —

Language skills:
Problems finding words to express him/herself —
Losing his/her vocabulary —
Problems pronouncing words —
Problems understanding others —
More frequently slurring words —
Problems clipping ends of words or sentences —
More frequently stuttering —

Problems finding names for common objects —
Problems forming any intelligible speech —

Memory functions:
Problems remembering previous actions on the same day —
Problems remembering past life events —
Asking questions repeatedly (despite answers) —
Problems recognizing faces of old friends or family —
Problems recognizing names of old friends or family —
Problems remembering newly introduced persons —
Problems leaving stove burners, water taps & light switches turned on —
Problems maintaining a train of thought —
Problems concentrating —
Problems remembering where he/she placed objects —
Increasingly frustrated over problems of remembering or thinking —
Increasingly defensive about problems remembering —
Problems remembering important personal dates —
Seemingly unaware of important current events —
Does not know own name —

Self-care functions:
Eating messily with spoon only —
Eating messily with spoon and with solid foods —
Has to be fed by someone else —
Problems dressing, e.g. occasional misplaced buttons —
Problems dressing, e.g. puts on clothes in wrong sequence —
Problems dressing, e.g. unable to dress self —
Problems with occasionally wetting bed —
Problems with frequently wetting bed —
Double incontinent —
Does not wash him/herself enough —
Must be bathed by someone else —
Grooming (combing of hair, etc.) inadequate —
Must be groomed by someone else —
Needs constant supervision in caring for self —

Functional Rating Scale (FRS)

	Healthy (1)	Questionable (2)	Mild (3)	Moderate (4)	Severe (5)
Memory	No deficit or inconsistent forgetfulness evident only on clinical interview	Variable symptoms reported by patient or relative; seemingly unrelated to level of functioning	Memory losses which intefere with daily living; more apparent for recent events	Moderate memory loss; only highly learned material retained, new material rapidly lost	Severe memory loss; unable to recall relevant aspects of current life; very sketchy recall of past life
Social/community and occupational	Neither patient nor relatives aware of any deficit	Variable levels of functioning reported by patient or relatives; no objective evidence of deficits in employment or social situations	Patient or relative aware of decreased performance in demanding employment or social settings; appears normal to casual inspection	Patient or relative aware of ongoing deterioration; does not appear normal to objective observer; unable to perform job; little independent functioning outside home	Marked impairment of social functioning; no independent functioning outside home
Home and hobbies	No changes noted by patient or relative	Slightly decreased involvement in household tasks and hobbies	Engages in social activities in the home but definite impairment on some household tasks; some complicated hobbies and interests abandoned	Only simple chores/hobbies preserved; most complicated hobbies/interests abandoned	No independent involvement in home or hobbies
Personal care	Fully capable of self-care	Occasional problems with self-care reported by patient/relatives or observed	Needs prompting to complete tasks adequately (i.e. dressing, feeding, hygiene)	Requires supervision in dressing, feeding, hygiene and keeping track of personal effects	Needs constant supervision and assistance with feeding, dressing, or hygiene, etc.
Language skills	No disturbance of language report by patient or relative	Subjective complaint of, or relative reports, language deficits; usually limited to word finding or naming	Patient or relative reports variable disturbances of such skills as articulation or naming; occasional language impairment evident during examination	Patient or relative reports consistent language disturbance, language disturbance evident on examination	Severe impairment of receptive and/or expressive language; production of unintelligible speech
Problem solving and reasoning	Solves everyday problems adequately	Variable impairment of problems solving, similarities, differences	Difficulty in handling complex problems	Marked impairment on complex problem solving tasks	Unable to solve problems at any level; trial and error behavior often observed
Affect	No change in affect reported by patient or relative	Appropriate concern with respect to symptomatology	Infrequent changes in affect (e.g. irritability) reported by patient or relative; would appear normal to objective observer	Frequent changes in affect reported by patient or relative; noticeable to objective observer	Sustained alterations of affect; impaired contact with reality observed or reported
Orientation	Fully oriented	Occasional difficulties with time relationships	Marked difficulty with time relationships	Usually disoriented to time and often to place	Oriented only to person or not at all

~duced with kind permission from Dr H Tuokko.

Dressing Performance Scale

Reference: Beck C (1988) Measurement of dressing performance in persons with dementia. *American Journal of Alzheimer's Care and Related Disorders and Research* 3: 21–5

Time taken 20 minutes (author's estimate)

Rating by carer

Main indications

To assess the dressing performance of people with dementia.

Commentary

The scale was developed specifically to address issues of dressing in people with dementia, noting that existing ADL instruments do not sufficiently encompass those aspects of function which are most often deficient in dementia, and thus not allowing for an appropriate measurement of the amount and type of assistance needed. The complex disabilities of people with dementia, such as those with apraxia, are, for example, helped if clothes are placed in the right sequence. Thus, the evaluation of ADL patients should be based on an instrument which is more discrete than simply having categories ranging from complete dependence to independence. The scale was developed following a task analysis of dressing using 34 separate components, derived from an analysis of the tasks of the types of assistance arranged into a hierarchy of categories of assistance based on the amount of caregiver involvement needed. A numerical value from 0 (no assistance) to 7 (complete assistance) was assigned. The initial study showed that changes in dressing performance could be assessed by the scale.

Content, validity and inter-rater reliability for the scale have been documented (Beck et al, 1992) and it has been shown to be sensitive to change in assessing improvements following a strategy to maximize self-care in people with dementia in nursing homes.

Additional references

Beck C, Heacock P, Mercer S, Walton C (1992) Decrease in caregiver assistance with older adults with dementia In: Funk S, Tornquist E, Champagne M (eds) Key aspects of elder care. New York: Springer, 309–19.

Beck C, Heacock P, Mercer S, Walls R, Rapp C, Volgelpohl T (1997) Improved dressing behaviour in cognitive impairment in nursing home residents. *Nursing Research* 46: 126–32.

Address for correspondence

Cornelia Beck RN PhD
Department of Psychiatry and Behavioral Sciences
College of Medicine
University of Arkansas for Medical Sciences
Little Rock, AR 72205
USA

Beck Dressing Performance Scale (Male)

Name: _____

Date: _____

Observer: _____

	Complete dependence	Complete physical guidance	Occasional physical guidance	Gestures or modeling	Repeated verbal prompt	Initial verbal prompt	Stimulus control	Independent	Not applicable
Selects appropriate clothes									
Picks up underpants									
Positions underpants appropriately									
Puts legs in underpants									
Pulls underpants to waist									
Fastens underpants									
Picks up t-shirt									
Positions t-shirt appropriately									
Puts head in opening and arms in sleeves									
Positions t-shirt correctly on body									
Picks up shirt									
Positions shirt appropriately									
Puts arms in sleeve									
Positions shirt correctly on body									
Buttons shirt									
Picks up trousers									
Positions trousers appropriately									
Puts legs in trousers									
Pulls trousers to waist									
Fastens trousers									
Puts on belt									
Fastens belt									
Picks up first sock									
Positions first sock appropriately									
Pulls first sock onto foot									
Picks up second sock									
Positions second sock appropriately									
Pulls second sock onto foot									
Picks up first shoe									
Puts first shoe on correct foot									
Picks up second shoe									
Puts second shoe on correct foot									
Ties or fastens first shoe									
Ties or fastens second shoe									

Source: Reprinted with permission from Beck C. *Am J Alzheimer's Care Rel Disord Res* 1988; **3:** 21–5.

Rapid Disability Rating Scale – 2 (RDRS-2)

Reference: **Linn MW, Linn BS (1982) The Rapid Disability Rating Scale – 2.** *Journal of the American Geriatrics Society* **30: 378–82**

Time taken 10 minutes (reviewer's estimate)

Rating anyone who knows the subject, preferably with one training session

Main indications

To assess disability in elderly people.

Commentary

The Rapid Disability Rating Scale (version 2) (RDRS-2) is a revision of the original scale described in 1967 (Linn, 1967). Changes were made, along with the clinical use of the instrument, over the intervening 15 years. In the main the changes were increasing the point rating from three to four, the emphasis was shifted to current activities and present behaviour (with the inference that it would then be more sensitive to change), and items were added about mobility, toileting and adaptive tasks. Global items relating to confusion and depression were also added. The scale measures 18 variables from none (=1) to severe (=4), giving a range of scores from 18 to 72. Elderly people living in the community with minimum disability would have a score of around 22, hospitalized elderly patients 32, and those in nursing homes 36. Some 100 patients were rated by two nurses independently, with intraclass correlation coefficients of between 0.62 and 0.98 and test/retest reliability (Pearson product moment correlation) of between 0.58 and 0.96. On factor analysis 120 institutionalized patients revealed the factors described in the scale – assistance with activities of daily living, degree of disability and degree of special problems. Validity was assessed by comparing ratings with independent physician ratings but self-report was used on health and mortality. An assessment over time was also made suggesting the scale is sensitive to change.

Additional reference

Linn MW (1967) A Rapid Disability Rating Scale. *Journal of the American Geriatrics Society* 15: 211.

Address for correspondence

MW Linn
Director, Social Science Research
Veterans Administration Medical Center
1201 Northwest 16th Street
Miami
FL 33125
USA

Rapid Disability Rating Scale – 2 (RDRS-2)

Directions: Rate what the person does to reflect current behavior. Circle one of the four choices for each item. Consider rating with any aids or prostheses normally used. None = completely independent or normal behavior. Total = that person cannot, will not, or may not (because of medical restriction) perform a behavior or has the most severe form of disability or problem.

Assistance with activities of daily living

Eating	None	A little	A lot	Spoon-feed; intravenous tube
Walking (with cane or walker if used)	None	A little	A lot	Does not walk
Mobility (going outside and getting about with wheelchair, etc., if used)	None	A little	A lot	Is housebound
Bathing (include getting supplies, supervising)	None	A little	A lot	Must be bathed
Dressing (include help in selecting clothes)	None	A little	A lot	Must be dressed
Toileting (including help with clothes, cleaning, or help with ostomy, catheter)	None	A little	A lot	Use bedpan or unable to care for ostomy/catheter
Grooming (shaving for men, hairdressing for women, nails, teeth)	None	A little	A lot	Must be groomed
Adaptive tasks (managing money/possessions; telephoning; buying newspaper, toilet articles, snacks)	None	A little	A lot	Cannot manage

Degree of disability

Communication (expressing self)	None	A little	A lot	Does not communicate
Hearing (with aid if used)	None	A little	A lot	Does not seem to hear
Sight (with glasses, if used)	None	A little	A lot	Does not see
Diet (deviation from normal)	None	A little	A lot	Fed by intravenous tube
In bed during day (ordered or self-initiated)	None	A little (<3 hrs)	A lot	Most/all of time
Incontinence (urine/feces, with catheter or prosthesis, if used)	None	Sometimes	Frequently (weekly +)	Does not control
Medication	None	Sometimes	Daily, taken orally	Daily; injection; (+ oral if used)

Degree of special problems

Mental confusion	None	A little	A lot	Extreme
Uncooperativeness (combats efforts to help with care)	None	A little	A lot	Extreme
Depression	None	A little	A lot	Extreme

Rating:

1 = none to 4 = severe
Score totals range from 18 (no disability) to 72 (most severe disabilities)

Reproduced, with permission, from Linn MW, Linn BS (1982) The Rapid Disability Rating Scale – 2. *Journal of the American Geriatrics Society*, Vol. 30, no. 6, pp. 378–82.

Functional Dementia Scale (FDS)

Reference: **Moore JT, Bobula JA, Short TB, Mischel M (1983) A Functional Dementia Scale.** *The Journal of Family Practice* **16: 499–503**

Time taken 15 minutes (reviewer's estimate)

Rating by carers

Main indications

An instrument used by families to monitor functional disability in dementia.

Commentary

The Functional Dementia Scale (FDS) contains 20 items in three subscales: activities of daily living, orientation and affect. The instrument was designed starting with 38 items in a pilot study which underwent further refinement. Cluster analysis reduced the number of items to 20, the final version being tested for reliability and validity. Inter-rater reliability was assessed on 40 patients, with agreement on over 80% of items. Test/retest reliability was 0.88, as was concurrent validity measured by existing cognitive tests, the Short Portable Mental Status Questionnaire (SPMSQ; page 64) and the SET Test (page 66).

Address for correspondence

James T Moore
Duke-Watts Family Medicine Program
407 Crutchfield Street
Durham
NC 27704–2799
USA

Functional Dementia Scale (FDS)

1. Has difficulty in completing simple tasks on own, e.g. dressing, bathing, doing arithmetic
2. Spends time either sitting or in apparently purposeless activity
3. Wanders at night or needs to be restrained to prevent wandering
4. Hears things that are not there
5. Requires supervision or assistance in eating
6. Loses things
7. Appearance is disorderly if left to own devices
8. Moans
9. Cannot control bowel function
10. Threatens to harm others
11. Cannot control bladder function
12. Needs to be watched so doesn't injure self, e.g. by careless smoking, leaving the stove on, falling
13. Destructive of materials around him, e.g. breaks furniture, throws food trays, tears up magazines
14. Shouts or yells
15. Accuses others of doing him bodily harm or stealing his possessions when you are sure the accusations are not true
16. Is unaware of limitations imposed by illness
17. Becomes confused and does not know where he/she is
18. Has trouble remembering
19. Has sudden changes of mood, e.g. gets upset, angered, or cries easily
20. If left alone, wanders aimlessly during the day or needs to be restrained to prevent wandering

Rating:
1 = None little of the time
2 = Some of the time
3 = Good part of the time
4 = Most/all of the time

Performance Test of Activities of Daily Living (PADL)

Reference: **Kuriansky J, Gurland B (1976) The Performance Test of Activities of Daily Living.** *International Journal of Aging and Human Development 7: 343–52*

Time taken 20 minutes (reviewer's estimate)

Rating by experienced interviewer

Main indications

To measure the self-care capacity of old-age psychiatry patients.

Commentary

The Performance Test of Activities of Daily Living (PADL) scale is a measure of actual performance on a series of activities in daily living functions, thus overcoming the drawback of the subjective nature of self or observer reports. Some 16 activities were measured on a total of 96 patients, 48 each in New York and London as part of the US/UK project (Copeland et al, 1976). Inter-rater reliability was 0.90 and face and content validity were apparent.

Additional reference

Copeland JRM, Kelleher MJ, Kellett JM et al (1976) A semi-structured clinical interview for the assessment of diagnosis and mental state in the elderly: the Geriatric Mental State Schedule. I. Development and reliability. *Psychological Medicine* **6**: 451–9.

Performance Test of Activities of Daily Living (PADL)

Tasks

Task requests	Props to be used
1. Drink from a cup	Cup
2. Use a tissue to wipe nose	Tissue box
3. Comb hair	Comb
4. File nails	Nail file
5. Shave	Shaver
6. Lift food onto spoon and to mouth	Spoon with candy on it
7. Turn faucet on and off	Faucet
8. Turn light switch on and off	Light switch
9. Put on and remove a jacket with buttons	Jacket
10. Put on and remove a slipper	Slipper
11. Brush teeth, including removing false ones	Toothbrush
12. Make a phone call	Telephone
13. Sign name	Paper and pen
14. Turn key in lock	Keyhole and key
15. Tell time	Clock
16. Stand up and walk a few steps and sit back down	

Sample items

Activity	Preparation	Interviewer instructions	Patient performance	Rating
Eating	Place candy on spoon and put spoon on flat surface in front of patient	'Show me how you eat'	Grasps spoon by handle	0 1 9
			Keep spoon horizontal	0 1 9
			Keeps candy balanced on spoon	0 1 9
			Aims at mouth	0 1 9
			Touches spoon to mouth	0 1 9
Grooming	Place comb on table in front of patient	'Show me how you comb your hair'	Takes comb in hand	0 1 9
			Grasps comb properly	0 1 9
			Brings comb to hair	0 1 9
			Makes combing motions	0 1 9
Dressing	Give patient jacket with sleeves	'Put this jacket on for me and then take it off'	Takes hold of jacket	0 1 9
			Slips one arm in jacket	0 1 9
			Pulls jacket over shoulders and back	0 1 9
			Slips other arm into sleeve	0 1 9
			Frees one arm	0 1 9
			Frees other arm	0 1 9
			Removes jacket from body	0 1 9

Reproduced from Kuriansky J, Gurland B (1976) The Performance Test of Activities of Daily Living. *International Journal of Aging and Human Development* **7**: 343–52, published by Baywood Publishing Co.

Structured Assessment of Independent Living Skills (SALES)

Reference: **Mahurin RK, DeBettignieis and Pirozzolo FJ (1991) Structured assessment of independent living skills: preliminary report of a peformance measure of functional abilities in dementia.** *Journal of Gerontology* **46: 58–66**

Time taken 60 minutes (reviewer's estimate)

Rating by trained interviewer

Main indications

Assessment of everyday activities affected in dementia.

Commentary

The Structured Assessment of Independent Living Skills (SALES) score is divided into a motor score (the addition of the four scales: fine motor skills, gross motor skills, dressing skills and eating skills) with a cognitive score representing the addition of expressive language, receptive language, time and orientation and money-related skills. Social interaction and mental activities are rated separately. SALES is divided into 10 subscales, each with five items rated on a three-point scale giving a maximum score of 150 points. A number of neuropsychological tests were carried out to act as markers of validity. The scale was administered to 18 patients with Alzheimer's disease and 18 controls. Test/retest for the total score was 0.81. Inter-rater reliability was 0.99. There were significant differences between the findings on the patients with Alzheimer's disease and the normal controls. Total score was correlated with the Mini-Mental State Examination (MMSE; page 36), the Global Deterioration Scale (page 236) and IQ test. There was no relation with the Geriatric Depression Scale (page 2).

Address for correspondence

Roderick K Mahurin
Alzheimer's Disease Research Center
Baylor College of Medicine
Department of Neurology
6550 Fannin – Suite 1801
Houston TX 77030
USA

Structured Assessment of Independent Living Skills (SALES)

SCORING FORM

Name: _____   Date: _____

Age: _____   Sex: _____   Handedness: _____   Education: _____   Examiner: _____

Diagnosis:

Note: If patient is unable to complete task, assign maximum time of 60" unless otherwise indicated

MOTOR TASKS

Fine Motor Skills	Time	Score

1. Picks up coins   0=drops two 1=drops one 2=slow 3=normal (8")
2. Removes wrappers   0=needs assistance 1=tears one or more 2=slow 3=normal (35")
3. Cuts with scissors   0=can't cut 1=off line 2=slow 3=normal (32")
4. Folds letter and places in envelope   0=can't fold 1=doesn't fit 2=slow 3=normal (16")
5. Uses key in lock   0=can't insert 1=can't unlock 2=slow 3=normal (13")
   Subtotal:

Gross Motor Skills	Time	Score

1. Stands up from sitting   0=unable 1=uses arms of chair 2=slow 3=normal (2")
2. Opens and walks through door   0=unable 1=needs door held open
   2=slow 3=normal (5")
3. Regular gait   0=unable 1=assistive device 2=slow 3=normal (6")
   Time 1) __ 2) __ Mean __ Steps 1) __ 2) __ Mean __
4. Tandem gait   0=unable, steps off 4 or more times 1=steps off 2–3 times
   2=slow (1 step off allowed) 3=normal (9")
   Time 1) __ 2) __ Mean __ Steps off line 1) __ 2) __ Mean __
5. Transfers object across room   0=drops 1=inaccurate placement 2=slow 3=normal (6")
   Time 1) __ 2) __ Mean __
   Subtotal:

Dressing Skills	Time	Score

1. Puts on shirt (maximum=120")   0=can't put on or button 1=misaligned
   2=slow 3=normal (86")
2. Buttons cuffs of shirt   0=unable 1=one cuff 2=slow 3=normal (45")
3. Puts on jacket   0=can't put on 1=needs help with zipper 2=slow 3=normal (27")
4. Ties shoelaces   0=unable/wrong feet 1=knot comes undone 2=slow 3=normal (9")
5. Puts on gloves   0=unable 1=one hand 2=slow 3=normal (21")
   Subtotal:

Eating Skills	Time	Score

1. Drinks from glass   0=unable 1=spits 2=slow 3=normal (3")
2. Transfers food with spoon   0=unable 1=drops 2=slow 3=normal (11")
3. Cuts with fork and knife   0=unable 1=drops 2=slow 3=normal (16")
4. Transfers food with fork   0=unable 1=drops 2=slow 3=normal (16")
5. Transfers liquid with spoon   0=unable 1=spills 2=slow 3=normal (13")
   Subtotal:

Total Motor Time _____   Total Motor Score _____

COGNITIVE TASKS

Expressive Language	Score

1. Quality of expression   0=severe < 25% 1=moderate 25–90% 2=mild 90-99% 3=intact
2. Repetition   0=no items 1=1 item 2=2 items 3=all 3 items
3. Object naming   0=3 or less 1=4 items 2=5 items 3=all 6 items
4. Writes legible note   0=illegible 1=1 item 2=2 items 3=all 3 items
5. Completes application form   0=3 or less 1=4 items 2=5 items 3=all 6 items
   Subtotal:

cont

Receptive language

Score

1. Reads and follows printed instructions   0=none 1=1 item 2=2 items 3=all 3 items
2. Understands written material   0=none 1=1-4 items 2=5 items 3=all 6 items
   Article 1: Correct 1) __ 2) __ 3)
   Article 2: Correct 1) __ 2) __ 3)
3. Understands common signs   0=none 1=1 item 2=2 items 3=all 3 items
4. Follows verbal directions   0=none 1=1 item 2=2 items 3=3 items
   1)Touch shoulder 2)Hands on table, close eyes 3)Draw circle, hand pencil, fold paper
5. Identifies named objects   0=none 1=1 item 2=2 items 3=all 3 items
   Subtotal:

Time and Orientation   Score

1. States time on clock (6:14) 0=off over 1 hour 1=off within 1 hour 2=off 10 minutes
   3=correct within 1 minute
2. Calculates time interval (until 7:30) 0=off 1 hour 1=off within 1 hour 2=off within 15 minutes
   3=correct within 1 minute
3. States time of alarm settIng (8:15) 0=off 1 hour 1=off within 1 hour 2=off within 15 minutes
   3=correct within 1 minute
4. Locates current date on calendar 0=incorrect month 1=correct month
   2=correct week 3=correct date
5. Correctly reads calendar 0=none 1=1 item 2=2 items 3=all 3 items
   1) Fridays 2) Day of 15th 3) 2nd Monday
   Subtotal:

Money-Related Skills   Score

1. Counts money 0=none 1=1 item 2=2 items 3=all 3 items
   1) 35 cents __ 2) 95 cents __ 3) $1.41 __
2. Makes change 0=none 1=1 item 2=2 items 3=all 3 items
   1) ($75 from $1.00)=S.25 __ 2) ($41 from $.50)=$.09 __
   3) ($2.79 from $5.00)=$2.21 __
3. Understands monthly utility bill 0=none 1=1 item 2=2 items 3=all 3 items
   1) (Light Co.) __ 2) ($38.46) __ 3) (3/6/87) __
4. Writes check 0=2 or less 1=3 items 2=4 items 3=all 5 items
   1)Date 2)Payee 3)Numerical amount 4)Written amount 5)Signature
5. Understands chequebook 0=none 1=1 item 2=2 items 3=all 3 items
   1)Checks on August 11 2)Check #355 3)Balance ($440.40)
   Subtotal:

Total Cognitive Score ___

Instrumental Activities   Score

1. Uses telephone book 0=none 1=1 item 2=2 items 3=all 3 items
2. Dials telephone number 0=cannot handle phone 1=misdials number
   2=needs help to read 3=correctly reads and dials
3. Understands medication label 0=none 1=1 item 2=2 items 3=all 3 items
4. Opens medication container 0=can't open two 1=can't open one 2=needs cue 3=normal
5. Follows simple recipe 0=unable 1=1 step 2=2 steps 3=all 3 steps

   Subtotal:

Social Interaction   Score

1. Responds to greeting and farewell 0=none 1=1 item 2=2 items 3=all 3 items
2. Responds to request for information 0=none 1=1 item 2=2 items 3=all 3 items
3. Responds to social directives 0=none 1=1 item 2=2 items 3=all 3 items
4. Requests needed information 0=none 1=1 item 2=2 items 3=all 3 items
5. Understanding non-verbal expression 0=none 1=1 item 2=2 items 3=all 3 items

   Subtotal:

GRAND TOTAL SCORE _____

Direct Assessment of Activities of Daily Living in Alzheimer's Disease

Reference: **Skurla E, Roger JC, Sunderland T (1988) Direct assessment of activities of daily living in Alzheimer's disease.** *Journal of the American Geriatrics Society* **36: 97–103**

Time taken 19.4 minutes

Rating by direct observation

Main indications

Assessment of activities of daily living by using a direct measure of self-care.

Commentary

Nine patients with Alzheimer's disease and nine matched normal controls were assessed using the four experimental tasks of dressing, meal preparation, telephoning and purchasing. Verbal prompts were given as necessary to help to initiate a task, as were visual and physical prompting. Each type of prompt was repeated twice. Two scores were obtained for each item. The first is a performance score rated 0–4, the second is the time required to complete each task. Significant positive correlations were found between the severity of dementia as measured by the Clinical Severity Rating and the ADL Situational Task, but a non-significant trend for a positive correlation between the latter and the test of cognitive function used the Short Portable Mental Status Questionnaire (SPMSQ; page 64). The Situational Task allowed the examiner to ascertain the nature of the impairment affecting performance and may have implications for caregiving strategies.

Performance of each subtask was scored 0–4 according to the following code: 4 = complete subtask independently; 3 = requires verbal prompting; 2 = requires verbal and visual prompting; 1 = requires verbal and physical prompting; 0 = does not complete the subtask. Maximum score for dressing is 40, for meal preparation is 36, for telephoning 44 and for purchasing 32. The subjects total raw score is then divided by the highest possible score to obtain a percentage for each ADL task. A higher percentage corresponds to better or more independent performances. Possible scores range from 0 to 152.

Direct Assessment of Activities of Daily Living in Alzheimer's Disease – ADL Situational Task

Dressing: Selecting and donning clothing for a cold, rainy day

1. Attempts to select clothing.
2. Selects appropriate clothing for weather conditions.
3. Selects adequate amount of clothing for weather.
4. Selects clothing of approximate size.
5. Attempts to put on clothing.
6. Puts on clothing in correct order.
7. Puts clothing on right side out and front forward.
8. Puts on reasonable layers of clothing.
9. Puts shoes on correct feet.
10. Buttons or snaps coat or sweater correctly.

Meal Preparation: Making a cup of instant coffee

1. Attempts to read the directions.
2. Puts an adequate amount of water in the pot.
3. Places pot on burner.
4. Turns burner on to correct temperature.
5. Opens jar.
6. Measures reasonable amount of coffee, sugar, and cream into cup.
7. Removes water from heat when hot and pours it into cup.
8. Uses caution around hot burner and pot.
9. Turns off burner.

Telephoning: Calling to find out pharmacy hours

1. Attempts to use phone book.
2. Uses alphabetized headings to find pharmacies.
3. Selects number from appropriate category.
4. Picks up the receiver before dialing.
5. Holds receiver correctly.
6. Attempts to dial the number.
7. Dials the number correctly.
8. Begins conversation when connection is made.
9. Asks appropriate questions to find out pharmacy hours.
10. Reports correct information.
11. Places receiver down correctly.

Purchasing: Using money to purchase a snack and gloves

1. Attempts to select a snack.
2. Selects an edible item for a snack.
3. Attempts to pay for snack.
4. Pays with the correct amount of change.
5. Attempts to select gloves.
6. Selects gloves that are the appropriate size.
7. Attempts to pay for the gloves.
8. Pays correct amount of money.

Refined ADL Assessment Scale (RADL)

Reference: **Tappen R (1994) Development of the refined ADL assessment scale for patients with Alzheimer's and related disorders.** *Journal of Gerontological Nursing* **20: 36–41**

Time taken 20 minutes

Rating by nurses

Main indications

Designed specifically for patients with Alzheimer's disease in the middle and later stages of the illness.

Commentary

The Refined ADL Assessment Scale (RADL) is composed of 14 separate tasks within 5 selected ADL areas (toileting, washing, grooming, dressing and eating). Each task is broken down into its component steps, the number of steps ranging from 5 to 21. The amount of time and help needed to complete the task is recorded. Reliability on 28 patients was between 50% and 90% without training and up to 100% agreement among nurse raters scoring a videotaped stimulation. Validity of the instrument was assessed by comparison with existing ADL scales (PSMS; page 221, and the Performance Test of Activities of Daily Living (PADL; page 210)). Correlations were moderate.

Additional References

Beck C (1988) Measurement of dressing performance in persons with dementia. *American Journal of Alzheimer's Care and Related Disorders and Research* **3**(3): 21–5.

Warzak WJ, Kilburn J (1990) A behavioral approach to activities of daily living. In Tupper DE, Cicerone KD (eds), *The neuropsychology of everyday life: Assessment and basic competences.* Boston: Kluwer Academic, 285–305.

Wiener JM, Hanley RJ, Clark R et al (1990) Measuring the activities of daily living: Comparisons across national surveys. *Journal of Gerontology* **45**: S229–37.

Address for correspondence

Ruth Tappen
School of Nursing
University of Miami
PO Box 248153 (5801 Red Road)
Coral Gables
FL 33124
USA

Sample Subscale from the Refined ADL Assessment Scale (RADL): Wash Hands

Given: Person standing or sitting at wheelchair-height sink. Bar of soap and paper towels at sink. Initial cue: 'Now, wash your hands.'

	Unassisted 6	Verbal Prompt 5	Nonverbal Prompt 4	Physical Guiding 3	Full Assist (Attempt Made) 2	Full Assist (No Attempt Made) 1	N/A*
Walk to sink							
Turn on water							
Place both hands in water							
Get soap							
Put soap on hands							
Put soap down							
Rub hands together							
Rinse hands							
Turn off water							
Get paper towel							
Dry hands							
Drop towel in wastebasket							
Leave bathroom							

Time to complete this action: _____ minutes.

*The N/A column (Not Applicable) is used only if the particular step is not necessary.

- Toileting: entering bathroom, using toilet facilities;
- Washing: washing hands, washing face;
- Grooming: brushing teeth, combing hair;
- Dressing: putting on pants, putting on shirt or blouse, putting on shoes; and
- Eating: cutting food, using a fork, using a spoon, drinking from a glass or cup, using a napkin.

Each of these tasks is broken down into its component steps. The number of steps ranges from 5 to 21 for a given task. The amount of time it takes the individual to complete each task is also recorded.

On the RADL, the cognitively impaired person's ability to perform each component step is rated in terms of the amount of assistance needed to complete the step successfully, ranging from unassisted to full assistance (Wiener et al, 1990).

Using a series similar to the one described by Beck (1988) and Warzak and Kilburn (1990), the individual is rated as having completed each step unassisted, with only a verbal prompt, with verbal and nonverbal prompts, with physical guiding, or with full assistance. Full assistance is rated as having been done with or without an attempt to perform the behavior. These five levels of assistance are defined as follows:

- Unassisted: done without further action on the part of the caregiver after initial cue;
- Verbal prompt: spoken directions only from caregiver;
- Nonverbal prompt: gestures, demonstration of correct behavior by caregiver;
- Physical guiding: caregiver provided some assistance with the behavior but patient participates in carrying out the step; and
- Full assistance: patient unable to contribute to carrying out the step (note whether the patient attempted the behavior).

Reproduced, with permission, from Tappen R (1994) Development of the refined ADL assessment scale for patients with Alzheimer's and related disorders. *Journal of Gerontological Nursing* 36–41.

Bayer Activities of Daily Living Scale (B-ADL)

Reference: **Hindmarch I, Lehfeld H, Jongh P (1998)** *Dementia and Geriatric Cognitive Disorders* **9 (Suppl 2): 20–6**

Time taken 20 minutes (reviewer's estimate)

Rating by caregiver

Main indications

Assessment of activities of daily living in people with mild to moderate dementia.

Commentary

The B-ADL scale was developed because of the need to measure changes in activities of daily living in the early stages of dementia. Sponsored by the pharmaceutical company Bayer, this scale was developed following an international series of field studies. One hundred and forty-one informant and 63 self-rated questionnaires were tested, and only those items sensitive to changes in early dementia and those without a significant gender of cultural bias were removed. Twenty-one items remained and a further four were added after the end of the pilot study, giving a total of 25 questions. The two introductory questions evaluate everyday activities, questions 3–20 assess direct problems in relation to specific tasks of everyday living, and the final five items relate to cognitive functions. The scoring is on a 10-point scale by asking the caregiver to draw a line through one of the appropriate circles marked 1–10. A global score is computed by summing the total score and dividing it by the number of answered items with a figure rounded to two decimal places, giving a total score of between 1.00 and 10.00. Further tests are underway to establish the reliability and validity of the scale.

Additional References

Erzigkeit H, Overall J, Stemmler M et al (1995) Assessing behavioural changes in anti-dementia therapy: perspectives of an international ADL project. In Bergener M, Brocklehurst J, Finkel S (eds), *Ageing, Health and Healing.* New York: Springer 1995, pp. 359–74.

Lehfeld H, Reisberg B, Finkel S et al (1997) Informant rated activities of daily living assessments. *Alzheimer's Disease and Associated Disorders* **1** (Suppl 4), S39–44.

Address for Correspondence

Professor Ian Hindmarch, HPRU Medical Research Centre, University of Surrey, Egerton Rd, Guildford GU2 7XP, UK

Bayer Activities of Daily Living Scale (B-ADL)

Does the person have difficulty

1. ...managing his/her everyday activities?
2. ...taking care of him/herself?
3. ...taking medication without supervision?
4. ...with personal hygiene?
5. ...observing important dates or events
6. ...concentrating on reading?
7. ...describing what he/she has just seen or heard?
8. ...taking part in a conversation?
9. ...using the telephone?
10. ...taking a message for someone else?
11. ...going for a walk without getting lost?
12. ...shopping?
13. ...preparing food?
14. ...correctly counting out money?
15. ...understanding his/her personal financial affairs?
16. ...giving directions if asked the way?
17. ...using domestic appliances?
18. ...finding his/her way in an unfamilar place?
19. ...using transportation?
20. ...participating his/her leisure activities?
21. ...continuing with the same task after a brief interruption?
22. ...doing two things at the same time?
23. ...coping with unfamiliar situations?
24. ...doing things safely?
25. ...performing a task when under pressure?

Instructions

The questions above are about everyday activities with which the patient might have difficulty. The frequency of occurrence of these difficulties are rated on a scale of 1–10 – with a rating of 1 indicating that the difficulty never arises and 10 indicating that it always arises. If the question is not applicable to the patient, or if the patient's experience of the difficulty is in anyway unclear, then these responses must be recorded too – as 'not applicable' and 'unknown' respectively. An example of this scoring is shown below:

	not applicable	unknown	SCORE
never ①②③④⑤⑥⑦⑧⑨⑩ always	☐	☐	☐

The Disability Assessment for Dementia (DAD)

Reference: **Gelinas I, Gauthier L, McIntyre M, Gauthier S (1999) Development of a functional measure for persons with Alzheimer's Disease: the Disability Assessment for Dementia.** *American Journal of Occupational Therapy* **53: 471–81**

Time taken less than 15 minutes

Rater by trained interviewer. A user guide is available to ensure proper administration and scoring of the instrument

Main indications

An assessment of functional disability for use of carers of community-dwelling persons who suffer from Alzheimer's disease. It helps clinicians and caregivers of populations with Alzheimer's disease. It helps make decisions regarding the choice of suitable interventions.

Commentary

The Disability for Assessment for Dementia Scale (DAD) has demonstrated a high degree of reliability over time and across different raters. It is practical and easy to administer, and avoids gender bias. It has a high degree of internal consistency and excellent inter-rater and test/retest reliability. It consists of 40 items, 17 related to self-care and 23 involving instrumental activities of daily living. As a research tool it is useful in describing the functional characteristics of populations with Alzheimer's disease and the course of the disease, and as an outcome variable in intervention studies.

Additional reference

Sclan SG, Reisberg B (1992) Functional Assessment Staging (FAST) in Alzheimer's disease: reliability, validity and ordinality. *International Psychogeriatrics* 4: 55–69

Address for Correspondence

Isabelle Gelinas
Assistant Professor
School of Physical and Occupational Therapy
McGill University
3654 Drummond Street
Montreal, Quebec
H3G 1Y5
Canada

The Alzheimer's Disease Functional Assessment and Change Scale (ADFACS)

Reference: Galasko D, Bennett D, Sano M et al (1997) An inventory to assess activities of daily living for clinical trials in Alzheimer's Disease. The Alzheimer's Disease co-operative study. *Alzheimer's Disease and Associated Disorders* 11 (Suppl 2): S33–9.

Time taken 20 minutes (reviewer's estimate)

Rating informant-based

Main indications

Assessment of ADL in patients with Alzheimer's Disease, with particular reference to outcomes in clinical trials.

Commentary

The Alzheimer's Disease Functional Assessment and Change Scale has been used in drug trials, and consists of 10 items for instrumental activities of daily living: ability to use the telephone, performing household tasks, using household appliances, handling money, shopping, preparing food, ability to get around both inside and outside the home, pursuing hobbies and leisure activities, handling personal mail and grasping situations or explanations.

These are rated on a five-point scale:

1 no impairment
2 mild impairment
3 moderate impairment
4 severe impairment
5 not assessable.

Basic activities of daily living are assessed on a six-point scale (an additional rating, very severe impairment, is included) – toileting, feeding, dressing, personal hygiene and grooming, physical ambulation and bathing.

The scale was developed from 45 ADL items, with the chosen items having been shown to be sensitive to change over 12 months, to correlate with the MMSE (page 36) and to have good test/retest reliability (Galasko et al, 1997).

Physical Self-Maintenance Scale (PSMS) and Instrumental Activities of Daily Living (IADL)

Reference: Lawton MP, Brody EM (1969) Assessment of older people: self-maintaining and instrumental activities of daily living. *Gerontologist 9: 179–86*

Time taken 5–10 minutes

Rater a trained rater interviewing a carer

Main indications

These two scales can be used in combination to assess both basic and more complex activities of daily living.

Commentary

The Physical Self-Maintenance Scale (PSMS) has six items, each ranked on a 0–5-point scale, with higher scores suggesting greater impairment. The items assessed are basic functions such as toileting, feeding and grooming. Loss of these abilities would suggest severe dementia. The IADL scale tends to assess abilities lost earlier in the course of dementia. The scale has eight items, three being scored on a three-point scale, three on a four-point scale and two on a five-point scale. Like the PSMS, higher scores suggest greater severity. The abilities specifically identified are lack of telephone skills, handling finances, and taking medication responsibly. The authors appreciate that this scale has items which are associated with gender stereotypes and can be difficult to assess between genders.

Physical Self-Maintenance Scale (PSMS)

Check one response to each of the following items that best describes this patient. Add the number of points and fill in the total score at the bottom.

A. Toilet
- ☐ 1. Cares for self at toilet completely; no incontinence.
- ☐ 2. Needs to be reminded, or needs help in cleaning self, or has rare (weekly at most) accidents.
- ☐ 3. Soiling or wetting while asleep more than once a week.
- ☐ 4. Soiling or wetting while awake more than once a week.
- ☐ 5. No control of bowels or bladder.

B. Feeding
- ☐ 1. Eats without assistance.
- ☐ 2. Eats with minor assistance at mealtimes and/or with special preparation of food, or helps in cleaning up after meals.
- ☐ 3. Feeds self with moderate assistance and is untidy.
- ☐ 4. Requires extensive assistance for all meals.
- ☐ 5. Does not feed self at all and resists efforts of others to feed him/her.

C. Dressing
- ☐ 1. Dresses, undresses, and selects clothes from own wardrobe.
- ☐ 2. Dresses and undresses self, with minor assistance.
- ☐ 3. Needs moderate assistance in dressing or selection of clothes.
- ☐ 4. Needs major assistance in dressing, but cooperates with efforts of others to help.
- ☐ 5. Completely unable to dress self and resists efforts of others to help.

D. Grooming (neatness, hair, nails, hands, face, clothing)
- ☐ 1. Always neatly dressed, well-groomed, without assistance.
- ☐ 2. Grooms self adequately with occasional minor assistance, e.g. shaving.
- ☐ 3. Needs moderate and regular assistance or supervision in grooming.
- ☐ 4. Needs total grooming care, but can remain well-groomed after help from others.
- ☐ 5. Actively negates all efforts of others to maintain grooming.

E. Physical Ambulation
- ☐ 1. Goes about grounds or city.
- ☐ 2. Ambulates within residence or about one block distant.
- ☐ 3. Ambulates with assistance of (check one)
  1 ( ) another person, b ( ) railing, c ( ) cane, d ( ) walker, e ( ) wheelchair
  1 _____ Gets in and out without help.
  2 _____ Needs help in getting in and out.
- ☐ 4. Sits unsupported in chair or wheelchair, but cannot propel self without help.
- ☐ 5. Bedridden more than half the time.

F. Bathing
- ☐ 1. Bathes self (tub, shower, sponge bath) without help.
- ☐ 2. Bathes self with help in getting in and out of tub.
- ☐ 3. Washes face and hands only, but cannot bathe rest of body.
- ☐ 4. Does not wash self but is cooperative with those who bathe him/her.
- ☐ 5. Does not try to wash self and resists efforts to keep him/her clean.

_____ **Total Score**

Dependence Scale

Reference: Stern Y, Albert SM, Sano M, Richards M, Miller L, Folstein M, Albert M, Bylsma FW, Laffeche G (1994) Assessing patient dependence in Alzheimer's disease. *Journal of Gerontology* 49: M216–M222

Time taken 5 minutes

Rater trained interviewer asking caregiver

Main indications

A structured scale developed for longitudinal studies of Alzheimer's dementia, to rate the degree of dependency of or assistance needed by a patient.

Commentary

There are 13 questions addressed to the caregiver. The dependence level is calculated using a separate scale that converts the scores of the 13 items into a score ranging from 0 to 5, with higher scores indicating greater dependency. A separate score can also be calculated to determine the equivalent level of institutional care needed for the patient. The score ranges from 1 (limited home care) to 3 (health-related facility). Sano et al (1997) conducted a study showing that a dependence level of 4 or 5 correlated well with dependency near the time when nursing home placement was required. The scale is sensitive to medication effects and, along with psychosis and extrapyramidal symptoms, has been used as a predictor for nursing home placement.

Additional references

Sano M, Ernesto C, Thomas RG et al (1997) A controlled trial of selegaline, alpha-tocopherol or both as treatment for Alzheimer's disease. The Alzheimer's Disease Cooperative Study. *New England Journal of Medicine* **336**: 1216–22.

Stern Y, Tang MX, Albert MS et al (1997) Predicting time to nursing home care and death in individuals with Alzheimer's disease. *Journal of the American Medical Association* **277**: 806–12.

Address for correspondence

Dr Y Stern
Department of Neurology
Columbia University College of Physicians and Surgeons
630 W 168th Street
New York
NY 10032
USA

The Alzheimer's Disease Activities of Daily Living International Scale (ADL-IS)

Reference: **Reisberg B, Finkel S, Overall J, Schmidt-Gollas N, Kanowski S, Lehfeld H, Hulla F, Sclan SG, Wilms HU, Heininger K, Hindmarch I, Stemmler M, Poon L, Kluger A, Cooler C, Bergener M, Hugonot-Diener L, Robert PH, Antipolis S, Erzigkeit H (2001) The Alzheimer's Disease Activities of Daily Living International Scale (ADL-IS).** *International Psychogeriatrics* **13: 163–81**

Time taken estimated 30 minutes

Rater caregiver completed

Main indications

An activities of daily living scale for pharmacological or other therapeutic trials in Alzheimer's disease and related dementing disorders.

Commentary

The scale consists of 40 items that include the categories of conversation; recreation; self-care; household activities; general activities; medication; social functioning; telephone; reading; organization; food preparation; travel; driving. Within each of these categories the least difficult items are listed first and the most challenging items are placed at the end. The scale is relatively free from gender and national bias and is sensitive to recipient and early (?) deficits. The 40-item scale is shown to have a 0.81 correlation with the Global Deterioration Scale, 0.81 with the Mental Status Assessment (Mini-Mental State Examination) and 0.81 with psychometric testing.

Address for correspondence

Dr Barry Reisberg
Department of Psychiatry
Ageing and Dementia Research Center
NYU Medical Center
550 First Avenue
New York 10016
USA
e-mail: barry.reisberg@med.nyu.edu

Chapter 2d

Global assessments/ quality of life

These are useful in describing, in broad terms, the severity of dementia. This can be of use in looking at a population and may be useful for measuring change. The assumption behind some of these tests is that dementia progresses in an orderly and linear form. This is clearly inaccurate, but there is still some use in identifying whether patients are mild, moderate or severely demented. The Clinical Dementia Rating (CDR; page 238) is the simplest scale, and is constructed from six domains, whereas the Global Deterioration Scale (GDS; page 236) emphasizes the signs and symptoms of dementia in the later stages of the illness. The Sandoz Clinical Assessment – Geriatric (SCAG; page 253) includes a seven-point severity rating scale after 18 questions covering a wide variety of features of dementia. The Hierarchic Dementia Scale (page 251) also rates global severity, but there has not been as much published work on it and functional and social capacity are not included. Some measures mix a variety of features together (e.g. the Mattis Dementia Scale (page 50), the Dementia Rating Scale (page 245), the GBS Scale (page 246), the PAMIE Scale (page 248), the Stockton Geriatric Rating Scale (page 250), the SCAG and the Psychogeriatric Dependency Rating Scales (PGDRS; page 243)).

Quality of life (QOL) is a difficult area to discuss because of the inherent problems in defining the term and the fact that it invariably means different things to different people. It is generally accepted that QOL in dementia is multi-faceted and one should try to individualize it. The concept of QOL for patients has been broken down into four domains: two objective and two subjective. Behavioural competence encompasses activities of daily living, cognitive performance and social behaviour, all of which can be measured. The second objective measure is the envionment, and scales such as the Social Care Environment Scale can evaluate the surroundings of a patient and rate them according to a set standard. The two subjective measures are the person's evaluation of their own environment in specific domains (e.g. housing, income, children, work) and finally a global measure of their evaluation of their own self within that environment. These two latter judgements are hard to sustain in the presence of significant cognitive impairment. As such, many of the measures in this book could be regarded as contributing to an overall QOL assessment which could be inferred from the absence of many of the disabilities measured in the scales. Specific measures of QOL

are included which attempt to summarize the concept but, in themselves, are probably not useful unless combined with other assessments of the self and the environment. The Quality of Life in Alzheimer's Disease: Patient and Caregiver Report (QOL-AD; page 232) attempts to measure QOL specifically in dementia. It is brief and addresses both the patient and the carer. Generic measures of QOL should be used with caution, although the scale described by Blau (Quality of Life in Dementia; page 229) has been used to show change in trials of drugs for Alzheimer's disease.

Global measures of change have become increasingly popular in drug trials, with the basic underlying assumption being that clinicians can detect a change in patients based on an interview without the need for formal scales. This is an inherently reasonable assumption, on which most of medicine is based. The first scale of this type was the Clinicians' Global Impression of Change (CGIC; page 240), in which patients were rated on a seven-point scale from very much improved to very much worse. This proved relatively insensitive to change, and structuring of the instruments began, driven in part by the pharmaceutical industry's attempt to provide a clinically meaningful assessment of real life change rather than relying on a change of a few points on a cognitive rating scale. This structuring spawned a number of scales (page 240), including the CIBIC and the CIBIC plus 9, in which information from an informant was provided in addition to the clinician interview. This structuring is helpful, but the downside is that the measures simply change into more rating scales rather than capturing the clinician's view of the patient. The CIBI has probably been most frequently tested and used in the recently published Aricept trials.

With the understandable emphasis on outcomes, it has become fashionable to look at changes over time in patients with cognitive impairment. Outcomes can be thought of as changes in a particular scale or scales, many of which were not designed to be sensitive to change but are used in that way in any case. Second (and easier to measure), are outcomes which are predetermined endpoints of disease such as admission to institutional care, progression to a predefined level of disability (such as the emergence of incontinence) or to a defined degree of dementia severity (say CDR 3 on the Clinical Dementia Rating). These are in addition to the ultimate outcome measure – death.

The Texas Functional Living Scale

Reference: Cullum CM, Saine K, Chan LD, Martin-Cook K, Cray KF, Weiner MF (2001) Performance-based instrument to assess functional capacity in dementia: the Texas Functional Living Scale. *Neurology, Neuropsychiatry and Behavioural Neurology* 14: 103–8

Time taken 15–20 minutes

Rating by experienced interviewer

Main indications

To measure functional abilities in dementia.

Commentary

This is a performance-based measure of functional abilities with an emphasis on instrumental activities of daily living skills. The TFLS consists of 21 items organized into five subscales: dressing, time, money, communication and memory. The ability to carry out specific activities is rated on a scale from 0 to 5.

Address for correspondence

C Munro Cullum
Department of Psychiatry
The University of Texas
Southwestern Medical Center
5323 Harry Hines Boulevard
Dallas
TX 75390-8898
USA

Sample Items from the Texas Functional Living Scale

Domain	Points	Task
Dressing	5	1. Puts on jacket
		2. Ties shoelaces
Time	15	1. States time on clock
		2. Calculates time interval on clock
		3. Sets clock
		4. Locates current date on calendar
		5. Reads calendar
Money	12	1. Counts money
		2. Pays specified amount
		3. Makes change
		4. Writes sample check
Communication	12	1. Addresses envelope
		2. Calls home
		3. Looks up designated telephone number
		4. Knows emergency telephone number
		5. Describes how to make peanut butter and jelly sandwich
Memory	8	1. Takes out three pills from bottle when timer sounds
		2. Recalls payee of check
		3. Recalls amount of check
Total	52	

Source: Cullum CM *et al. Neuropsychiatry Neuropsychology Behav Neurol* 2001; **14**: 103–8. Reproduced by permission.

EuroQol

Reference: **Brooks R (1996) EuroQol: the current state of play.** *Health Policy* **37: 53–72**

Time taken 10–15 minutes (reviewer's estimate)

Rating by self-assessment

Main indications

A non-disease specific instrument used to measure health-related quality of life.

Commentary

The EuroQol instrument is intended to complement other quality-of-life measures and to aid the collection of a common dataset for reference purposes. The instrument was devised by a small group of researchers and centres in five European countries. Studies were conducted in the UK, The Netherlands and in Sweden whereby the questionnaires were mailed to individuals selected at random on the general population. In each case Spearman's ρ was close to 1.0 and Kendal's coefficient of concordance w for the rank ordering of states across all three studies was high and significant ($w = 0.984$, $p<0.001$) – indicating broad agreement regarding the ranking of states. No specific studies have examined validity in the elderly.

Additional references

Bergner M, Bobitt RA et al (1976) The Sickness Impact Profile: conceptual formulation and methodology for the development of a health status measure. *International Journal of Health Services* **6**: 393–415.

Hunt SM, McEwen J, McKenna SP (1986) *Measuring health status.* London: Croom Helm.

Patrick DL, Bush JW, Chen MM (1973) Toward an operational definition of health. *Journal of Health and Social Behaviour* **14**: 6–23.

Rosser RM, Watts VC (1972) The measurement of hospital output. *International Journal of Epidemiology* **1**: 361–8.

The EuroQol Group (1990) EuroQol – a new facility for the measurement of health-related quality of life. *Health Policy* **16**: 199–208.

Address for correspondence

Alan Williams
Centre for Health Economics
University of York
York YO1 5DD
UK
www.euroqol.org

EuroQol Health Questionnaire

By placing a tick in one box in each group below, please indicate which statements best describe your own health state today.

Mobility
I have no problems in walking about ☐
I have some problems in walking about ☐
I am confined to bed ☐

Self-Care
I have no problems with self-care ☐
I have some problems washing or dressing myself ☐
I am unable to wash or dress myself ☐

Usual Activities (*e.g. work, study, housework, family or leisure activities*)
I have no problems with performing my usual activities ☐
I have some problems with performing my usual activities ☐
I am unable to perform my usual activities ☐

Pain/Discomfort
I have no pain or discomfort ☐
I have moderate pain or discomfort ☐
I have extreme pain or discomfort ☐

Anxiety/Depression
I am not anxious or depressed ☐
I am moderately anxious or depressed ☐
I am extremely anxious or depressed ☐

Reproduced from The EuroQol Group (1990) EuroQol – a new facility for the measurement of health-related quality of life. *Health Policy* **16**: 199–208.

Quality of Life in Dementia

Reference: **Blau TH (1977) Quality of life, social indicators, and criteria of change.**
***Professional Psychology* November, 464–73**

Time taken 15 minutes (reviewer's estimate)

Rating self-rated

Main indications

Assessment of quality of life.

Commentary

The Quality of Life in Dementia rating scale was developed to assess quality of life, based on a theoretical model of trying to distinguish between the variety of approaches to quality of life: social, economic and psychological approaches and attempts to operationalize quality of life itself. The scale was developed to assess those features regarded as important by people undergoing psychotherapy. The main reason for its inclusion here is that it has been used (adapted slightly) to measure change in quality of life in patients with Alzheimer's disease undergoing clinical trials (Rogers et al, 1996).

Additional reference

Rogers S, Friedhoff L et al (1996) The efficacy and safety of donepezil in patients with Alzheimer's disease. *Dementia* **7**: 293–303.

Quality of Life in Dementia

Evaluation

1. Working	5. Social contact
2. Leisure	6. Earning
3. Eating	7. Parenting
4. Sleeping	8. Loving
	9. Environment
	10. Self-acceptance

Score:
Rated on a line score of 0–50
 0 = Non-existent or no opportunity
10 = Minimal
30 = Adequate
50 = Best possible score

Lancashire Quality of Life Profile (Residential)

Reference: Oliver J, Mohamad H (1996) The quality of life of the chronic mentally ill: a comparison of public, private and voluntary residential provisions. *British Journal of Social Work* 22: 391–404

Time taken 90 minutes (estimate for review of component scales)

Rating by trained interviewer

Main indications

Measurement of quality of life in older people in residential care.

Commentary

The Lancashire Quality of Life Profile is an extensive instrument assessing quality of life in a number of different populations. It has been adapted for use in residential care, and work currently underway (Huxley, Challis, Burns et al, Quality of Life in Residential and Nursing Home Care, University of Manchester) will provide further information specifically on its use for elderly people in these settings.

The Quality of Life Profile is divided into objective and subjective wellbeing. A number of well accepted measures have been incorporated into the scale: life domains (Lehman, 1983), social indicators (Campbell et al, 1976; Lehman, 1983), a quality-of-life uni-scale (Spitzer and Dobson, 1981), Cantrill's ladder (Cantrill, 1965), delighted–terrible scale (Lehman, 1983), affect balance scale (Bradburn, 1969), critical incidence and disability adaptation (Flannigan, 1982), self-esteem scale (Rosenberg, 1965) and happiness scale (Bradburn, 1969).

Additional references

Bagley H, Cordingley L, Burns A, Godlove Mozley C, Sutcliffe C, Challis D, Huxley P (2000) Recognition of depression by staff in nursing and residential homes. *Journal of Clinical Nursing* 9: 445–50.

Bradburn N (1969) *The structure of psychological wellbeing.* Chicago, IL: Aldheim Publishing.

Campbell A et al (1976) Subjective measures and wellbeing. *American Psychologist* 31: 117–24.

Cantrill H (1965) *The pattern of human concerns.* New Brunswick, NJ: Rutgers.

Challis D, Godlove Mozley C, Sutcliffe C (2000) Dependency in older people recently admitted to care homes. *Age and Ageing* 29: 255–60.

Flannigan J (1982) Measurement of quality of life: current state of the art. *Archives of Physical Medicine and Rehabilitation* 63: 56–9.

Godlove Mozley C, Challis D, Sutcliffe C et al (2000) Psychiatric symptomatology in elderly people admitted to nursing and residential homes. *Aging and Mental Health* 4(2): 136–41.

Lehman A (1983) The wellbeing of chronic mental patients. *Archives of General Psychiatry* 40: 4369–73.

Oliver J, Huxley P, Bridges K et al (1996) *Quality of life in mental health Services.* London: Routledge.

Rosenberg M (1965) *Society and the adolescent image.* Princeton, NJ: Princeton University Press.

Spitzer W, Dobson A (1981) Measuring the quality of life in cancer patients. *Journal of Chronic Diseases* 34: 585–97.

Address for correspondence

Professor Peter Huxley
Institute of Psychiatry
De Crespigny Park
Denmark Hill
London SE5 8AF
UK

Lancashire Quality of Life Profile

Items included are:
Leisure/participation
Family relations
Religion
Living situation
Social relations
Health
General wellbeing

Section 1: General Wellbeing Today
Can you tell me how you feel about your life as a whole today?

Section 2: Leisure/Participation
10 questions regarding being outside, watching TV or listening to the radio. Rating of pleasure (5-point scale) associated with that.

Section 3: Family Relations
7 questions about family, children, grandchildren and contact with them.

Section 4: Religion
5 questions concerning importance of and practice of religion.

Section 5: Living Situation
10 questions regarding living arrangements, independence, privacy, food, opportunities for occupation.

Section 6: Social Relations
5 questions about friends and contacts in and outside the home.

Section 7: Health
11 questions about depression, walking, hearing and vision.

Section 8: Cantrill's Ladder
Bottom = 'Life is as bad as it could possibly be'
Top = 'Life is as good as it could possibly be'
Measured in millimetres.

Section 9: General Wellbeing
Most questions rated as 1 (very dissatisfied) – 5 (very satisfied).
Ratings of confidence in interveiew responses (reliable/mixed/unreliable) made at the end of every section.

Reproduced from Oliver J, Mohamad H (1996) The quality of life of the chronic mentally ill: a comparison of public, private and voluntary residential provisions. *British Journal of Social Work* **22**: 391–404, by permission of Oxford University Press.

Quality of Life in Alzheimer's Disease: Patient and Caregiver Report (QOL-AD)

Reference: Logsdon RG, Gibbons LE, McCurry SM, Teri L (1999) Quality of life in Alzheimer's disease: patient and caregiver reports. *Journal of Mental Health and Aging* 5: 21–32

Time taken 10 minutes each (reviewer's estimate)

Rating self and caregiver reports

Main indications

Assessment of quality of life in dementia.

Commentary

The Quality of Life in Alzheimer's Disease: Patient and Caregiver Report (QOL-AD) is a 13-item self and and caregiver measure of quality of life. Seventy-seven patients with Alzheimer's disease were assessed and ratings made of quality of life, Mini-Mental State Examination (MMSE; page 36), Activities of daily living, PSMS (page 221), depression (the Hamilton Depression Rating Scale; page 6), the Geriatric Depression Scale (page 2), and the Pleasant Events Schedule (page 341). The 13 items are rated on a 4-point scale, with 1 being poor and 4 being excellent, with a total score of between 13 and 52. To give a composite score which weights the patient rating more heavily than that of the caregiver, the patient's score is multiplied by 2, the caregiver score is multiplied by 2, the caregiver score added and the sum divided by 3. Internal consistency of the scale was good (Cronbach's alpha 0.88). Acceptable validity was found in comparison with the other instruments. Patient and caregiver quality of life were correlated, and moderate levels of cognitive impairment did not compromise reliability or validity.

Address for correspondence

Rebecca Logsdon
Psychosocial & Community Health
Box 357263
University of Washington
Seattle
WA 98195-7263
USA

Quality of Life in Alzheimer's Disease

Instructions for Interviewers

The QOL-AD is administered in interview format to individuals with dementia, following the instructions below.

Hand the form to the participant, so that he or she may look at it as you give the following instructions (instructions should closely follow the wording given in **bold type**):

I want to ask you some questions about your quality of life and how you rate different aspects of your life using one of four words; poor, fair, good, or excellent.

Point to each word (poor, fair, good, and excellent) on the form as you say it.

When you think about your life, there are different aspects, like your physical health, energy, family, money, and others. I'm going to ask you to rate each of these areas. We want to find out how you feel about your current situation in each area.

If you're not sure about what a question means, you can ask me about it. If you have difficulty rating any item, just give it your best guess.

It is usually apparent whether an individual understands the questions, and most individuals who are able to communicate and respond to simple questions can understand the measure. If the participant answers all questions the same, or says something that indicates a lack of understanding, the interviewer is encouraged to clarify the question. However, under no circumstances should the interviewer suggest a specific response. Each of the four possible responses should be presented, and the participant should pick one of the four.

If a participant is unable to choose a response to a particular item or items, this should be noted in the comments. If the participant is unable to comprehend and/or respond to two or more items, the testing may be discontinued, and this should be noted in the comments.

As you read the items listed below, ask the participant to circle her/his response. If the participant has difficulty circling the word, you may ask her/him to point to the word or say the word, and you may circle it for him or her. You should let the participant hold his or her own copy of the measure, and follow along as you read each item.

cont.

1. First of all, how do you feel about your physical health? Would you say it's. poor, fair, good, or excellent? Circle whichever word you think beat describes your physical health right now.

2. How do you feel about your energy level? Do you think it is poor, fair, good, or excellent? If the participant says that some days are better than others, ask him or her to rate how she/he has been feeling most of the time lately.

3. How has your mood been lately? Have your spirits been good, or have you been feeling down? Would you rate your mood as poor, fair, good, or excellent?

4. How about your living situation? How do you feel about the place you have now? Would you say it's poor, fair, good, or excellent?

5. How about your memory? Would you say it is poor, fair, good, or excellent?

6. How about your family and your relationship with family members? Would you describe it as poor, fair, good, or excellent? If the respondent says they have no family, ask about brothers, sisters, children, nieces, nephews.

7. How do you feel about your marriage? How is your relationship with (spouse's name). Do you feel it's poor, fair, good, or excellent? Some participants will be single, widowed, or divorced. When this is the case. ask how they feel about the person with whom they have the closest relationship, whether it's a family member or friend. If there is a family caregiver, ask about their relationship with this person. If there is no one appropriate, or the participant is unsure, score the item as missing.

8. How would you describe your current relationship with your friends? Would you say it's poor, fair, good, or excellent? If the respondent answers that they have no friends, or all their friends have died, probe further. Do you have anyone you enjoy being with besides your family? Would you call that person a friend? It the respondent still says they have no friends, ask how do you feel about having no friends – poor, fair, good, or excellent?

9. How do you feel about yourself – when you think of your whole self and all the different things about you, would you say it's poor, fair, good, or excellent?

10. How do you feel about your ability to do things like chores around the house or other things you need to do? Would you say it's poor, fair, good, or excellent?

11. How about your ability to do things for fun, that you enjoy? Would you say it's poor, fair, good, or excellent?

12. How do you feel about your current situation with money, your financial situation? Do you feel it's poor, fair, good, or excellent? If the respondent hesitates, explain that you don't want to know what their situation is (as in amount of money), just how they feel about it

13. How would you describe your life as a whole. When you think about your life as a whole, everything together, how do you feel about your life? Would you say it's poor, fair, good, or excellent?

UWMC/ADPR/QOL
Aging and Dementia: Quality of Life in AD
Quality of Life: AD
(Participant Version)

ID Number   Assessment Number   Interview Date
☐☐☐☐☐☐   ☐☐   ☐☐   ☐☐   ☐☐
                                                                 Month   Day   Year

Instructions: Interviewer administer according to standard instructions.
Circle participant responses.

1.	Physical health.	Poor	Fair	Good	Excellent
2.	Energy.	Poor	Fair	Good	Excellent
3.	Mood.	Poor	Fair	Good	Excellent
4.	Living situation.	Poor	Fair	Good	Excellent
5.	Memory.	Poor	Fair	Good	Excellent
6.	Family.	Poor	Fair	Good	Excellent
7.	Marriage.	Poor	Fair	Good	Excellent
8.	Friends.	Poor	Fair	Good	Excellent
9.	Self as a whole.	Poor	Fair	Good	Excellent
10.	Ability to do chores around the house	Poor	Fair	Good	Excellent
11.	Ability to do things for fun.	Poor	Fair	Good.	Excellent
12.	Money.	Poor	Fair	Good	Excellent
13.	Life as a whole.	Poor	Fair	Good	Excellent

Comments:

Scale continued overleaf

UWMC/ADPR/QOL
Aging and Dementia: Quality of Life in AD
Quality of Life: AD
(Family Version)

ID Number

☐☐☐☐☐☐

Assessment Number

☐☐

Interview Date

☐☐   ☐☐   ☐☐
Month   Day   Year

Instructions: Please rate your relative's current situation, as you see it.
Circle your responses.

1.	Physical health.	Poor	Fair	Good	Excellent
2.	Energy.	Poor	Fair	Good	Excellent
3.	Mood.	Poor	Fair	Good	Excellent
4.	Living situation.	Poor	Fair	Good	Excellent
5.	Memory.	Poor	Fair	Good	Excellent
6.	Family.	Poor	Fair	Good	Excellent
7.	Marriage.	Poor	Fair	Good	Excellent
8.	Friends.	Poor	Fair	Good	Excellent
9.	Self as a whole.	Poor	Fair	Good	Excellent
10.	Ability to do chores around the house	Poor	Fair	Good	Excellent
11.	Ability to do things for fun.	Poor	Fair	Good	Excellent
12.	Money.	Poor	Fair	Good	Excellent
13.	Life as a whole.	Poor	Fair	Good	Excellent

Comments:

Reproduced with kind permission from Dr L Teri.

Functional Assessment Staging (FAST)

Reference: **Reisberg B (1988) Functional assessment staging (FAST).** *Psychopharmacology Bulletin* **24:** 653–9

Time taken 2 minutes (once all the information is gathered)

Rating by clinician, after interview with informant

Main indications

Assessment of funtional change in ageing and dementia.

Commentary

The Functional Assessment Staging (FAST) is a rating scale which can be used as part of the Global Deterioration Scale (GDS; page 236). It rates functional change in seven major stages with a total of 16 successive stages and substages. Reliability of the FAST has been demonstrated with intraclass correlations of above 0.85. Concurrent validity has been assessed against the GDS and a number of neuropsychological tests (Reisberg et al, 1994). It has been shown that functional detriments in Alzheimer's disease proceed in a hierarchial ordinal pattern reflecting the FAST stages (Sclan and Reisberg, 1992). A particular advantage of the FAST is that it identifies a total of 11 substages according to the later stages

of the GDS and so is particularly useful in the detailed staging and substaging of severe Alzheimer's disease.

Additional references

Reisberg B (1986) Dementia: a systematic approach to identifying reversible causes. *Geriatrics* **41:** 30–46.

Reisberg B et al (1994) Dementia staging in chronic care populations. *Alzheimer Disease and Associated Disorders* **8:** S188–S205.

Sclan S, Reisberg B (1992) FAST in Alzheimer's disease; reliability, validity and ordinality. *International Psychogeriatrics* **4** (Suppl 1): 55–69.

Address for correspondence

Barry Reisberg
Department of Psychiatry
Aging and Dementia Research Center
NYU Medical Center
550 First Avenue
NY 10016, USA
www.geriatric-resources.com/html/fast.html

Functional Assessment Staging (FAST)

Yes	Months[1]	No.		
—	——	—	1.	No difficulties, either subjectively or objectively.
—	——	—	2.	Complains of forgetting location of objects; subjective work difficulties.
—	——	—	3.	Decrease job functioning evident to coworkers; difficulty in traveling to new locations.
—	——	—	4.	Decreased ability to perform complex tasks (e.g. planning dinner for guests; handling finances; marketing)
—	——	—	5.	Requires assistance in choosing proper clothing.
—	——	—	6a.	Difficulty putting clothing on properly.
—	——	—	6b.	Unable to bathe properly; may develop fear of bathing.
—	——	—	6c.	Inability to handle mechanics of toileting (i.e. forgets to flush, doesn't wipe properly).
—	——	—	6d.	Urinary incontinence.
—	——	—	6e.	Fecal incontinence.
—	——	—	7a.	Ability to speak limited (1 to 5 words a day).
—	——	—	7b.	All intelligible vocabulary lost.
—	——	—	7c.	Nonambulatory.
—	——	—	7d.	Unable to sit up independently.
—	——	—	7e.	Unable to smile.
—	——	—	7f.	Unable to hold head up.

TESTER: _____ COMMENTS: _____

Note: Functional staging score = Highest ordinal value. [1]Number of months FAST stage deficit has been noted.

Reproduced from Reisberg B (1988) Functional assessment staging (FAST). *Psychopharmacology Bulletin* **24:** 653–9.

Global Deterioration Scale (GDS)

Reference: **Reisberg B, Ferris SH, de Leon MJ, Crook T (1982) The Global Deterioration Scale (GDS) for assessment of primary degenerative dementia.** *American Journal of Psychiatry* 139: 1136–9

Time taken 2 minutes (once information has been collected)

Rating by clinician

Main indications

A staging instrument indicating deterioration in dementia.

Commentary

The Global Deterioration Scale (GDS) is the main part of a clinical rating system called the Global Deterioration Scale Staging System. Three independent measures are included in the Staging System: the GDS, the Brief Cognitive Rating Scale (BCRS; page 61) and the Functional Assessment Staging measure (FAST; page 235). The GDS is made up of detailed clinical descriptions of seven major clinically distinguishable stages, ranging from normal cognition to very severe dementia. Concurrent validity of the GDS has been demonstrated by a highly significant correlation between ratings and other neuropsychological tests such as the Mini-Mental State Examination (MMSE; page 36) (Reisberg et al, 1988). Content validity of the GDS was demonstrated independently by developing a 30-item questionnaire which, following a principal components analysis, clustered naturally into stages corresponding with GDS descriptions (Overall et al, 1990).

Inter-rater and test/restest reliability has been demonstrated regularly at over 0.90 in terms of both test/retest and inter-rater reliability (Reisberg et al, 1996). It has a wide number of uses as a staging measure in descriptive and intervention studies.

Additional references

Overall J, Scott J, Rhodes H, Lesser J (1990) Empirical scaling of the stages of cognitive decline in senile dementia. *Journal of Geriatric Psychiatry and Neurology* **3**: 212–20.

Reisberg B, Ferris S, Schulman E et al (1986) Longitudinal course of normal aging and progressive dementia of the Alzheimer's type: a prospective study of 106 subjects over a 3.6 year mean interval. *Progress in Neuro-psychopharmacology and Biological Psychiatry* **10**: 571–8.

Reisberg B et al (1988) Stage specific behavioural cognitive and in vivo changes in community residing subjects with AAMI and AD. *Drug Development Research* **15**: 101–4.

Reisberg B et al (1993) Clinical stages of normal ageing in Alzheimer's disease: the GDS staging system. *Neuroscience Research Communications* **13**: 551–4.

Reisberg B et al (1996) Overview of methodologic issues for pharmacologic trials in mild, moderate and severe Alzheimer's disease. *International Psychogeriatrics* **8**: 159–93.

Address for correspondence

Barry Reisberg
Department of Psychiatry
Aging and Dementia Research Center
NYU Medical Center
550 First Avenue
New York 10016
USA

e-mail: barry.reisberg@med.nyu.edu

Global Deterioration Scale (GDS)

1. No subjective complaints of memory deficit. No memory deficit evident on clinical interview.

2. Subjective complaints of memory deficit, most frequently in following areas:
   (a) forgetting where one has placed familiar objects.
   (b) forgetting names one formerly knew well.

3. Earliest clear-cut deficits.

   Manifestations in more than one of the following areas:
   (a) patient may have gotten lost when travelling to an unfamiliar location.
   (b) co-workers become aware of patient's relatively poor performance.
   (c) word and/or name finding deficit become evident to intimates.
   (d) patient may read a passage or book and retain relatively little material.
   (e) patient may demonstrate decreased facility remembering names upon introduction to new people.
   (f) patient may have lost or misplaced an object of value.
   (g) concentration deficit may be evident on clinical testing.

4. Clear-cut deficit on careful clinical interview.
   Deficit manifest in following areas:
   (a) decreased knowledge of current and recent events.
   (b) may exhibit some deficit in memory of one's personal history.
   (c) concentration deficit elicited on serial subtractions.
   (d) decreased abilty to travel, handle finances, etc.

   Frequently no deficit in following areas:
   (a) orientation to time and place.
   (b) recognition of familiar persons and faces.
   (c) ability to travel to familiar locations.

5. Patient can no longer survive without some assistance.

   Patient is unable during interview to recall a major relevant aspect of their current life, e.g.:
   (a) their address or telephone number of many years.
   (b) the names of close members of their family (such as grandchildren).
   (c) the name of the high school or college from which they graduated.

6. May occasionally forget the name of the spouse upon whom they are entirely dependent for survival.
   Will be largely unaware of all recent events and experiences in their lives.
   Retain some knowledge of their surroundings; the year, the season, etc.
   May have difficulty counting by 1s from 10, both backward and sometimes forward.

   Will require some assistance with activities of daily living:
   (a) may become incontinent.
   (b) will require travel assistance but occasionally will be able to travel to familiar locations.

   Diurnal rhythm frequently disturbed.
   Almost always recall their own name.
   Frequently continue to be able to distinguish familiar from unfamiliar persons in their environment.

   Pesonality and emotional changes occur. These are quite variable and include:
   (a) delusional behavior, e.g. patients may accuse their spouse of being an imposter; may talk to imaginary figures in the environment , or to their own reflection in the mirror.
   (b) obsessive symptoms, e.g. person may continually repeat simple cleaning activities.
   (c) anxiety symptoms, agitation, and even previously non-existent violent behavior may occur.
   (d) cognitive abulia, e.g. loss of willpower because an individual cannot carry a thought long enough to determine a purposeful course of action.

7. All verbal abilities are lost over the course of this stage.
   Early in this stage words and phrases are spoken but speech is very circumscribed.
   Later there is no speech at all – only grunting.

   Incontinent; requires assistance toileting and feeding.

   Basic psychomotor skills (e.g. ability to walk) are lost with the progression of this stage.
   The brain appears to no longer be able to tell the body what to do.
   Generalized and cortical neurologic signs and symptoms are frequently present.

Source: *American Journal of Psychiatry*, Vol. 139, pp. 1136–1139, 1982. Copyright 1982, the American Psychiatric Association. Reprinted by permission. The GDS is copyrighted. Copyright © 1983 by Barry Reisberg, MD. All rights reserved.

Clinical Dementia Rating (CDR)

Reference: **Hughes CP, Berg L, Danziger WL, Coben LA, Martin RL (1982) A new clinical scale for the staging of dementia.** *British Journal of Psychiatry* **140: 566–72; updated by Morris J (1993) The CDR: current version and scoring rules.** *Neurology* **43: 2412–3.**

Time taken the scale is usually completed in the setting of a detailed knowledge of the individual patient. As such, much of the information will already have been gathered, either as part of normal clinical practice or as part of a research study. If a separate interview is carried out, about 40 minutes is needed to gather the relevant information.

Rating by a clinician using information gathered as part of clinical practice

Main indications

A global measure of dementia.

Commentary

The Clinical Dementia Rating (CDR) has now become one of the gold standards of global ratings of dementia in trials of patients with Alzheimer's disease. Six domains are assessed: memory; orientation; judgement and problem solving; community affairs; home and hobbies; and personal care. CDR ratings are 0 for healthy people, 0.5 for questionable dementia and 1, 2 and 3 for mild, moderate and severe dementia as defined in the scale. The total CDR rating is made from the sum of boxes which represents an aggregate score of each individual's areas. Inter-rater reliability was excellent (correlation coefficient 0.89). The original study included 58 healthy controls and 59 people with dementia. A number of different scales were used in an interview with the spouse and subject, taking about 90 minutes in total. The Blessed Dementia Scale (page 46) (Blessed et al, 1968), the Face–Hand Test (FHT; page 75) (Zarit et al, 1978) and the Short Portable Mental Status Questionnaire (SPMSQ; page 64) were used, and highly significant correlation was found between these tests and the final CDR rating.

The reliability of the CDR has been further established (Berg et al, 1988). Longitudinal data are available on its use (e.g. Berg et al, 1992; Galasko et al, 1995) and it has been validated against neuropathological information (Morris et al, 1988).

Additional references

Berg L, Miller J, Baty A et al (1992) Mild senile dementia of Alzheimer type. *Annals of Neurology* **31**: 242–9.

Berg L, Miller JP, Storandt M et al. (1988) Mild senile dementia of the Alzheimer type: 2. Longitudinal assessment. *Annals of Neurology* **23**: 497–84.

Blessed G, Tomlinson B, Roth M (1968) The association between quantitative measures and dementia and senile change in the cerebral grey matter of elderly subjects. *British Journal of Psychiatry* **114**: 797–811.

Burke W, Miller P, Rueben E et al (1988) Reliability of the Washington University Clinical Dementia Rating. *Archives of Neurology* **45**: 31–2.

Galasko D, Edland S, Morris J et al (1995) The consortium to establish a registry for Alzheimer's disease. Part 11. Clinical milestones in patients with Alzheimer's disease followed over 3 years. *Neurology* **45**: 1451–5.

Morris J, McKeel D, Fulling K et al (1988) Validation of clinical diagnostic criteria for Alzheimer's disease. *Annals of Neurology* **24**: 17–22.

Pfeiffer E (1975) A short portable mental state questionnaire for the assessment of organic brain deficit in elderly patients. *Journal of the American Geriatrics Society* **23**: 433–41.

Zarit S, Miller N, Khan R (1978) Brain function, intellectual impairment and education in the aged. *Journal of the American Geriatrics Society* **26**: 58–67.

Address for correspondence

J Morris
Memory and Aging Project
Washington University School of Medicine
660 South Euclid Avenue
PO Box 8111
St Louis
MO 63110
USA
www.adrc.wustl.edu/adrc/cdrScale.html

Clinical Dementia Rating (CDR)

	Impairment				
	None 0	Questionable 0.5	Mild 1	Moderate 2	Severe 3
Memory	No memory loss or slight inconstant forgetfulness	Consistent slight forgetfulness; partial recollection of events; 'benign' forgetfulness	Moderate memory loss; more marked for recent events; defect interferes with everyday activities	Severe memory loss; only highly learned material retained; new material rapidly lost	Severe memory loss; only fragments remain
Orientation	Fully oriented	Fully oriented except for slight difficulty with time relationships	Moderate difficulty with time relationships; oriented for place at examination; may have geographic disorientation elsewhere	Severe difficulty with time relationships; usually disoriented to time, often to place	Oriented to person only
Judgment and Problem Solving	Solves everyday problems and handles business and financial affairs well; judgment good in relation to past performance	Slight impairment in solving problems, similarities, and differences	Moderate difficulty in handling problems, similarities, and differences; social judgment usually maintained	Severely impaired in handling problems, similarities, and differences; social judgment usually impaired	Unable to make judgments or solve problems
Community Affairs	Independent function at usual level in job, shopping, and volunteer and social groups	Slight impairment in these activities	Unable to function independently at these activites although may still be engaged in some; appears normal to casual inspection	No pretense of independent function outside home Appears well enough to be taken to functions outside a family home	Appears too ill to be taken to functions outside a family home
Home and Hobbies	Life at home, hobbies, and intellectual interests well maintained	Life at home, hobbies, and intellectual interests slightly impaired	Mild but definite impairment of function at home; more difficult chores abandoned; more complicated hobbies and interests abandoned	Only simple chores preserved; very restricted interests, poorly maintained	No significant function in home
Personal Care	Fully capable of self-care		Needs prompting	Requires assistance in dressing, hygiene, keeping of personal effects	Requires much help with personal care; frequent incontinence

Rating:

Score only as decline from previous usual level due to cognitive loss, not impairment due to other factors

Reproduced from the *British Journal of Psychiatry*, Hughes CP, Berg L, Danziger WL, Coben LA, Martin RL (1982) A new clinical scale for the staging of dementia. Vol. 140, pp. 566–72. © 1982 Royal College of Psychiatrists. Reproduced with permission.

Clinicians' Global Impression of Change

Reference: **Guy W (ed) (1976) Clinical Global Impressions (CGI). In:** *ECDEU Assessment Manual for Psychopharmacology.* **US Department of Health and Human Services, Public Health Service, Alcohol Drug Abuse and Mental Health Administration, NIMH Psychopharmacology Research Branch, 218–22.**

Time taken varies: 10–40 minutes

Rating by trained rater

Main indications

Global ratings.

Commentary

These measures depend on the ability of a clinician to detect change. By definition, they are global ratings of a patient's clinical condition, and inevitably draw information from a wide variety of sources. These scales have been used extensively in clinical trials of anti-dementia drugs, and assess change from a specified baseline. Only minimal conditions are provided, and the rating is made by choosing and response. The various scales are summarized in the table.

Additional references

Knopman D et al (1994) The Clinician Interview-Based Impression (CIBI): a clinician's global change rating scale in Alzheimer's disease. *Neurology* **44**: 2315–21.

Schneider LS, Olin JT (1996) Clinical global impressions in Alzheimer's clinical trials. *International Psychogeriatrics* **8**: 277–88.

Schneider LS et al (1997) Validity and reliability of the Alzheimer's Disease co-operative study – clinical global impression of change. *Alzheimer Disease and Associated Disorders* **11**: S22–32.

Selected Global Impressions of Change scales used in clinical trials

Clinicians' Global Impression of Change (CGIC) (Guy, 1976)
- Also used as a general term for various impressionistic measures, rated by the clinician, based on interviews with or without a collateral source, with or without reference to mental status examination, and with or without reference to cognitive assessment results
- Rated on 7 points: 1 = very much improved; 2 = much improved; 3 = minimally improved; 4 = no change; 5 = minimally worse; 6 = much worse; 7 = very much worse.

FDA Clinicians' Interview-Based Impression of Change (CIBIC)
- FDA modifications to the CGIC suggested that clinical change should be patient interview only
- Access to other sources of information is prevented to minimize bias and maintain independence. During a 10-minute interview, the clinician should systematically assess the domains ordinarily considered part of a clinical examination.
- Rationale: if an experienced clinician can perceive clinical change on the basis of an interview, then such change is likely to be clinically meaningful.
- Various constructions have been made by different companies.

Clinicians' Interview-Based Impression of Change – Plus (CIBIC+)
- A CIBIC as described above except conducted by interviewing both the patient and informant has come to be known as CIBIC+.

CIBI (Parke–Davis) (Schneider and Olin, 1997; Knopman et al, 1997)
- Thorough interviews of the patient and caregiver by a clinician

experienced in managing AD patients, require that 8 specific items be addressed, including assessment of mental status.
- A follow-up interview solely with the patient prior to making a change rating.
- Rating is made on a 7-point ordinal scale similar to the CGIC.
- Interviewer is required to assess patient's history, strengths and weaknesses, language, behaviors sensitive to change, motivation, activities of daily living, and anything else of apparent importance.

ADCS-CGIC (Schneider et al, 1997)[1]
- Assesses 15 areas under the domains of cognition, behavior, and social and daily functioning.
- Using a form as a guideline, both patient and caregiver are interviewed; order is not specified.
- Under each area is a list of sample probes and space for notes. There are few requirements for the interviews – an assessment of mental status must be made; clinicians are not permitted to ask about side effects, nor to discuss the patient's functioning with others.
- Change rating is made on the 7-point CGIC scale.

NYU CIBIC+
- Relatively more structured than the previous instruments, requiring separate interviews with the patient to assess cognition and with the caregiver to assess functional activities.
- Uses elements of previously validated assessments of cognition, daily functional activities, and behavior.
- Additional descriptors are provided for the 7-point scale so that for a 1-point minimal rating, change must be 'detectable'; for a 2-point moderate rating, change must be 'clearly apparent', and for a 3-point marked rating, change must be 'dramatic'.

From Schneider LS (1997) An overview of rating scales used in dementia reseaerch, *Alzheimer Insights* – Special Edition, pp. 8–14.

Crichton Royal Behavioural Rating Scale (CRBRS)

Reference: **Robinson RA (1961) Some problems of clinical trials in elderly people.**
Gerontologia Clinica **3: 247–57**

Time taken 10–15 minutes (reviewer's estimate)

Rating by informant

Main indications

For the assessment of psychogeriatric patients.

Commentary

The original paper by Robinson (1961) was a description of a scale used in clinical practice. It contains no data but is a masterpiece of clinical description. The Crichton Royal Behavioural Rating Scale (named after Crichton Royal Hospital in Dumfries, Scotland) has been used in a number of different studies and is available in a self-completed version or one to be used with informants (Wilkin and Thompson, 1989). The main scale items are: mobility, memory, orientation, communication, cooperation, restlessness, dressing, feeding, bearing and continence. A confusion subscale has been described which is the sum of the memo-ry orientation and communication scales, and has been found separately to be a reliable and easy method to identify the presence of dementia (Vardon and Blessed, 1986). Validity has been shown to be good when compared to cognitive tests, and construct validity and internal consistence have also been measured (Wilkin and Thompson, 1989). Inter-rater reliability is excellent (Cole, 1989).

Additional references

Cole M (1989) Inter-rater reliability of the Crichton Geriatric Behaviour Rating Scale. *Age and Ageing* 18: 57–60.

Vardon VM, Blessed G (1986) Confusion ratings and abbreviated mental test performance: a comparison. *Age and Ageing* 15: 139–44.

Wilkin D, Thompson C (1989) Crichton Royal Behavioural Rating Scale. In *User's guide to dependency measures in elderly people. Social Services Monographs.* Sheffield: University of Sheffield.

Crichton Royal Behavioural Rating Scale (CRBRS)

Score	1 Mobility	2 Orientation	3 Communication	4 Co-operation	5 Restlessness
1	Fully ambulant (including stairs)	Complete	Always clear and retains information	Actively co-operative	None
2	Usually independent (not stairs)	Orientated in ward and identifies persons correctly	Can indicate needs. Can understand simple verbal directions. Can deal with simple information	Passively co-operative	Intermittent
3	Walks with supervision	Misidentifies persons and surroundings but can find way about	Understands simple verbal and non-verbal information but does not indicate needs	Requires frequent encouragement and/or persuasion	Persistent by day
4	Walks with artificial aids or under careful supervision	Cannot find way to bed or to toilet without assistance	Cannot understand simple verbal or non-verbal information but retains some expressive ability	Rejects assistance and shows some independent but poorly directed activity	Persistent by day with frequent nocturnal restlessness
5	Bedfast or mainly so, Chairfast	Lost	No effective contact	Completely resistive or withdrawn	Constant

6 Dressing	7 Feeding	8 Cotinence	9 Sleep	10 Mood Objective	11 Subjective
Dresses correctly unaided	Feeds correctly unaided at appropriate times	Fully continent	Normal (hypnotic not required)	Normal and stable affective response and appearance	Well-being or euphoria
Dressing imperfect but adequate	Feeds adequately with minimum supervision	Nocturnal incontinence unless toileted. Occasional accident (urine or faeces)	Requires occasional hypnotic; or occasionally restless	Fair affective response; or not always appropriate or stable	Self-reproachful, listless, dejected, indecisive, lacks interest. (Not completely well though no specific complaints)
Dressing adequate with minimum supervision	Does not feed adequately unless continually supervised	Continent by day if regularly toileted	Sleeps well with regular hypnotic; or usually restless for a period every night	Marked blunting or impairment of mood or inappropriateness of affect	Marked somatic or hypochondriacal concern. Preoccupation
Dressing inadequate unless continually supervised	Defective feeding because of physical handicap or poor appetite	Urinary incontinence in spite of regular toileting	Occasionally disturbed in spite of regular standard hypnotic	Emotional lability or incontinence of affect. Retarded, lacks spontaneity but can respond	Severe retardation or agitation. Marked withdrawal though responds to questioning
Unable to dress or retain clothing because of mental impairment	Unable to feed because of mental impairment	Regularly/ frequently doubly incontinent	Disturbed even with heavier sedation	Hallucinations or nihilistic delusions of guilt or somatic dysfunction	Suicidal or death wishes. Mute, or agitated to the point of incoherence

Psychogeriatric Dependency Rating Scales (PGDRS)

Reference: **Wilkinson IM, Graham-White J (1980) Psychogeriatric Dependency Rating Scales (PGDRS). A method of assessment for use by nurses.** *British Journal of Psychiatry* 137: 558–65

Time taken 20 minutes (reviewer's estimate)

Rating by staff

Main indications

Measure of dependency in elderly patients.

Commentary

The rationale behind the development of the Psychogeriatric Dependency Rating Scales (PGDRS) was specifically to use the knowledge of nurses dealing with psychogeriatric patients in as informed a way as possible to measure orientation, behaviour and physical problems in inpatients, emphasizing the need to define dependency (i.e. nursing time demanded by the patient). Reliability and validity information were presented on over 600 patients. Inter-rater reliability was 0.61 for the orientation items, 0.48 for the behaviour and 0.58 for the physical items. The scales have good face validity and reliability validated against independent judgements of nursing time demanded against diagnosis. A shorter version of the scales was also devised.

Psychogeriatric Dependency Rating Scales (PGDRS)

1. Orientation

Yes	No	
☐	☐	Name in full
☐	☐	Age (years)
☐	☐	Relatives – recognize
☐	☐	Realtives – name
☐	☐	Staff – recognize
☐	☐	Staff – name
☐	☐	Bedroom
☐	☐	Dining room
☐	☐	Bathroom
☐	☐	Belongings

2. Behaviour

N	O	F	
☐	☐	☐	Disruptive
☐	☐	☐	Manipulating
☐	☐	☐	Wandering
☐	☐	☐	Socially Objectionable
☐	☐	☐	Demanding Interaction
☐	☐	☐	Communication Difficulties
☐	☐	☐	Noisy
☐	☐	☐	Active Aggression
☐	☐	☐	Passive Aggression
☐	☐	☐	Verbal Aggression
☐	☐	☐	Restless
☐	☐	☐	Destructive – Self
☐	☐	☐	Destructive (Property)
☐	☐	☐	Affect – Elated
☐	☐	☐	Delusions/Hallucinations
☐	☐	☐	Speech Content

3. Physical

Hearing
- ☐ Full
- ☐ Slight
- ☐ Severe
- ☐ Deaf

Visual
- ☐ Full
- ☐ Slight
- ☐ Severe
- ☐ Blind

Speech
- ☐ Full
- ☐ Slight
- ☐ Severe
- ☐ Dumb

Mobility
- ☐ Full
- ☐ Stairs
- ☐ Aids
- ☐ Assistance
- ☐ Chairfast
- ☐ Bedfast

Dressing
- ☐ Full
- ☐ Verbal
- ☐ Partial
- ☐ Assistance

Personal Hygiene

Verbal guidance

		Physical assistance
☐	Oral	☐
☐	Washes	☐
☐	Cleans*	☐
☐	Hair	☐
☐	Bath entry	☐

*after toileting

N	O	F	
☐	☐	☐	Requires Toiletting
☐	☐	☐	Urine – Day
☐	☐	☐	Urine – Night
☐	☐	☐	Faeces – Day
☐	☐	☐	Faeces – Night
☐	☐	☐	Feeding

Special Physical Disabilities: (specify)

Rating:

N = Never
O = Occasionally = 2/5 days or less
F = Frequently = 3/5 days or more

Reproduced from the *British Journal of Psychiatry*, Wilkinson IM, Graham-White J (1980) Psychogeriatric Dependency Rating Scales (PGDRS). A method of assessment for use by nurses. Vol. 137, pp. 558–65. © 1980 Royal College of Psychiatrists. Reproduced with permission.

Dementia Rating Scale

Reference: **Lawson JS, Rodenburg M, Dykes JA (1977) A Dementia Rating Scale for use with psychogeriatric patients.** *Journal of Gerontology* **32: 153–9**

Time taken 20–25 minutes (reviewer's estimate)

Rating by observer

Main indications

Evaluation of global functioning in dementia.

Commentary

The Dementia Rating Scale is a 27-item scale rated on a simple yes/no response. Inter-rater reliability was 0.95. Test/retest reliability was above 0.59 (depending on time lapse), and internal consistency was assessed using split half reliability and found to be 0.86. A factor analysis revealed eight factors, four accounting for 50% of the variance. The scale was able to differentiate between patients with organic and functional illness.

Dementia Rating Scale

1. Disorientation to place
    (Where are you now? If the patient fails to reply or gives irrelevant reply – Are you in a school, a church, a hospital or a house? Only the alternative 'hospital' earns a zero score.)
2. Disorientation to people
    (Ability to distinguish staff from patients scores zero.)
3. Disorientation to time
    (Year.)
4. Disorientation to time
    (Month.)
5. Disorientation to time
    (Day.)
6. Disorientation to time of day
    (Morning, afternoon, evening. Consider meals – lunch and supper as cut-off points.)
7. Disorientation to inside surroundings
    (Inability to find bathroom.)
8. Disorientation to own age
    (Within five years earns zero score.)
9. Loss of personal identity
    (Patient does not know whom he is.)
10. Eating
    (Inability to feed himself without assistance for reasons other than physical illness.)
11. Dressing
    (Inability to dress himself without assistance for reasons other than physical illness.)
12. Incontinence
    (Incontinence of urine during the day.)
13. Sleep
    (Repeat of PRN hypnotic required.)
14. Wandering
    (Patient roams aimlessly through the hospital or ward.)
15. Motor restlessness
    (Pacing or agitated behavior for other than physical reasons.)
16. Slowing of motor function
    (For other than physical reasons.)
17. Motor perseveration
    (Purposeless repetition of a movement.)
18. Verbal perseveration
    (Purposeless repetition of a syllable, word or phase.)
19. Echopraxia
    (Copies the movement of others.)
20. Echoalia
    (Copies verbal utterances of others.)
21. Emotional lability
    (Inappropriate and sudden change of emotional expression.)
22. Catastrophic reaction
    (Affect of inappropriate intensity in response to inconsequential events.)
23. Aggression
24. Inability to write own name
    (Cannot sign name for other than physical reasons.)
25. Inability to read
    (Cannot read 'The grass is green' for other than physical reasons.)
26. Linguistic expression
    (Noticeable difficulty in word finding or object naming.)
27. Understanding
    (Inability to understand spoken word.)

Rating:
Score 'I' if pathology is present; otherwise score '0'

GBS Scale

Reference: **Gottfries CG, Bråne G, Steen G (1982) A new rating scale for dementia syndromes. *Gerontology* 28: 20–31**

Time taken 30 minutes

Rating by trained observer

Main indications

To rate the degree of physical inactivity, impairment of intellectual and emotional capacities and behavioural symptoms common in dementia.

Commentary

The GBS Scale is divided into four subscales in order to estimate the motor, intellectual and emotional functions and symptom characteristics of the dementia syndromes. Its aim is that information is collected for a quantitative measure of dementia rather than a diagnosis. The reliability of the scale was tested on 100 patients and found to be between 0.83 and 0.93. Validity was from correlation with another geriatric rating scale (the Gottfries–Gottfries Scale, quoted by the authors).

Address for correspondence

CG Gottfries
Department of Psychiatry and Neurochemistry
St Jörgens Hospital
S-422 03 Hisings Backa
Sweden

GBS Scale

MOTOR FUNCTIONS

1. Motor insufficiency in undressing and dressing
2. Motor insufficiency in taking food
3. Impaired physical activity
4. Deficiency of spontaneous activity
5. Motor insufficiency in managing personal hygiene
6. Inability to control bladder and bowel

INTELLECTUAL

1. Impaired orientation in space
2. Impaired orientation in time
3. Impaired personal orientation
4. Impaired recent memory
5. Impaired distant memory
6. Impaired wakefulness
7. Impaired concentration
8. Inability to increase tempo
9. Absentmindedness
10. Longwindedness
11. Distractability

EMOTIONAL FUNCTIONS

1. Emotional blunting
2. Emotional lability
3. Reduced motivation

DIFFERENT SYMPTOMS COMMON IN DEMENTIA

1. Confusion
2. Irritability
3. Anxiety
4. Agony
5. Reduced mood
6. Restlessness

Instructions: Assess the condition of the patient as it has been during the most recent period, using the following questionnaire (__ weeks __ days). For each question the patient can score 0, 2, 4 or 6 points. Mark with a cross the alternative answer which in your view corresponds to the condition of the patient. If the condition of the patient does not correspond to any one of the defined alternatives but lies somewhere between them, mark alternative 1, 3 or 5. For three variables, it is also possible to mark 9 = patient not testable. By repeated ratings – do it every day at the same time.

Geriatric Rating Scale (GRS)

Reference: Plutchik R, Conte H, Lieberman M, Bakur M, Grossman J, Lehrman N (1970) Reliability and validity of a scale for assessing the functioning of geriatric patients. *Journal of the American Geriatrics Society* 18: 491–500

Time taken 20–25 minutes (reviewer's estimate)

Rating by observer, no special training needed

Main indications

The assessment of behavioural problems and functional ability of geriatric patients.

Commentary

The Geriatric Rating Scale (GRS) was developed after identification of key areas by professionals and review of existing scales, in particular the Stockton Geriatric Rating Scale (page 250). The study was carried out on 281 in-patients, data being obtained on 207. Inter-rater reliability was 0.87, and validity was assessed by the ability of the individual items to differentiate between the 30 highest ranking and 30 lowest ranking subjects in terms of overall functioning in comparing the results with non-geriatric patients. Independent ratings by clinicians confirmed the accuracy of the scale in evaluating functioning of patients.

Geriatric Rating Scale (GRS)

1. When eating, the patient requires.
2. The patient is incontinent.
3. When bathing or dressing, the patient needs.
4. The patient will fall from his bed or chair unless protected by side rails.
5. With regard to walking, the patient.
6. The patient's vision, with or without glasses, is.
7. The patient's hearing is.
8. With regard to sleep, the patient.
9. During the day, the patient sleeps.
10. With regard to restless behavior at night, the patient is.
11. The patient's behavior is worse at night than in the daytime.
12. When not helped by other people, the patient's appearance is.
13. The patient masturbates or exposes himself publicly.
14. The patient is confused (unable to find his way around the ward, loses his possessions, etc.).
15. The patient knows the names of.
16. The patient communicates in any manner (by speaking, writing, or gestering) well enough to make himself easily understood.
17. The patient reacts to his own name.
18. The patient plays games, has hobbies, etc.
19. The patient reads books or magazines on the ward.
20. The patient will begin conversations with others.
21. The patient is willing to do things asked of him.
22. The patient helps with chores on the ward.
23. Without being asked, the patient physically helps other patients.
24. With regard to friends on the ward, the patient.
25. The patient talks with other people on the ward.
26. The patient has a regular work assignment.
27. The patient is destructive of materials around him (breaks furniture, tears up magazines, etc.)
28. The patient disturbs other patients or staff by shouting or yelling.
29. The patient steals from other patients or staff members.
30. The patient *verbally* threatens to harm other patients or staff.
31. The patient *physically* tries to harm other patients or staff.

Patients are scored on a scale of 0–2, with 0 indicating never, none or no, and 2 indicating often, many or extremely

---

PAMIE Scale

Reference: **Gurel L, Linn MW, Linn BS (1972) Physical and mental impairment-of-function evaluation in the aged: the PAMIE Scale.** *Journal of Gerontology* 27: 83–90

Time taken 45 minutes

Rating by a nurse familiar with the patient

Main indications

The quantitative description of behaviours in geriatric patients and those with mental illness.

Commentary

The PAMIE Scale was developed to meet the need for an instrument which would allow a comprehensive behavioural evaluation of the disabilities of a heterogeneous group of patients going from hospital to nursing home care. The instrument was based on two previous scales, the Self-Care Inventory (SCI) (Gurel and Davis, 1967), which looked at the areas of ambulation, feeding, dressing, toileting and bathing; and the 43-item Patient Evaluation Scale (PES) (Gurel, 1968), which looked at particular dimensions such as impairment in ambulation,

self-care, dependency, verbal hostility, bedfastness, sensory motor impairment, mental disorganization and co-operation. The PAMIE Scale focused on information from both these scales, but also included deteriorated appearance, withdrawal and apathy, anxiety, depression and paranoia. Factor analysis revealed 10 factors (self-care, irritability, confusion, anxiety-depression, bedridden-moribund, behavioural deterioration, paranoid ideas, psychomotor disability, withdrawal-apathy, mobility) plus a special items section. Validation was with the Cumulative Illness Rating Scale.

Additional references

Gurel L (1968) Community resources and VA outplacement. In *Proceedings of 13th Annual Conference VA Cooperative Studies in Psychiatry*. Denver, April 1968. Washington DC: Veterans Administration, 85–9.

Gurel L, Davis JE Jr (1967) A survery of self-care dependency in psychiatric patients. *Hospital and Community Psychiatry* 18: 135–8.

PAMIE Scale

1. **Which of the following best fits the patient?**
   Has no problem in walking
   Slight difficulty in walking, but manages. May use cane
   Great difficulty in walking, but manages. May use crutches or stroller
   Uses wheelchair to get around by himself
   Uses wheelchair pushed by others
   Doesn't get around much, mostly or completely bedfast, or restricted to chair

2. **As far as you know, has the patient had one or more strokes (C.V.A.)**
   No stroke
   Mild stroke(s)
   Serious stroke(s)

3. **Which of the following best fits the patient?**
   In bed all almost all day
   More of the waking day in bed, than out of bed
   About half of the waking day in bed, and about half out of bed
   More of the waking day out of bed than in bed
   Out of bed all or almost all day

4.	Eats a regular diet	YES	NO
5.	Is given bed baths	YES	NO
6.	Gives sarcastic answers	YES	NO
7.	Takes a bath/shower without help or supervision	YES	NO
8.	Leaves his clothes unbuttoned	YES	NO
9.	Is messy in eating	YES	NO
10.	Is irritable and grouchy	YES	NO
11.	Keeps to himself	YES	NO
12.	Say he's not getting good care and treatment	YES	NO

scale continued opposite

13.	Resists when asked to do things	YES	NO
14.	Seems unhappy	YES	NO
15.	Doesn't make much sense when talks to you	YES	NO
16.	Acts as though he has a chip on his shoulder	YES	NO
17.	Is IV or tube fed once a week or more	YES	NO
18.	Has one or both hands/arms missing or paralyzed	YES	NO
19.	Is cooperative	YES	NO
20.	Is toileted in bed by catheter and/or enema	YES	NO
21.	Is deaf or practically deaf, even with hearing aid	YES	NO
22.	Ignores what goes on around him	YES	NO
23.	Knows who he is and where he is	YES	NO
24.	Gives the staff a 'hard time'	YES	NO
25.	Blames other people for his difficulties	YES	NO
26.	Says, without good reason, that he's being mistreated or getting a raw deal	YES	NO
27.	Gripes and complains a lot	YES	NO
28.	Says other people dislike him, or even hate him	YES	NO
29.	Says he has special or superior abilities	YES	NO
30.	Has hit someone or been in a fight in last six months	YES	NO
31.	Eats without being closely supervised or encouraged	YES	NO
32.	Says he's blue and depressed	YES	NO
33.	Isn't interested in much of anything	YES	NO
34.	Has taken his clothes off at the wrong time or place during the last six months	YES	NO
35.	Makes sexually suggestive remarks or gestures	YES	NO
36.	Objects or gives you an argument before doing what he's told	YES	NO
37.	Is distrustful and suspicious	YES	NO
38.	Looks especially neat and clean	YES	NO
39.	Seems unusually restless	YES	NO
40.	Says he's going to hit people	YES	NO
41.	Receives almost constant safety supervision (for careless smoking, objects in mouth)	YES	NO
42.	Looks sloppy	YES	NO
43.	Keeps wandering off the subject when you talk with him	YES	NO
44.	Is noisy, talks very loudly	YES	NO
45.	Does things like brush teeth, comb hair, and clean nails without help or urging	YES	NO
46.	Has shown up drunk or brought a bottle on the ward	YES	NO
47.	Cries for no obvious reason	YES	NO
48.	Says he would like to leave the hospital	YES	NO
49.	Wets or soils once a week or more	YES	NO
50.	Has trouble remembering things	YES	NO
51.	Has one or both feet/legs missing or paralyzed	YES	NO
52.	Walks flight of steps without help	YES	NO
53.	When needed, takes medication by mouth	YES	NO
54.	Is easily upset when little things go wrong	YES	NO
55.	Uses the toilet without help or supervision	YES	NO
56.	Conforms to hospital routine and treatment program	YES	NO
57.	Has much difficulty in speaking	YES	NO
58.	Sometimes talks out loud to himself	YES	NO
59.	Chats with other patients	YES	NO
60.	Is shaved by someone else	YES	NO
61.	Seems to resent it when asked to do things	YES	NO
62.	Dresses without any help or supervision	YES	NO
63.	Is often demanding	YES	NO
64.	When left alone, sits and does nothing	YES	NO
65.	Says others are jealous of him	YES	NO
66.	Is confused	YES	NO
67.	Is blind or practically blind, even with glasses	YES	NO
68.	Decides things for himself, like what to wear, items from canteen (or canteen cart), etc	YES	NO
69.	Swears, uses vulgar or obscene words	YES	NO
70.	When you try to get his attention, acts as though lost in a dream world	YES	NO
71.	Looks worried and sad	YES	NO
72.	Most people would think him a mental patient	YES	NO
73.	Shaves without any help or supervision, other than being given supply	YES	NO
74.	Yells at people when he's angry or upset	YES	NO
75.	Is dressed or has his clothes changed by someone	YES	NO
76.	Gets own tray and takes it to eating place	YES	NO
77.	Is watched closely so he doesn't wander	YES	NO

Stockton Geriatric Rating Scale

Reference: **Meer B, Baker JA (1966) The Stockton Geriatric Rating Scale.** *Journal of Gerontology* **21: 392–403**

Time taken 10–15 minutes

Rating by nurse carer

Main indications

Rating of needs based on behaviour, physical and mental functioning.

Commentary

The Stockton Geriatric Rating Scale was designed to assess behaviour of a geriatric patient in a hospital setting. The original paper also wished to describe the significant dimensions of the behaviour of patients on a long-stay ward. Over 1000 patients in the Stockton State Hospital were assessed using the scale, and a factor analysis was carried out identifying four factors: physical disability, apathy, communication failure and socially irritating behaviour. Inter-rater reliability of the four factors ranged from 0.7 (communication failure) to 0.88 (physical disability). Validity has been assessed according to outcome.

Stockton Geriatric Rating Scale

1. The patient will fall from his bed or chair unless protected by side rails or soft ties (day or night).
2. The patient helps out on the ward (other than a regular work assignment).
3. The patient understands what you communicate to him (you may use speaking, writing, or gesturing).
4. The patient is objectionable to other patients *during the day* (loud or constant talking, pilfering, soiling furniture, interfering in affairs of others).
5. Close supervision is necessary to protect the patient, due to feebleness, from other patients.
6. The patient keeps self occupied in constructive or useful activity (works, reads, play games, has hobbies, etc.).
7. The patient communicates in any manner (by speaking, writing, or gesturing).
8. The patient engages in repetitive vocal sounds (yelling, moaning, talking, etc.) which are directed to no one in particular or to everyone.
9. When bathing or dressing, the patient requires.
10. The patient socializes with other patients.
11. The patient knows his own name.
12. The patient threatens to harm other patients, staff, or people outside the hospital *either* verbally (e.g. 'I'll get him') *or* physically (e.g. raising of fist).
13. The patient is able to walk.
14. The patient, without being asked, physically helps one or more patients in various situations (pushing wheel chair, helping with food tray, assisting in shower, etc.).
15. The patient wants to go home or leave the hospital.
16. The patient is objectionable to other patients *during the night* (loud or constant talking, pilfering, soiling furniture, interfering in affairs of others, wandering about, getting into some other patient's bed, etc.).
17. The patient is incontinent of urine and/or feces (day or night).
18. The patient takes the initiative to *start* conversations with others (exclude side remarks not intended to open conversations).
19. The patient *accuses* others (patients, staff, or people outside the hospital) of doing him bodily harm or stealing his personal possessions (if you are *sure* the accusations are true, rate zero; otherwise rate one or two).
20. The patient is able to feed himself.
21. The patient has a regular work assignment.
22. The patient is destructive of materials around him (breaks furniture, tears up magazines, sheets, clothes, etc.).

Patients are scored on a scale of 0–2, with 0 indicating never, none or no, and 2 indicating often, many or extremely

---

Hierarchic Dementia Scale

Reference: **Cole MG, Dastoor DP, Koszycki D (1983) The Hierarchic Dementia Scale.** *Journal of Clinical Experimental Gerontology* **5: 219–34**

Time taken 15–30 minutes

Rating by observer

Main indications

To assess cognitive performance over a wide range of disabilities including reflexes and comprehension.

Commentary

The Hierarchic Dementia Scale allows the rapid identification of the highest level of performance for each of 20 mental functions. Being able to start at an appropriate level to that of patient allows problems arising from the presence of physical, sensory or emotional handicaps, fatigue and irritability to be overcome. Validation studies were performed on 50 patients with dementia (Alzheimer's disease and multi-infarct dementia) against the Blessed Dementia Scale (page 46) and the Crichton Royal Geriatric Rating Scale (page 241). Inter-rater reliability was 0.89 and test/retest reliability 0.84. Cronbach's alpha was 0.97. The maximum score for the whole scale is 200. A person with very mild dementia would score around 160; someone with very severe dementia scores less than 40.

Additional reference

Cole M, Dastoor D (1987) A new hierarchic approach to the management of dementia. *Psychosomatics* **28**: 258–304.

Ronnberg L, Ericsson K (1994) Reliability and validity of the Hierarchic Dementia Scale. *International Psychogeriatrics* **6**: 87–94.

Address for correspondence

Martin G Cole
St Mary's Hospital Center
3830 Avenue Lacombe
Montreal PQ
H3T 1M5
Canada

The Hierarchic Dementia Scale

1. Orienting
10. No impairment
8. Shakes examiner's hand
6. Reacts to auditory threat
4. Reacts to visual threat
2. Reacts to tactile threat

2. Prefrontal
10. None
8. Tactile prehension
6. Cephalobuccal reflex
4. Orovisual reflex
2. Oral tactile reflex

3. Ideomotor
10. Reversed hands
9. Double rings
8. Double fingers
7. Opposed hands
6. Single ring
5. Single finger
4. Clap hands
3. Wave
2. Raise hands
1. Open mouth

4. Looking
10. Finds images
8. Searches for images
6. Grasps content of picture
4. Scans picture
2. Looks at picture

5. Ideational
10. Imaginary match and candle
9. Imaginary nail and hammer
8. Imaginary scissors
7. Imaginary comb
6. Match and candle
5. Nail and hammer
4. Scissors
3. Comb
2. Put on shoes
1. Open door

6. Denomination
10. No errors
9. Nominal aphasia – parts

cont.

8. Nominal aphasia – objects
7. Use of parts
6. Use of objects
5. Conceptual field – parts
4. Conceptual field – objects
3. Sound alike – parts
2. Sound alike – objects
1. Deformed words

7. Comprehension
Verbal:
5. Close eyes and touch left ear
4. Clap hands three times
3. Touch your right eye
2. Touch your nose
1. Open mouth
Written:
5. Close eyes and touch left ear
4. Clap hands three times
3. Touch your right eye
2. Touch your nose
1. Open mouth

8. Registration
10. Spoon, candle, scissors, button whistle
8. Spoon, candle, scissors, button
6. Spoon, candle, scissors
4. Spoon, candle
2. Spoon

9. Gnosis
10. Superimposed words
9. Sumperimposed images
8. Digital gnosis
7. Right-left – examiner
6. Right-left – self
5. Body parts – examiner
4. Body parts – self
3. Touch (pinch) 5 cm
2. Touch (pinch) 5 to 15 cm
1. Response to touch (pinch)

10. Reading
10. Paragraph
8. Paragraph with error(s)
6. The cat drinks milk
4. Receive
2. M

11. Orientation
10. Date
8. Month
6. Year of birth
4. Morning or afternoon
2. First name

12. Construction
10. Four blocks diagonal
8. Four blocks square
6. Two blocks diagonal
4. Two blocks square
2. Form board circle

13. Concentration
10. Serial 7s (100, 93,...)
9. Serial 3s (30, 27,...)
8. Months of year backward
7. Days of week backward
6. 93 to 85
5. 10 to 1
4. Months of year forward
3. Days of week forward
2. 1 to 10

1. Actual counting

14. Calculation
10. 43 – 17
9. 56 + 19
8. 39 – 14
7. 21 + 11
6. 15 – 6
5. 18 + 9
4. 9 – 4
3. 8 + 7
2. 2 – 1
1. 3 + 1

15. Drawing
10. Cube
9. Cube (difficulty with perspective)
8. Two rectangles
7. Circle and square
6. Rectangle
5. Square
4. Circle inside circle
3. Circle
2. Line
1. Scribble

16. Motor
10. No impairment
9. Increased muscle tone – repeated
8. Increased muscle tone – initial
7. Loss of rhythm
6. Loss of associated movements
5. Contractures of legs
4. Kyphosis
3. Vertical restriction of eye movement
2. Nonambulatory
1. Lateral restriction of eye movement

17. Remote memory
10. Amount of pension
8. Number of grandchildren
6. Year of marriage or of first job
4. Father's occupation
2. Place of birth

18. Writing
Form:
5. Flowing style
4. Loss of flow
3. Letters misshapen
2. Repetition or substitution of letters
1. Scribble
Content:
5. No error
4. Word substitution
3. Missing preposition
2. Missing verb or noun
1. Missing 3 or 4 words

19. Similarities
10. Airplane – bicycle
8. Gun – knife
6. Cat – pig
4. Pants – dress
2. Orange – banana

20. Recent memory
10. All five
8. Any four
6. Any three
4. Any two
2. Any one

Reprinted from Cole MG, Dastoor DP, Koszycki D, *Journal of Experimental Gerontology*, **5**, 219–234, by courtesy of Marcel Dekker Inc.

Sandoz Clinical Assessment – Geriatric (SCAG)

Reference: **Shader RI, Harmatz JS, Salzman C (1974) A new scale for clinical assessment in geriatric populations: Sandoz Clinical Assessment – Geriatric (SCAG).** *Journal of the American Geriatrics Society* **22:** 107–13

Time taken 15–20 minutes (reviewer's estimate)

Rating by anyone familiar with the patient; training is required

Main indications

Assessment of psychopathology in older people.

Commentary

The Sandoz Clinical Assessment – Geriatric (SCAG) represents one of the early scales for the assessment of older people based on the assumption that many similar scales used for geriatric psychopharmacologic research are not used specifically with the elderly (Salzman et al, 1972). The original study was described in two parts. One was on 51 geriatric subjects (25 volunteers and 26 hospital inpatients) where the SCAG was rated against an existing measure, the Mental Status Examination Record (Spitzer and Endicott, 1971). The second was an assessment of inter-rater reliability on eight subjects by four psychiatrists. The first study showed good differentiation using the SCAG scale between four groups of individuals: health, minimum dementia, depression and severe dementia. Good separation was found between the groups. Inter-rater reliability resulted in an average intraclass correlation coefficient of 0.75.

Additional references

Salzman C, Kochansky GE, Shader IR (1972) Rating scales for geriatric psychopharmacology – a review. *Psychopharmacology Bulletin* **8**: 3.

Spitzer R, Endicott IJ (1971) An integrated group of forms for automated psychiatric case records. *Archives of General Psychiatry* **24**: 540.

Address for correspondence

Richard I Shader
Department of Pharmacology and Experimental Therapeutics
Tufts University School of Medicine
136 Harrison Avenue
Boston
MA 02111
USA

Sandoz Clinical Assessment – Geriatric (SCAG)

1. CONFUSION: Lack of proper association for surroundings, persons and time not with it. Slowing of thought processes and impaired comprehension, recognition and performance; disorganization. Rate on patient's response and on reported episodes since last interview.
2. MENTAL ALERTNESS: Reduction of attentiveness, concentration, responsiveness, alacrity, and clarity of thought, impairment of judgement and ability to make decisions. Rate on structured questions and response at interview.
3. IMPAIRMENT OF RECENT MEMORY: Reduction in ability to recall recent events and actions of importance to the patient, e.g. visits by members of family, content of meals, notable environmental changes, personal activities. Rate on structured pertinent questions and not on reported performance.
4. DISORIENTATION: Reduced awareness of place and time, identification of persons including self. Rate on response to questions at interview only.
5. MOOD DEPRESSION: Dejected, despondent, helpless, hopeless, preoccupation with defeat or neglect by family or friends, hypochondriacal concern, functional somatic complaints, early waking. Rate on patient's statements, attitude and behavior.
6. EMOTIONAL LABILITY: Instability and inappropriateness of emotional response, e.g. laughing or crying or other undue positive or negative response to non provoking situations as the interviewer sees them.
7. SELF CARE: Impairment of ability to attend to personal hygiene, dressing, grooming, eating and getting about. Rate on observation of patient at and outside interview situation and not on statements of patients.
8. ANXIETY: Worry, apprehension, overconcern for present or future, fears, complaints of functional somatic symptoms, e.g. headache, dry mouth, etc. Rate on patient's own subjective experience and on physical signs, e.g. trembling, sighing, sweating, etc. if present.
9. MOTIVATION INITIATIVE: Lack of spontaneous interest in initiating or completing task, routine duties and even attending to individual needs. Rate on observed behavior rather than patient's statements.
10. IRRITABILITY (Cantankerousness): Edgy, testy, easily frustated, low tolerance threshold to aggravation and stress or challenging situations. Rate on patient's statements and general attitude at interview.
11. HOSTILITY: Verbal aggressiveness, animosity, contempt, quarrelsome, assaultive. Rate on impression at interview and patient's observed attitude and behavior towards others.
12. BOTHERSOME: Frequent unnecessary requests for advice or assistance, interference with others, restlessness. Rate on behavior at and outside the interview situation.
13. INDIFFERENCE TO SURROUNDINGS: Lack of interest in everyday events, pasttimes and environment where interest previously existed, e.g. news, TV, heat, cold, noise. Rate on patient's statements and observed behavior during and outside the interview situation.
14. UNSOCIABILITY: Poor relationships with others, unfriendly, negative reaction to social and communal recreational activities, aloof. Rate on observed behavior and not patient's own impression.
15. UNCOOPERATIVENESS: Poor compliance with instructions or requests for participation. Performance with ill-grace, resentment or lack of consideration for others. Rate on attitudes and responses at interview and observed behavior outside interview situation.
16. FATIGUE: Sluggish, listless, tired, weary, worn out, bushed. Rate on patient's statements and observed responses to normal daily activities outside interview situation.
17. APPETITE (Anorexia): Disinclination for food, inadequate intake, necessity for dietary supplements, loss of weight. Rate on observed attitude towards eating, food intake encouragement required and loss of weight.
18. DIZZINESS: In addition to true vertigo, dizziness in this context includes spells of uncertainty of movement and balance, subjective sensations in the head apart from pain, e.g., lightheadedness. Rate on physical examination as well as patient's subjective experience.
19. OVERALL IMPRESSION OF PATIENT: Considering your total clinical experience and knowledge of the patient, indicate the patient's status at this time, taking into account physical, psychic and mental functioning.

Rating:
1 = not present
2 = very mild
3 = mild
4 = mild to moderate
5 = moderate
6 = moderatly severe
7 = severe

Reproduced from Shader RI, Harmatz JS, Salzman C, A new scale for clinical assessment in geriatric populations: Sandoz Clinical Assessment – Geriatric (SCAG). *Journal of the American Geriatrics Society*, Vol. 22, no. 3, pp. 107–113.

Comprehensive Psychopathological Rating Scale (CPRS)

Reference: **Bucht G, Adolfsson R (1983) The Comprehensive Psychopathological Rating Scale in patients with dementia of Alzheimer type and multiinfarct dementia.** *Acta Psychiatrica Scandinavica* **68: 263–70**

Time taken 20 minutes (reviewer's estimate)

Rating by clinician

Main indications

The assessment of neuropsychiatric features of dementia in patients with Alzheimer's disease and multi-infarct dementia.

Commentary

The Comprehensive Psychopathological Rating Scale (CPRS) is an extensive scale measuring a wide range of symptoms and signs. A subscale of items commonly seen in dementia was taken from the larger scale and two additional items – recent memory and long-term memory – were added. A three-point severity rating scale was used on 18 patients with Alzheimer's disease and 20 with multiinfarct dementia.

Additional reference

Åsberg M, Perris CP, Schalling D et al (1978) The CPRS – development and applications of a psychiatric rating scale. *Acta Psychiatrica Scandinavica* **(Suppl)**: 271.

Address for correspondence

G Bucht
Umea Dementia Research Group
Department of Geriatric Medicine and Geriatric Psychiatry
University Hospital
Umea
Sweden

Comprehensive Psychopathological Rating Scale (CPRS)

Reported items

1.	Sadness
2.	Elation
4.	Hostile feelings
5.	Inability to feel
6.	Pessimistic thoughts
7.	Suicidal thoughts
14.	Lassitude
15.	Fatiguability
16.	Concentration difficulties
17.	Failing memory
19.	Reduced sleep
20.	Increased sleep
24.	Aches and pains
26.	Loss of sensation or movement
31.	Ideas of persecution
38.	Other auditory hallucinations
40.	Other hallucinations

Observed items

41.	Apparent sadness
42.	Elated mood
43.	Hostility
44.	Labile emotional response
47.	Sleepiness
48.	Distractability
50.	Perplexity
52.	Disorientation
55.	Specific speech defects
58.	Perseveration
59.	Overactivity
60.	Slowness of movement
61.	Agitation
62.	Involuntary movements
64.	Mannerisms and postures
65.	Hallucinatory behaviour
66.	Global rating of illness
68.	Recent memory
69.	Long-term memory

Scaling from 0 to 3 on all items. Use of half-steps recommended

---

Validity and Reliability of the Alzheimer's Disease Co-operative Study – Clinical, Global Impression of Change (ADCS-CGIC)

Reference: **Schneider L, Olin J, Doody R et al (1997) Validity and reliability of the Alzheimer's Disease co-operative study – clinical global impression of change.** *Alzheimer's Disease and Associated Disorders* 11 (suppl 2): S22–33

Time taken about 40 minutes

Rating by trained rater, with at least one year's experience in clinical trials

Main indication

Rating of global changes in Alzheimer's disease.

Commentary

The ADCS-CGIC consists of three parts: a baseline interview with the patient and informant, a follow-up interview and a rating review by the clinician. Raters are required to

have one year's experience of making global ratings in clinical trials. The rating is made on a seven point scale:

1 marked improvement
2 moderate improvement
3 minimal improvement
4 no change
5 minimal worsening
6 moderate worsening
7 marked worsening

Validity and reliability data presented for the ADCS-CGIC are excellent, and satisfactory correlations are found between the instrument and The MMSE (page 36), CDR (page 238), Global Deterioration Scale (page 236) and FAST (page 235).

Instructions for Administration of the Alzheimer's Disease Cooperative Study-Clinical Global Impression of Change (ADCS-CGIC)

The ADCS-GCIC consists of two parts: Part I, baseline evaluation (includes information from both subjects and informant); Part II, ADCS-GCIC forms for both subject and informant.

The overall intent of the ADCS-CGIC is to provide a reliable means to assess global change from baseline in a clinical trial. It provides a semistructured format to enable clinicians to gather necessary clinical information from both the patient and informant to make a global impression of clinical change.

Part I is used to record baseline information to serve as a reference for future ratings. Part II is composed of two sections, a subject interview form and an informant interview form. These forms are used to record information from separate interviews with both subject and informant from which an impression of change score is made.

Method of Administration

Baseline Evaluation:
At baseline, the clinician interviews the patient and caregiver, recording onto Part I notes about baseline status for later reference. At baseline only, clinical information about the subject from any source can be used. The clinician indicates on a checklist the sources of information compiled during the baseline evaluation.

Parts I and II share a similar format for recording relevant clinical information. The column headed "Areas" identifies various areas that a clinician might consider while evaluating a patient for potential clinical change, including what might be expected to be assessed in performing an ordinary but brief comprehensive office interview to determine a subject's baseline status and eligibility for a clinical trial.

The "Probes" column provides sample items that a clinician might find useful in assessing an area, and these are intended as guides for collecting relevant information. The last column provides space for notes. For the baseline form, there are separeate spaces for notes taken from the informant and patient interviews.

There is no specified amount of time to complete the baseline form.

Follow-up visits:
Part II is administered at each follow-up visit. At each follow-up visit, the order of interviews should be the same for all participants, with all subjects being interviewed first or, alternatively, all informants being interviewed first.

After completing the interviews, the clinician records the clinical impression of change on a 7-point Likert-type scale (from marked improvement to marked worsening). The ADCS-CGIC is a rating of change and not of severity. The clinician may refer to the baseline data in Part I.

The clinician, alone, must make decisions about change, without consulting other staff. The clinician should avoid asking opinions of the interviewee, which may contaminate the ratings, such as opinions regarding change in symptoms or side effects. At the beginning of the interview, the clinician may wish to caution the informant to refrain from mentioning this information.

The time allotted for the subsequent ratings of change is 20 min each per subject or informant interview. This time was chosen on the basis of the mean time reported by clinicians who often assess clinical charge.

Source: Schneider L, Olin J, Doody R et al (1997) Validity and reliability of the Alzheimer's Disease co-operative study – clinical global impression of change. *Alzheimer's Disease and Associated Disorders* 11 (suppl 2): 322–33. Reproduced with permission from Lippincott–Raven Publishers.

Echelle Comportement et Adaptation (ECA) Scale

Reference: Ritchie K, Ledesert B (1991) Measurement of incapacity in the severely demented elderly: the validation of a behavioural assessment scale. *International Journal of Geriatric Psychiatry* 6: 217–26

Time taken 10–20 minutes

Main indications

The study describes the development and validation of a French scale, Echelle Comportement et Adaptation (ECA), for the observation of behavioural changes in older people.

Commentary

The content of the scale included items from a number of previous activities of daily living scales and 52 items were selected. A pilot study to assess inter-rater reliability and item acceptability was conducted and items were deleted that had a low test/retest coefficient, and the wording and order of some of the other items were assessed. The final scale consisted of 32 items, of which 23 are scaled and require evaluation of the person's performance on a scale of severity; nine are dichotomous items that are scored as being either present or absent. The French translation of the instrument was translated and backtranslated into English. A total of 322 people over the age of 60 with a diagnosis of dementia were assessed with the different sub-scales of the instrument and the results agreed with the assessments on the Clinical Dementia Rating (see page 238), and to a lesser extent with tests of cognitive function. There is a high correlation between scores on the ECA and Mini-Mental State Examination. Cronbach's α coefficients showed a high degree of internal reliability.

Address for correspondence

Dr Karen Ritchie
Directeur de Recherche
INSERM E0361
Pathologies du Système Nerveux:
Recherche Epidémiologique et Clinique
Hôpital la Colombière
39 Ave Charles Flahault
34093 Montpellier Cedex 5
France
e-mail: Ritchie@montp.inserm.fr

CarenapD

Reference: **McWalter GJ, Toner HL, Eastwood J, Corser AS, Marshal MT, Turvey AA, Howie C (1996) CarenapD – User manual for the Care Needs Assessment Pack for Dementia (CarenapD). University of Stirling, Stirling FK9 4LA**

Time taken approximately I hour

Rating by trained healthcare professional

Main indications

The CarenapD was developed to provide a needs assessment for older people with dementia.

Commentary

The CarenapD is an assessment tool for trained health, social care and voluntary sector practitioners working with people in the community. It was stimulated by the philosophy that a proper assessment of need, with associated good case management, is the cornerstone for high-quality care. The CarenapD does not assess what specific services are appropriate, but rather what services have to do. The aim is that the instrument should be useful in the development of care plans, and it is emphasised that it is not meant to be a replacement for a professional assessment but more of an aid to that process. The instrument was developed by examining theories of need, surveying existing assessments, consultation with users and piloting an early draft and, finally, field studies. Information on these is available from the Dementia Services Development Centre in Stirling. (www.stir.ac.uk/Departments/Human Sciences/AppSocSci/DS/publications/trainingpacks.htm)

There are four sections:

Sections 1 and 2
- Basic information/referral sheet and screen (contains information needed prior to an assessment to allow a judgement to be made as to whether the person meets the criteria for a CarenapD assessment or not
- Needs assessment (a person with dementia). This has a number of pages, including a record of perceived needs, what the person is currently receiving, and questions about finance
- Needs assessment, including sections on health and mobility, self-care and toileting, social interaction, behaviour and mental state, house-care and community living.

- There then follows a list of the types of help that may be needed:
  Social stimulation/activity
  Prompting/supervision
  Physical assistance, aids and adaptations
  Specialist assessment
  Counselling for person
  Behaviour management
  Carer advice/training.
  The last part of the needs assessment are checklists for nutrition and housing.

Section 3 Needs assessment for the carer
This consists of questions regarding the frequency of contact, their perceived needs, and assessments of health, daily difficulties, support, breaks from caring, feelings, information, intentions and carers' needs.

Section 4 Personal history
This includes questions to record personal details such as family, personality, religious beliefs, social life, hobbies and interests, routines and habits, favourite food and drinks, and pets.

The CarenapD should not be completed without training.

Additional references

McWalter G, Toner H, Corsar A, Eastwood J, Marshall M, Turvey T (1994) Needs and needs assessment: their components and definitions with reference to dementia. *Health and Social Care in the Community* **2**: 213–19.

Address for correspondence

Dr G McWalter
Dementia Services Development Centre
University of Stirling
Stirling FK9 4LA
UK

http://www.dementia.stir.ac.uk/training/softwareapp.htm

The FSAB Battery

Reference: Rothlind JC, Brandt J (1993) A brief assessment of frontal and subcortical functions in dementia. *Journal of Neuropsychiatry and Clinical Neurosciences* 5: 73–7

Time taken 5 minutes

Main indications

The authors describe three brief assessment procedures administered to patients with Huntington's disease, Parkinson's disease, Alzheimer's disease and to healthy controls which assess specifically frontal and subcortical functions (the FSAB Battery).

Commentary

The Frontal and Subcortical Assessment Battery (FSAB) consists of three brief, standardized tasks. The first is a verbal fluency test that requires worklist generation, with the added requirement that subjects retrieve words from different semantic categories, alternating categories after each third response. Thus, the subject is asked to name three animals, then three vegetables, then three different animals, then three different vegetables, and so on, for 60 seconds. Total correct words and total triads correctly spoken are tabulated, with a point being deducted from the total score for each failure to shift categories.

The second test is standardization of Luria's hand-position sequencing task. Following a practice period of 30 seconds, production of sequential hand postures, (fist, palm, side) is evaluated over a period of 60 seconds.

Subjects perform with their dominant hand. The number of correct hand movements, completed sets of three and correct sets of three are recorded. A correct hand movement is scored for each movement from one correct hand position to the next expected hand position based on the order fist-palm-side-fist-palm-side etc. Thus, a sequence of 'fist-palm-side-fist-palm *fist*-side fist' would receive a score of 5 correct hand movements but only 1 correct set.

The final test is a motor go/no-go task in which the subject is instructed to tap the table twice in response to a single tap by the examiner (out of the subject's view) and not to tap the table all in response to two taps by the examiner. Ten trials are administered, and performance is scored as either correct or incorrect for each trial.

The FSAB requires paper, a pencil and a stopwatch or other timing device and takes about 5 minutes to administer and score. Detailed administration and scoring information on all three tasks is available from the authors.

Address for correspondence

Dr JC Rothlind
University of Maryland School of Medicine
Walter P Carter Center
630 West Fayette Street
Baltimore
MD 21201
USA

Milan Overall Dementia Assessment

Reference: **Brazzelli M, Capitani E, Della Sala S, Spinnier H, Zuffi M (1994) A neuropsychological instrument adding to the description of patients with suspected cortical dementia: the Milan Overall Dementia Assessment.** *Journal of Neurology, Neurosurgery and Psychiatry* **57: 1510–17**

Time taken 30 minutes (reviewer estimate)

Rating by trained assessor

Main indications

The main use of the Milan Overall Dementia Assessment is as a screening tool for dementia.

Commentary

This is a brief neuropsychologically oriented test for dementia assessment. There are three sections, a behavioural scale and two neuropsychological testing sections. The behavioural part measures every day coping skills based on collateral information from a reliable source. It gathers information on walking, dressing, personal hygiene, control of sphincters and eating. The score on each of the questions on the above items ranges from 0 (in need of total supervision) to 3 (total autonomy).

The second section is orientation enquiry which is made up of four different sets of items including temporal orientation, spatial orientation, personal orientation and family orientation.

The final section is a series of brief neuropsychological tests which assess attention, intelligence, memory, language, space cognition and visual perception.

It has been validated against the MMSE and has a higher sensitivity and specificity in individuals with cognitive deficits than the MMSE.

Autonomy Scale

This scale measures everyday coping skills and is the only non-neuropsychological section of the MODA. As it is predicted that performance on this section will be hampered only in the later stages of the dementia, it should enable us to score even the most deteriorated patients. The examiner needs the collaboration of someone who is able to provide information about the subject's present behaviour. The section considers 5 aspects of everyday living: walking, dressing, personal hygiene, control of sphincters and eating. The score for each queston ranges from 0 (in need of total supervision) to 3 (total autonomy). The overall score range is 0–15.

Orientation enquiry

This section is made up of four different sets of items. The items require the subject to produce information that either changes (for example, age) or remains the same (for example, date of birth) over time. An answer is accepted when checked against the 'truth' (documents or witnesses). The score range of the entire section is 0–35. The four sets of items are:

Temporal orientation – Five questions are asked: the day of the week, the date of the month, the month, the year and the time of day, following the procedure of Benton et al the score ranges from 0–10.

Spatial orientation – Three questions requiring topographical information on town and country are asked. The score ranges from 0–3.

Personal orientation – Seven questions regarding personal background are asked. Standardized items are weighted differently according to face value difficulty. The score ranges from 0–10.

Family orientation – The subject is asked the name and age (±5 years) of four different family members, and whether they are alive or dead. The score ranges from 0–12.

Neuropsychological tests

All tests are drawn from an Italian standardized series of formal, currently employed, neuropsychological tests. Only the easiest items have been chosen to avoid, as far as possible, a 'floor performance' in demented patients. The score range for the whole section is 0–50.

Tests assess attention (digit cancellation; reversal learning), intelligence (logical reasoning), memory (prose memory), language (verbal comprehension; fluency), space cognition (finger agnosia: constructional apraxia), and visual perception (figure completion). These are detailed opposite in the order of administration.

Additional reference

Benton AL (1983) *Benton Visual Retention Test Stimulus Booklet* 5th edition. San Antonio (CA): Psychological Corp. Harcourt Brace and Company.

Address for correspondence

Dr Hans Spinnier
Clinica Neurologica III
University of Milan
Polo Didattico dell'Ospedale San Paolo alla Barona
via A Starabba Di Rudini
20142 Milan
Italy

Milan Overall Dementia Assessment

Test	No of items	Score range
Reversal learning	5	0–5
Digit cancellation test	10	0–10
Logical reasoning	2	0–6*
Prose memory	16 units	0–8
Semantic word fluency (names of animals)		0–5†
Token test	5	0–5
Finger agnosia	5	0–5
Construction apraxia	3	0–3
Street completion test	3	0–3

*Subjects are requested to say what is different between a truck and a coach and the meaning of a well known proverb. The scoring system accounts for norms.
†Score is categorized according to the number of words produced in two minutes and weighted against norms.

Source: Reproduced by permission of the BMJ Publishing Group, from Brazzelli M *et al. J Neurol Neurosurg Psychiatry* 1994; **57:** 1510–17.

Cognitively Impaired Life Quality Scale (CILQ)

Reference: **DeLetter MC, Tully CL, Wilson JF, Rich EC (1995) Nursing Staff Perceptions of Quality of Life of Cognitively Impaired Elders: Instrumental Development.** *Journal of Applied Gerontology* 14: 426–43

Time taken long version – 25 minutes (reviewer's estimate); short version – 10–15 minutes (reviewer's estimate)

Main indications

To assess quality of life in older people with dementia.

Commentary

The authors describe the development of a quality of life scale focusing on cognitively impaired older people. Two studies are described. The first developed a 29-item version of the Cognitively Impaired Life Quality Scale (CILQ) with a number of focus groups. It was then tested on caregivers (*n* = 83) and Cronbach's alpha used to assess the internal consistency of the scale. Items were assessed on a five-point Likert Scale (0–4) to indicate the importance of the quality of life study. A factor analysis was carried out, revealing the factors as indicated opposite. The second study was described when the 29-item version and several items were combined and was slimmed down to a 14-item scale; 67 nursing caregivers completed this scale and a similar factor analytic analysis was carried out.

Address for correspondence

Dr Mary DeLetter RN
315 CON/HSLC
University of Kentucky
Lexington
KY 40536-0232
USA

Factors and items of CILQ

Factor label	Item label	Factor label	Item label
Social interaction	Talk about present *Recognize family Interact with other while eating *Recognise staff *Talk about/remember past Taste/enjoy food Improve Help transfer	Appearance of patient to others	*Be remembered fondly by family *Be remembered fondly by staff *Be free of disfigurement *Be free of visible lines/tubes
		Nutrition	Be alive but losing weight Be minimally nourished Be alive
Basic physical care	*Move freely in bed *Have no restraints *Be clean *Have no skin breakdown Help turn in bed Be free of choking/strangling Maintain eye contact	Pain	Be free of discomfort *Look comfortable *Be free of pain
		Items not loading on a single factor	Be free of any lines/tubes Maintain attention *Be well nourished *Be well hydrated

* These questions represent the 14-item scale.

Source: Reproduced with permission from DeLetter MC *et al. J Appl Gerontol* 1995; **14:** 426–43.

Quality of Life Assessment Schedule (QoLAS)

Reference: **Selai CE, Trimble MR, Rossor M, Harvey RJ (2001) Assessing quality of life in dementia: preliminary psychometric testing of the Quality of Life Assessment Schedule (QOLAS).** *Neuropsychological Rehabilitation* **11: 219–43**

Time taken estimated 5 minutes

Rating by trained interviewer who will need to prompt answers

Main indications

Questionnaire to identify the relationship between patients current health condition and their quality of life.

Commentary

Questionnaire consists of five domains of quality of life:

physical, psychological, social, daily activities and cognitive function. Each domain has two constructs to specifically identify and prompt with symptoms. The schedule can be used with longitudinal trials.

Address for correspondence

Professor Michael Trimble
Institute of Neurology
Queen Square
London WC1N 3DG
UK

Quality of Life Assessment Schedule

The streamlined QOLAS – most simpole version:

1. The patient is interviewed and the following areas are covered:
   (i) Introduction and rapport-building;
   (ii) Patient is invited to recount what is important for his/her QOL and way in which their current health condition is affecting their QOL. Key constructs are extracted from this narrative. Prompting is occasionally required.
   (iii) A total of ten 'constructs' are elicited: 2 for each of the following domains of QOL: physical, psychological, social, work/economic and cognitive functioning (or wellbeing).
   (iv) The patient is asked to rate how much of a problem each of these is NOW on a 0–5 scale where: 0 = no problem; 1 = very slight problem; 2 = mild problem; 3 = moderate problem; 4 = big problem and 5 = it could not be worse.
2. The scoring
   The scores for each of the 10 constructs rated for 'NOW' are summed to give an overall score out of 50. A profile of scores can be drawn up by summing the scores for the 2 constructs in each domain.

Example

Domain	Construct	Score
Physical:	**1.** Headache	☐
	2. Tiredeness	☐
Psychological:	**1.** Anxiety	☐
	2. Depression	☐
Social:	**1.** Never go out any more	☐
	2. Friends disappear	☐
Daily activities:	**1.** Can't work any more	☐
	2. Can no longer do shopping	☐
Cognitive:	**1.** Memory	☐
	2. Confused	☐
Total:		☐

The Dementia Quality of Life Instrument (DqoL)

Reference: Brod M, Stewart AL, Sands L, Walton P (1999) Conceptualization and measurement of quality of life in dementia: the Dementia Quality of Life Instrument (DqoL). *Gerontologist* 39: 25–35

Time taken author's estimate 30–40 minutes

Rating by trained interviewer

Main indications

A direct assessment of quality of life of persons with dementia.

Commentary

A 29-item instrument designed to assess quality of life by direct interview with dementia patients was developed and tested on 99 participants. The data show the instrument to be reliable and evidence of validity. Patients with mild to moderate dementia can be considered good informants for their own subjective states, as 96% of participants were able to respond to questions appropriately. Domains considered included physical functioning, daily activities, discretionary activities such as hobbies, mobility, social interaction, interaction capacity (ability to interact with the environment), bodily wellbeing, sense of wellbeing and sense of aesthetics (sensory awareness and enjoyment of surroundings and overall perceptions).

Address for correspondence

Meryl Brod
Center for Clinical and Aging Services Research
Goldman Institute of Aging
3330 Geary Boulevard 2E
San Francisco
CA 94118
USA
mbrod@gioa.org

An Instrument for Assessing Health-Related Quality of Life in Persons with Alzheimer's Disease (ADRQL)

Reference: **Rabins PV, Kasper JD, Kleinman L, Black BS (1999) Concepts and methods in the development of the ADRQL: an instrument for assessing health-related quality of life in persons with Alzheimer's disease.** *Journal of Mental Health and Aging* **5: 33–48**

Time taken unknown

Main indications

To measure the health-related quality of life in patients with Alzheimer's disease.

Commentary

The ADRQL is a measure made up of responses to 5 questionnaires consisting of a total of 47 statements comprising 5 domains: Social Interaction, Awareness of Self, Feeling and Mood, Enjoyment of Activities, and Response to Surroundings. The instrument is copyright and further information is available from Betty Black (see opposite).

Additional references

Lyketsos CG, Gonzales-Salvador T, Chin JJ, Baker A, Black P, Rabins P (2003) A follow-up study of change in quality of life among persons with dementia residing in a long-term care facility. *International Journal of Geriatric Psychiatry* **18**: 275–81.

Gonzales-Salvador T, Lyketsos CG, Baker A, Hovanec L, Roques C, Brandt J, Steele C (2000) Quality of life in dementia patients in long-term care. *International Journal of Geriatric Psychiatry* **15**: 181–9.

Address for correspondence

Betty Black
600 North Wolfe Street/Meyer 2-279
Baltimore
MD 21287-7279
USA

Cornell–Brown Scale for Quality of Life in Dementia

Reference: **Ready RE, Ott BR, Grace J, Fernandez I (2002) The Cornell–Brown Scale for Quality of Life in Dementia.** *Alzheimer Disease and Associated Disorders* 16: 109–15

Time taken 10–12 minutes

Rating by experienced interviewer

Main indications

To measure the quality of life in patients with dementia.

Commentary

The quality of life of dementia patients is measured in terms of mood-related signs and ideational disturbance, and is based on a brief interview with both patients and caregivers. The ratings are based on symptoms and signs during the week prior to interview. It would appear that the reliability and validity of the scale are not adversely affected by the degree of the patient's cognitive impairment.

Address for correspondence

Rebecca E Ready
Memorial Hospital of Rhode Island
Department of Medical Rehabilitation
111 Brewster Street
Pawtucket
RI 02860
USA
rebecca_ready@brown.edu

Cornell–Brown Scale for Depression and Quality of Life in Dementia

Name _____ Age _____ Sex _____ Date _____

Circle one: Inpatient   Nursing Facility Resident   Outpatient

User this measurement scale to document quality of life in dementia patients.

Scoring system

−1 = mild or intermittent	0 = absent	+1 = mild or intermittent
−2 = severe or constant	a = unable to evaluate	+2 = very or constant

Ratings should be based on symptoms and signs occurring during the week prior to interview. No score should be given if symptoms result from physical disability or illness.

Mood-related signs

1. **Anxiety** (anxious expression, ruminations, worrying)   **Comfort** (relaxed expression, assured, no worries)
   −2   −1   0/a   +1   +2

2. **Sadness** (sad expression, sad voice, tearfulness)   **Happiness** (happy expression or voice, smiles, and laughs)
   −2   −1   0/a   +1   +2

3. **Lack of reactivity to pleasant events**   **Enjoyment of life's pleasant events**
   −2   −1   0/a   +1   +2

4. **Irritability** (easily annoyed, short tempered)   **Tolerance** (easily pleased, mild mannered)
   −2   −1   0/a   +1   +2

Ideational Disturbance

5. **Suicide** (feels life is not worth living, has suicidal wishes, or makes suicide attempt)   **Value of life** (feels life is worth living, has no suicidal thoughts, makes plans for future)
   −2   −1   0/a   +1   +2

6. **Self-deprecation** (self blame, poor self-esteem, feelings of failure)   **Self-esteem** (feelings of pride and accomplishment; high self-regard)
   −2   −1   0/a   +1   +2

7. **Pessimism** (anticipation of the worst)   **Optimism** (anticipation of the best)
   −2   −1   0/a   +1   +2

8. **Mood congruent delusions** (delusions of poverty, illness, or loss)   **Secure feelings** (feelings of wealth, good health, or better off than others)
   −2   −1   0/a   +1   +2

Source: Ready E *et al. Alzheimer's Dis Assoc Disord* 2002; **16**: 109–15. Reproduced by permission.

The Bedford Alzheimer Nursing Severity Scale for the Severely Demented

Reference: Volicer L, Hurley AC, Lathi DC, Kowall NW (1994) Measurement of the severity in advanced Alzheimer's disease. *Journal of Gerontology* 49: M223–226

Time taken 2–3 minutes

Rating by nursing staff

Main indications

An assessment scale for severe dementia patients in nursing homes

Commentary

The Bedford Alzheimer Nursing Severity Scale (BANS-s) evaluates the cognitive abilities (speech, eye contact), basic day to day living (dressing, eating, ambulating) and also pathological symptoms (sleep, wake, psycho disturbances, muscle rigidity) in people severely affected by dementia. The scale has been validated against other standardized scales.

Additional references

Bellelli G, Frisoni GB, Bianchetti A, Trabucchi M (1997) The Bedford Alzheimer Nursing Severity Scale for the severely demented: validation study. *Alzheimer Disease and Associated Disorders* 11: 71–7.

Address for correspondence

Dr L Volicer
Geriatric Research
Education and Clinical Center
EN Rogers Memorial Veterans Hospital
Bedford
Massachusetts
USA

Quality of Well-Being Scale

Reference: **Kerner DN, Patterson TL, Grant I, Kaplan RM (1998) Validity of the Quality of Well-Being Scale for patients with Alzheimer's disease.** *Journal of Aging and Health* **10: 44–61**

Time taken 25 minutes (reviewer's estimate)

Main indications

To measure health-related QoL.

Commentary

The Quality of Well-Being Scale (QWB) is a comprehensive measure of health-related quality of life. It has been used in a variety of clinical and population studies in people with a number of medical conditions. A total of 159 patients and 52 controls were assessed. Satisfactory reliability with the Mattis Dementia Rating Scale, Memory and Behavioural Problems Checklist and the Brief Symptom Interview were all satisfactory. They scored between 0.0 (the patient being dead) and 1, and the mean value for the patients was 0.5 meaning that each year of survival in the state described is counted as 0.5 in quality of life years. Observable levels of functioning over the previous 6 days form separate scales, mobility, physical activity and social activity. These scales each carry a variety of items.

In the second stage, each patients identifies his or her most undesirable symptom or problem from a list of 27 items. The observed levels of function and subjective symptomatic complaint are weighted by preference or utility for the state on a scale ranging from 0 (for dead) to 1.0 (for optimum function).

Address for correspondence

Professor Robert M Kaplan
102 Ash Building (MOD1)/SOM
Mail Code 0622
University of California, San Diego
9500 Gilman Drive
La Jolla
CA 92093
USA
rkaplan@ucsd.edu

Community Screening Instrument for Dementia (CSI 'D')

Reference: **Hall KS, Hendrie HH, Brittain HM et al. (1993) The development of a dementia screening interview in two distinct languages.** *International Journal of Methods in Psychiatric Research* 3:1–28

Time taken 30 minutes (reviewer's estimate)

Indications

Screening for dementia

Summary

The Community Screening Instrument for Dementia (CSI 'D') (Hall et al, 1993) is unusual in two respects. First, it combines culture and education-fair cognitive testing of the participant and an informant interview into a single predictive algorithm. Second, it was from the outset intended to be used across cultures with the minimum of necessary adaptation. It was developed and first validated among Cree American Indians (Hendrie et al, 1993; Hall et al, 1993) , further validated and used in population-based research (The NIA US-Nigeria Study) among Nigerians in Ibadan and African-Americans in Indianapolis (Hendrie et al, 1995), and has also been validated among white Canadians in Winnipeg, and in Jamaica (Hall et al, 2000). The addition of the informant interview significantly improved upon the predictive power of the CSI 'D' cognitive test component in Ibadan, Winnipeg and Jamaica (Hall et al, 2000). The CSI 'D' test score distributions among those with dementia and controls, and the degree of discrimination provided were remarkably consistent across these five very different cultural settings (Hall et al, 2000). In a wider validation exercise it demonstrated the same desirable properties in 24 centres across Latin America, India, China and SE Asia and Africa (Prince et al, 2003).

CSI 'D' consists of a 32-item cognitive test administered to the participant (20 minutes) and a 26-item informant interview, enquiring after the participant's daily functioning and general health (15 minutes). Three summary scores can be generated from the CSI 'D': (a) The cognitive score (COGSCORE), an item-weighted total score from the participant cognitive test; (b) The informant score (RELSCORE), an unweighted total score from the informant interview; (c) The discriminant function score (DFSCORE), a weighted score combining COGSCORE and RELSCORE. For the COGSCORE and DFSCORE there are validated cutpoints suggestive of probable and possible cases of dementia.

Additional references

Hall KS, Gao S, Emsley CL et al. (2000) Community screening interview for dementia (CSI 'D') performance in five disparate study sites. *International Journal of Geriatric Psychiatry* **15**: 521–31.

Hendrie HC, Hall KS, Pillay N et al. (1993) Alzheimer's disease is rare in Cree. *Int Psychogeriatr* **5**: 5–14.

Prince M, Acosta D, Chiu H et al (2003) Dementia diagnosis in developing countries: a cross-cultural validation study. *Lancet* **361**: 909–17.

Chapter 3

Global mental health assessments

There are some situations in which a global rating of symptoms is required in elderly patients without any particular reason to suspect or to be looking for a specific diagnosis such as depression or dementia. These measures may be useful in the setting of general practice where a relatively quick global assessment may help in pointing toward the need for a further assessment for depression or dementia. They can also be very useful in nursing and residential home care where a global rating of a resident (or group of residents) is necessary. The Sandoz Clinical Assessment – Geriatric (SCAG; page 253) and the Brief Psychiatric Rating Scale (BPRS; page 272) are early examples of this type of scale. Later ones include the Neurobehavioral Rating Scale (NRS; page 146), the Global Assessment of Psychiatric Symptoms (GAPS; page 276), the Multidimensional Observation Scale for Elderly Subjects (MOSES; page 284) (Helmes et al, 1987) and the Crichton Royal Behaviour Rating Scale (CRBRS; page 241). The SCAG, NRS and CRBRS are discussed in Chapter 2 in view of their association with dementia. More lengthy interviews are the Geriatric Mental State Schedule (GMSS; page 279) and, derived from that, the Comprehensive Assessment and Referral

Evaluation schedule (CARE; page 290), which itself has a shortened version, and the two subscales of the depression and cognitive impairment items codified in the Brief Assessment Schedule. The GMSS is used predominantly outside the USA, and has a diagnostic algorithm (AGECAT) allowing computerized diagnoses.

The Canberra Interview for the Elderly (page 280), the Structured Interview for the Diagnosis of the Alzheimer's Type and Multi-infarct Dementia and Dementias of other Aetiology (SIDAM; page 275), the Cambridge Mental Disorders of the Elderly Examination (CAMDEX; page 286) and the Pittsburgh Agitation Scale (PAS; page 163) are relatively lengthy interviews similar to the GMSS and CARE.

The NRS, SCAG, CRBRS and MOSES have sections which are relevant to people with mild to moderate cognitive impairment and would be of use where a high risk of impairment is thought to be present, while the BPRS and GAPS are more general. There is evidence that the SCAG and BPRS are sensitive to measure change. Therefore, if a drug trial or change in service were planned, these would be the instruments of choice.

Brief Psychiatric Rating Scale (BPRS)

Reference: Overall JE, Gorham DR (1962) The Brief Psychiatric Rating Scale. *Psychological Reports* 10: 799–812

Time taken 18 minutes

Rating by trained interviewer

Main indications

A rapid assessment of global psychiatric symptomatology particularly suited to the evaluation of patient change.

Commentary

The Brief Psychiatric Rating Scale (BPRS) is a 16-item, seven-point ordered category rating scale which has been developed through previous versions (Gorham and Overall, 1960). The questions are completed in 2 or 3 minutes following the interview. The ratings are divided into those based on observation of the patient (tension, emotional withdrawal, mannerisms and posturing, motor retardation and uncooperativeness) and all the others based on verbal report. Product moment correlation tested inter-rater reliability, and this varied from 0.56 to 0.87 for the 16-item scale. Data were presented to allow a 'total pathology' score using independent ratings from 20 psychiatrists.

Additional references

Gorham DR, Overall JE (1960) Drug action profiles based upon an abbreviated psychiatric rating scale. *Journal of Nervous and Mental Disease* **132**: 528–35.

Gorham DR, Overall JE (1961) Dimensions of change in psychiatric symptomatology. *Diseases of the Nervous System* **22**: 576–80.

Address for correspondence

JE Overall
Department of Psychiatry and Behavioral Sciences
University of Texas Medical School at Houston
PO Box 20708
Houston
TX 77225
USA
www.priory.com/psych/bprs.htm

Brief Psychiatric Rating Scale (BPRS)

Directions: Draw a circle around the term under each symptom which best describes the patient's present condition.

1. SOMATIC CONCERN – Degree of concern over present bodily health. Rate the degree to which physical health is perceived as a problem by the patient, whether complaints have realistic basis or not.

    Not present   Very mild   Mild   Moderate   Moderate, severe   Severe   Extremely severe

2. ANXIETY – Worry, fear, or over-concern for present or future. Rate solely on the basis of verbal report of patient's own subjective experiences. Do not infer anxiety from physical signs or from neurotic defense mechanisms.

    Not present   Very mild   Mild   Moderate   Moderate, severe   Severe   Extremely severe

3. EMOTIONAL WITHDRAWAL – Deficiency in relating to the interviewer and the interview situation. Rate only degree to which the patient gives the impression of failing to be in emotional contact with other people in the interview situation.

    Not present   Very mild   Mild   Moderate   Moderate, severe   Severe   Extremely severe

4. CONCEPTUAL DISORGANIZATION – Degree to which the thought processes are confused, disconnected or disorganized. Rate on the basis of integration of the verbal products of the patient; do not rate on the basis of the patient's subjective impression of his own level of functioning.

    Not present   Very mild   Mild   Moderate   Moderate, severe   Severe   Extremely severe

5. GUILT FEELINGS – Over-concern or remorse for past behavior. Rate on the basis of the patient's subjective experiences of guilt as evidenced by verbal report with appropriate affect; do not infer guilt feelings from depression, anxiety, or neurotic defenses.

    Not present   Very mild   Mild   Moderate   Moderate, severe   Severe   Extremely severe

cont.

6. TENSION – Physical and motor manifestations of tension, 'nervousness', and heightened activation level. Tension should be rated solely on the basis of physical signs and motor behavior and not on the basis of subjective exprinces of tension reported by the patient.

Not present   Very mild   Mild   Moderate   Moderate, severe   Severe   Extremely severe

7. MANNERISMS AND POSTURING – Unusual and unnatural motor behavior, the type of motor behavior which causes certain mental patients to stand out in a crowd of normal people. Rate only abnormality of movements; do not rate simple heightened motor activity here.

Not present   Very mild   Mild   Moderate   Moderate, severe   Severe   Extremely severe

8. GRANDIOSITY – Exaggerated self-opinion, conviction of unusual ability or powers. Rate only on the basis of patient's statements about himself or self-in-relation-to-others, not on the basis of his demeanor in the interview situation.

Not present   Very mild   Mild   Moderate   Moderate, severe   Severe   Extremely severe

9. DEPRESSIVE MOOD – Despondency in mood, sadness. Rate only degree of despondency; do not rate on the basis of inferences concerning depression based upon general retardation and somatic complaints.

Not present   Very mild   Mild   Moderate   Moderate, severe   Severe   Extremely severe

10. HOSTILITY – Animosity, contempt, belligerence, disdain for other people outside the interview situation. Rate solely on the basis of the verbal report of feelings and actions of the patient toward others; do not infer hostility from neurotic defenses, anxiety nor somatic complaints. (Rate attitude toward interviewer under 'uncooperativeness'.)

Not present   Very mild   Mild   Moderate   Moderate, severe   Severe   Extremely severe

11. SUSPICIOUSNESS – Belief (delusional or otherwise) that others have now, or have had in the past, malicious or discriminatory intent toward the patient. One the basis of verbal report, rate only those suspicions which are currently held whether they concern past or present circumstances.

Not present   Very mild   Mild   Moderate   Moderate, severe   Severe   Extremely severe

12. HALLUCINATORY BEHAVIOR – Perceptions without normal external stimulus correspondence. Rate only those experiences which are reported to have occurred within the last week and which are described as distinctly different from the thought and imagery processes of normal people.

Not present   Very mild   Mild   Moderate   Moderate, severe   Severe   Extremely severe

13. MOTOR RETARDATION – Reduction in energy level evidenced in slowed movements and speech, reduced body tone, decreased number of movements. Rate on the basis of observed behavior of the patient only; do not rate on basis of patient's subjective impression of own energy level.

Not present   Very mild   Mild   Moderate   Moderate, severe   Severe   Extremely severe

14. UNCOOPERATIVENESS – Evidence of resistance, unfriendliness, resentment, and lack of readiness to cooperate with the interviewer. Rate only on the basis of the patient's attitude and responses to the interviewer and the interview situation; do not rate on basis of reported resentment or uncooperativeness outside the interview situation.

Not present   Very mild   Mild   Moderate   Moderate, severe   Severe   Extremely severe

15. UNUSUAL THOUGHT CONTENT – Unusual, odd, strange, or bizarre thought content. Rate here the degree of unusualness, not the degree of disorganization of thought processes.

Not present   Very mild   Mild   Moderate   Moderate, severe   Severe   Extremely severe

16. BLUNTED AFFECT – Reduced emotional tone, apparent lack of normal feeling or involvement.

Not present   Very mild   Mild   Moderate   Moderate, severe   Severe   Extremely severe

Source: Overall JE, Gorham DR 'The Brief Psychiatric Rating Scale.' *Psychological Reports*, 1962, **10**, 799–812. © Southern Universities Press.

Relative's Assessment of Global Symptomatology (RAGS)

Reference: **Raskin A, Crook T (1988) Relative's assessment of global symptomatology (RAGS).** *Psychopharmacology Bulletin* **24: 759–63**

Time taken 15 minutes (reviewer's estimate)

Rating by observer, no training required

Main indications

Specifically designed for use by a close relative or friend of a patient to assess his or her behaviour in the community.

Commentary

This is a 21-item scale assessing psychiatric symptoms and behaviour. It emerges from a series of papers reflecting analyses of psychopathology at interview (Raskin et al, 1967, 1969; Shulterbrandt et al, 1974). The RAGS was administered to 456 individuals. Construct validity was shown by successful discrimination of 14 of the 21 RAGS items in distinguishing patients with senile dementia from other groups. It correlated with ratings on a mood scale and a memory scale of other self-administered instruments. A 'total pathology' score can be derived by reversing the score for item 2.

Additional references

Raskin A (1985) Validation of a battery of tests designed to assess psychopathology in the elderly. In Burrows GD, Norman TR, Dennerstein L, eds. *Clinical and pharmacological studies in psychiatric disorders.* London: John Libbey, 337–43.

Raskin A, Schulterbrandt JG, Reatig N et al (1967) Factors of psychopathology in interview, ward behavior and self-report ratings of hospitalized depressives. *Journal of Consulting and Clinical Psychology* **31**: 270–8.

Raskin A, Schuterbrandt JG, Reatig N et al (1969) Replication of factors of psychopathology in interview, ward behavior and self-report ratings of hospitalized depressives. *Journal of Nervous and Mental Disease* **148**: 87–98.

Schulterbrandt JG, Raskin A, Reatig N (1974) Further replications of factors of psychopathology in the interview, ward behavior and self-report ratings of hospitalized depressed patients. *Psychological Reports* **34**: 23–32.

Address for correspondence

Allen Raskin
7658 Water Oak Point Road
Pasadena
MD 21122
USA

Relative's Assessment of Global Symptomatology (RAGS)

To what extent does he or she:

1. Need help in caring for personal needs and appearance?
2. Participate in social and recreational activities?
3. Appear depressed, blue, or despondent?
4. Appear tense, anxious, and inwardly distressed?
5. Display irritability, annoyance, impatience, or anger?
6. Appear suspicious of people?
7. Report peculiar or strange thoughts or ideas?
8. Appear to be hearing or seeing things that are not there?
9. Show mood swings or changes?
10. Appear excited or 'high' emotionally?
11. Have difficulty in sleeping at night?
12. Appear slowed-down, fatigued, and lacking in energy?
13. Lack motor coordination?
14. Have difficulty speaking?
15. Express concern with own bodily health?
16. Appear inattentive?
17. Appear confused, perplexed, or otherwise seem to be having difficulty organizing his/her thoughts?
18. Seem disoriented?
19. Appear forgetful?
20. Appear agitated?
21. Show variability in mental functioning?

Score:
1 = Not at all; 2 = A little; 3 = Moderately; 4 = Quite a bit; 5 = Extremely

---

Structured Interview for the Diagnosis of the Alzheimer's Type and Multi-infarct Dementia and Dementias of other Aetiology (SIDAM)

Reference: **Zaudig M, Mittelhammer J, Hiller W, Pauls A, Thora C, Morinigo A, Mombour W (1991) SIDAM – a structured interview for the diagnosis of dementia of the Alzheimer type, multi-infarct dementia and dementias of other aetiology according to ICD-10 and DSM-III-R.** *Psychological Medicine* **21: 225–36**

Time taken 30 minutes

Rating by clinician addressed to the patient and carer

Main indications

A structured interview for the diagnosis of dementia according to ICD-10 and DSM-III-R criteria.

Commentary

The Structured Interview for the Diagnosis of the Alzheimer's Type and Multi-infarct Dementia and Dementias of other Aetiology (SIDAM) was constructed primarily to differentiate patients with dementia from non-demented individuals according to the DSM-III-R and ICD-10 criteria. The SIDAM is divided into the following sections: (1) a brief semi-structured clinical overview with the patient or information concerning aspects of the subject's past and present medical history; (2) a cognitive examination (when scored separately, this is designated the SISCO, with a range of 0–55 (no cognitive impairment)); all items of the Mini-Mental State Examination (MMSE; page 36) are contained in the SISCO; (3) a structured schedule for the recording of clinical judgement in relation to the aetiology of dementia and differentiation from other psychiatric conditions; (4) a severity grading for dementia; (5) a list of present and past medical disorders; (6) a summary sheet; (7) a diagnostic algorithm. Sixty subjects underwent the reliability study, with measures of test/retest reliability with agreements of over 95% and very good kappa values for all subtypes of dementia, the lowest being for multi-infarct dementia (0.64).

Address for correspondence

M Zaudig
Psychosomatic Hospital
Schuetzemstreet 16
86949 Windach
Germany

e-mail: zaudig@klinik-windach.de

Global Assessment of Psychiatric Symptoms (GAPS)

References: Raskin A, Gershon S, Crook TH, Sathananthan G, Ferris S (1978) The effects of hyperbaric and normobaric oxygen on cognitive impairment in the elderly. *Archives of General Psychiatry* 35: 50–6

Raskin A, Crook T (1988) Global Assessment of Psychiatric Symptoms (GAPS). *Psychopharmacology Bulletin* 24: 721–5

Time taken approximately 15–20 minutes (reviewer's estimate)

Rating by trained observers

Main indications

A global assessment of psychiatric symptoms for use in older people, designed to detect change.

Commentary

The Global Assessment of Psychiatric Symptoms (GAPS) is a 19-item abbreviated version of a larger inventory used in a study of the effects of hyperbaric oxygen in older people (Raskin et al, 1978): the Observer Rated Inventory of Psychic and Somatic Complaints – Elderly, modelled after the Brief Psychiatric Rating Scale (BPRS; page 272). The GAPS has been administered to 509 people over the age of 60 in institutions in the USA and 290 normal elderly control subjects. Intraclass correlation coefficients ranged from 0.43 to 0.72. Mean differences on the scale calculated across different diagnostic groups showed successful differentiation between the groups. Raskin (1985) produced validity measures of the GAPS showing correlations between both independent measures of memory and depression and self-report.

Additional reference

Raskin A (1985) Validation of a battery of tests designed to assess psychopathology in the elderly. In Burrows GD, Norman TR, Dennerstein L, eds. *Clinical and pharmacological studies in psychiatric disorders.* London: John Libbey, 337–43.

Address for correspondence

Allen Raskin
7658 Water Oak Point Road
Pasadena
MD 21122
USA

Global Assessment of Psychiatric Symptoms (GAPS)

To what extent does the patient:

1. Appear sloppy or unkempt in appearance?
2. Lack motor coodination?
3. Appear slowed-down, fatigued and lacking in energy?
4. Have difficulty speaking?
5. Appear confused, perplexed, or otherwise seem to be having difficulty organizing his/her thoughts?
6. Seem disoriented?
7. Appear inattentive?
8. Appear forgetful?
9. Appear unfriendly or unsociable?
10. Display irritability, annoyance; impatience, or anger?
11. Appear depressed, blue, or despondent?
12. Appear tense, anxious and inwardly distressed?
13. Appear agitated?
14. Appear suspicious of people?
15. Report peculiar or strange thoughts or ideas?
16. Appear to be hallucinating?
17. Appear excited or 'high' emotionally?
18. Complain of difficulty in sleeping at night?
19. Express concern with bodily health?

Score:
1 = Not at all
2 = A little
3 = Moderately
4 = Quite a bit
5 = Extremely

The Core Assessment and Outcomes Package for Older People

Reference: **FACE Recording and Measurement Systems**

Rating by experienced interviewer

Commentary

Holistic assessment of older people.

Main indications

The Core Assessment and Outcomes Package for Older People is designed to support routine practice and the implementation of the *National Service Framework for Older People*. It provides a number of tools which:

- Ensure accurate multiprofessional assessment of health and social needs
- Support risk assessment and risk management
- Support clinical governance and performance management
- Support the integration of health and social care
- Engage service users and carers
- Measure health, social and risk outcomes
- Provide information for benchmarking.

A triage assessment is used as a screening assessment to provide an overview. This is followed by four specialist assessments:

- Physical wellbeing and activities of daily living (assessment of health and disability, impairment)
- Self-care (functioning inside and outside the home)
- Psychological wellbeing (mental health, cognitive function, behaviour)
- Social
- Risk profile.

Some information is provided about the profiles of scores on the various domains as well as monitoring progress but no information is given about any reliability or validity studies. Training is available and the licence is purchased from FACE Recording and Measurement Systems.

Address for correspondence

FACE Recording and Measurement Systems
King John Chambers
13-15 Bridlesmith Gate
Nottingham NG1 2GR
UK
Tel: +44 115 950 8300, Fax: +44 115 911 0375
www.facecode.com

Psychogeriatric Assessment Scales (PAS)

Reference: Jorm AF, MacKinnon AJ, Henderson AS, Scott R, Christensen H, Korten AE, Cullen JS, Mulligan R (1995) The Psychogeriatric Assessment Scales: a multidimensional alternative to categorical diagnoses of dementia and depression in the elderly. *Psychological Medicine* 25: 447–60

Time taken 10 minutes (reviewer's estimate)

Rating by trained lay interviewer or clinician, after familiarization with the manual

Main indications

The Psychogeriatric Assessment Scales (PAS) provide an assessment of the clinical changes seen in dementia and depression. It is easy to administer, can be used by lay interviewers and is intended for use in research and service evaluation.

Commentary

The PAS has the benefits of assessing both dementia and depression. There are three scales derived from an interview with the subject (cognitive impairment, depression and stroke) and three from an interview with an informant (cognitive decline, behavioural change and stroke). The scales cover the clinical domain as defined in ICD-10 and DSM-III-R and are based on the Canberra Interview for the Elderly (CIE; page 280). The results are described using data from three samples – two clinical samples and one population sample, the latter having about 1000 people and the two others about 60. Five factors emerged from the principal components analysis of each item: cognitive decline, cognitive impairment, behaviour change, stroke and depression. Internal consistency ranged from 0.58 to 0.86, test/retest correlations between 0.47 and 0.66, and validity was proven against other mood and cognitive scales.

Additional reference

Jorm AF, MacKinnon AJ, Christensen H et al (1997) The Psychogeriatric Assessment Scales (PAS): further data on psychometric properties and validity from a longitudinal study of the elderly. *International Journal of Geriatric Psychiatry* 12: 93–100.

Address for correspondence

AF Jorm
NH and MRC Social Psychiatry Research Unit
The Australian National University
Canberra
ACT 0200
Australia

Geriatric Mental State Schedule (GMSS)

References: **Copeland JRM, Kelleher MJ, Kellett JM, Gourlay AJ, Gurland BJ, Fleiss JL, Sharpe L (1976) A semi-structured clinical interview for the assessment of diagnosis of mental state in the elderly: the Geriatric Mental State Schedule. I. Development and reliability.** *Psychological Medicine* **6: 439–49**

Gurland BJ, Fleiss JL, Goldberg K, Sharpe L, Copeland JRM, Kelleher MJ, Kellett JM (1976) A semi-structured clinical interview for the assessment of diagnosis of mental state in the elderly: the Geriatric Mental State Schedule. II. A factor analysis. *Psychological Medicine* **6: 451–9**

Time taken 40–45 minutes

Rating by trained interviewer

Main indications

Assessment of psychopathology in elderly people.

Commentary

The Geriatric Mental State Schedule (GMSS) is one of the most widely used and respected assessment instruments for measuring a wide range of psychopathology in elderly people both in institutionalized settings and, more importantly, in community settings. It is based on the Present State Examination (Wing et al, 1974) and the Psychiatric Status Schedule (Spitzer et al, 1970), and consists of a number of detailed questions concerning psychopathology and behaviour in the last month. Literature on the GMSS is extensive, and a number of different factors can be derived from the results. The instrument was used in the original US/UK project (Cowan et al, 1975), and there is a computerized algorithm of proven reliability and validity, the AGECAT (Copeland et al, 1986). A history and aetiology schedule is also available. The GMSS can conveniently be given via a laptop computer, and it has been translated into a number of different languages.

Additional references

Copeland JRM, Kelleher MJ, Kellett JM et al (1975) Cross-national study of diagnosis of the mental disorders: a comparison of the diagnoses of elderly psychiatric patients admitted to mental hospitals serving Queens County, New York, and the former Borough of Camberwell, London. *British Journal of Psychiatry* **126**: 11–20.

Copeland JRM, Dewey ME, Griffiths-Jones HM (1986) A computerized psychiatric diagnostic system and case nomenclature for elderly subjects: GMS and AGECAT. *Psychological Medicine* **16**: 89–99.

Cowan DW, Copeland JRM, Kelleher MJ et al (1975) Cross-national study of diagnosis of the mental disorders: a comparative psychometric assessment of elderly patients admitted to mental hospitals serving Queens County, New York, and the former Borough of Camberwell, London. *British Journal of Psychiatry* **126**: 560–70.

Spitzer RL, Endicott J (1969) DIAGNO II: further developments in a computer program for psychiatric diagnosis. *American Journal of Psychiatry* **125**: 12–21.

Spitzer RL, Endicott J, Fleiss JL et al (1970) Psychiatric Status Schedule: a technique for evaluating psychopathology and impairment in role functioning. *Archives of General Psychiatry* **23**: 41–55.

Spitzer RL, Fleiss JL (1974) A re-analysis of the reliability of psychiatric diagnosis. *British Journal of Psychiatry* **125**: 341–7.

Wing JK, Cooper JE, Sartorius N (1974) *The measurement and classification of psychiatric symptoms: an instruction manual for the PSE and Catego program.* Cambridge: Cambridge University Press.

Factors derived from the Geriatric Mental State Schedule (GMSS)

1. Depression
2. Anxiety
3. Impaired memory
4. Retarded speech
5. Hypomania
6. Somatic concerns
7. Observed belligerence
8. Reported belligerence
9. Obsessions
10. Drug–alcohol dependence
11. Cortical dysfunction
12. Disorientation
13. Lack of insight
14. Depersonalization–derealization
15. Paranoid delusion
16. Subjective experience of disordered thought
17. Visual hallucination
18. Auditory hallucination
19. Abnormal motor movements
20. Non-social speech
21. Incomprehensibility

Canberra Interview for the Elderly (CIE)

Reference: Henderson AS et al (1992) The Canberra Interview for the Elderly: a new field instrument for the diagnosis of dementia and depression by ICD-10 and DSM-III-R. *Acta Psychiatrica Scandinavica* 85: 105–13

Time taken 69 minutes with subjects, 37 minutes with informant (average values)

Rating designed to be administered by lay interviewers

Main indications

An instrument for identifying cases of dementia and depression for research purposes.

Commentary

An instrument was designed in which items systematically represented the elements for depression and dementia in DSM-III-R and ICD-10 diagnostic criteria. A computer algorithm of the diagnoses was then constructed, leading to a diagnosis. The Canberra Interview for the Elderly (CIE) is particularly useful for epidemiological studies and acceptable to the elderly. The instrument involves some pictorial material which could not be stored on disk and is available in booklet form. Test/rerest reliability is high and comparison with cognitive function tests and diagnostic categories (ICD-10 and DSM-III-R) is excellent.

Address for correspondence

AS Henderson
Director
NH and MRC Psychiatric Epidemiology Research Centre
The Australian National University
Canberra
ACT 0200
Australia

Canberra Interview for the Elderly (CIE)

Memory functioning
    Long-term memory
    Short-term verbal memory
    Short-term nonverbal memory
    History of deterioration

Intellectual performance
    Premorbid intelligence
    Orientation to time and place
    Vocabulary
    Similarities

Sentence verification
Verbal fluency
Phrase repetition
Object naming
Mental concentration
Copying, writing, pointing, following simple and complex commands (dyspraxia)
Perceptual identification
Perceptual motor speed and intelligence
History of deterioration

Survey Psychiatric Assessment Schedule (SPAS)

Reference: **Bond J, Brooks P, Carstairs V, Giles L (1980) The reliability of a Survey Psychiatric Assessment Schedule for the elderly.** *British Journal of Psychiatry* **137: 148–62**

Time taken 20–30 minutes (reviewer's estimate)

Rating by qualified observer

Main indications

Intended to assess the prevalence of the whole range of psychiatric disorders affecting elderly people.

Commentary

Orignally derived from a short version of the Geriatric Mental State Schedule (GMSS; page 279) the Survey Psychiatric Assessment Schedule (SPAS) consists of 51 items divided into three groups: organic disorders (scores vary from 0 to 12), affective disorders/psychoneurosis (scores vary from 0 to 65) and schizophrenia/paranoid

disorders (scores vary from 0 to 10). Cut-off points are available to indicate the severity from each of the global scores.

Additional reference

Bond J (1987) Psychiatric illness in later life. A study of the prevalance in a Scottish population. *International Journal of Geriatric Psychiatry* **2**: 39–57.

Address for correspondence

John Bond
Centre for Health Services Research
University of Newcastle
21 Claremont Place
Newcastle upon Tyne NE2 4AA
UK

Survey Psychiatric Assessment Schedule (SPAS)

1. I'd like to begin by checking that I have got a few details correct.

Both names correct	1

    Could you spell your last name for me? And your first name?

Both names not correct	0

    (Check against spelling of name provided from records. One minor spelling error allowed.)

No reply/don't know	0

2a. What is the full postal address here?

    (Check with records)

Both number and street (or name of institution) correct	1
Number and/or street (or name of institution) incorrect	0
No reply/don't know	0

b.

Town or district correct	1
Town or district incorrect	0
No reply/don't know	0

3. My name is .... (Give last name only) I'd like you to remember that.

Correct or almost correct	1

    Can you repeat that please. (Spell and repeat name 3 times or until

Totally incorrect	0

    correctly repeated. Accept only approximation to correct pronunciation).

No reply	0

4. How old were you on your last birthday? (If vague ask) About how old are you?

Same as record	1
Different from records	0
No reply/don't know	0

5. What year were you born in?

Same as records	1
Different from records	0
No reply/don't know	0

    Other survey questions about general health of subject.

6. Do you remember my name? What is it? (Accept any approximation to correct pronunciation).

7. What is the date today? (Allow error of one day).

8. What month is this? (Allow error of one week, e.g. March in first week of April).

9. What year is this? (Allow error of one month, e.g. 1977 in January 1978).

10. Who is the Prime Minister?

cont.

11. Who was the Prime Minister before this?

Questions 6–11 score 1 for correct name; 0 for incorrect or no reply/don't know
I should now like to get some idea of how you yourself have been getting along lately – how your general health has been, and how you have been feeling about things. Some of the things I am now going to ask you may not apply to you but I am just making sure that everything has been mentioned. Most of the questions I shall ask you will apply to how you have been feeling in the last month.

12. Most people have some sort of worries or troubles from time to time. Have you worried a great deal about any of the following recently: money, ill health, housing, people you live with, relatives, neighbours, what people think of you, having done something wrong, not doing things properly, not being able to cope.
(If worries about any of these ask 13–15)

	Score 1 for every positive reply	**Score**
13. How often do you worry?	Never	0
	Some days	1
	Most days	2

14. When you worry about these things is it unpleasant or not?		
	Not unpleasant	0
	Unpleasant	1

15. Can you stop yourself worrying?		
	Can stop	0
	If I do something	1
	Cannot stop worrying	2

16. Have there been times lately when you have been nervous or anxious for no good reason? Is this no more than usual or more than usual?

	None	0
	No more than usual	1
	More than usual	2

17. **If yes at 16.** Does this happen from time to time or most of the time?

	Not anxious	0
	From time to time	1
	Most of the time	2

18. Are you troubled with frightening dreams?

	No	0
	Yes	1

19. Do you wake in fear or panic?

	No	0
	Yes	1

20. **If yes at 18 or 19**. Does this happen occasionally, some nights or most nights?

	Never	0
	Occasionally	1
	Some nights	2
	Most nights	3

21. Do you feel tense and restless?

	No	0
	Yes	1

22. People sometimes have fears that they know don't make sense, like being afraid of crowds or certain activities. Do you have any fears like this? For instance, do you tend to get very frightened: when you are alone; in a small room; when you are in a crowd; when you travel by bus; when you are in a shop; in open spaces; when in an enclosed space.
Probe to establish whether or not fear is reasonable.
Score 1 for only fears which are unreasonable.

Score 1 for all unreasonable fears

23. Does this fear/these fears ever prevent you from doing things you want to do? Is there anything you can do to overcome this like taking someone with you?

	No	0
	Can overcome	1
	Cannot overcome	2

24. Do you ever feel your heart pounding? (If yes) Is this because you get frightened or is it for some other reason?

	No	0
	Not frightened	1
	Frightened	2

25. Do ever feel yourself trembling? (If yes) Is this because you get frightened or is it for some other reason?

	No	0
	Not frightened	1
	Frightened	2

26. Do you ever get dizzy? (If yes) Is this because you get frightened or is it for some other reason?

	No	0
	Not frightened	1
	Frightened	2

27. Do you ever get hot or cold all over? (If yes) Is this because you get frightened or is it for some other reason?

	No	0
	Not frightened	1
	Frightened	2

28. Do you ever faint or lose consciousness? (If yes) Is this because you get frightened or is it for some other reason?

	No	0
	Not frightened	1
	Frightened	2

29. Do you ever get a sinking feeling in your stomach? (If yes) Is this because you get frightened or is it for some other reason?

	No	0
	Not frightened	1
	Frightened	2

30. Have you been depressed or miserable during the past month for no good reason? (If yes) Is this no more than usual or more than usual?

	No	0
	No more than usual	1
	More than usual	2

31. (If yes at 30). Does this come and go or is it constant?

	Come and go	0
	Constant	1

32. (If yes at 30). Does it interfere with your life or not?

Does not interfere	0
Interferes	1

33. How much have you cried lately?

Not at all	0
Once or twice a month	1
More often than this	2

34. How much have you felt like crying or have wanted to cry, without actually weeping, for no good reason?

Not at all	0
Once or twice a month	1
More often than this	2

35. How do you see your future?

All right	0
Avoids thinking about it	1
Seems bleak/dark/hopeless	2

36. Have there been times lately when you wish you were dead?

No	0
Yes	1

37. Have you had trouble sleeping?

No	0
Yes	1

38. Do you have difficulty getting off to sleep?

No	0
Yes	1

39. Do you lie awake during the night for an hour or more?

No	0
Yes	1

40. Do you wake early and lie awake?

No	0
Yes	1

41. Do you regularly take tablets to make you sleep?

Never	0
Some nights	1
Most nights	2

42. Is anyone interfering with your thoughts in a strange way which you cannot understand? (If yes) In what way?

No	0
Yes	1

43. Can other people read your thoughts in some strange way which you cannot understand? (If yes) In what way?

No	0
Yes	1

44. Do you feel people are putting thoughts into your head in some strange way which you cannot understand? (If yes) In what way?

No	0
Yes	1

45. Do you feel people are controlling your mind against your will? (If yes) In what way?

No	0
Yes	1

46. Do you get a peculiar feeling that people are taking thoughts out of your head? (If yes) In what way?

No	0
Yes	1

47. Are there people you do not trust? (If yes) Who and why don't you trust them?

No	0
Yes	1

48. Do people laugh at you and say unpleasant things about you behind your back? (If yes) What do they say?

No	0
Yes	1

49. Do you feel that people are trying to upset or harm you in any way for no good reason? (If yes) Who and how are they trying to harm you?

No	0
Yes	1

50. Do you ever see or hear something on television or on radio or in the papers which is directed at you or has a special meaning for you and nobody else? (If yes) What do you see or hear?

No	0
Yes	1

51. Do you ever think you hear a voice when there is nobody there? (If yes) Where does the voice come from? What does it say?

No	0
Yes	1

Section 1 – Additive scores derived

No organic disorder	9–12
Mild organic disorder	7–8
Severe organic disorder	0–6

Section 2 – Summate responses

Non-case	0–10
Case	11–22

Section 3 – Any positive answer indicates a possible case

Reproduced from *The British Journal of Psychiatry*, Bond J, Brooks P, Carstairs V, Giles L, The reliability of a Survey Psychiatric Assessment Schedule for the elderly, Vol. 137, pp. 148–62. © 1980 Royal College of Psychiatrists. Reproduced with permission.

Multidimensional Observation Scale for Elderly Subjects (MOSES)

Reference: **Helmes E, Csapo KG, Short J-A (1987) Standardization and validation of the Multidimensional Observation Scale for Elderly Subjects (MOSES).** *Journal of Gerontology* **42: 395–405**

Time taken 25 minutes (reviewer's estimate)

Rating by observers trained in the subject

Main indications

Assessment of behaviours in elderly people.

Commentary

The Multidimensional Observation Scale for Elderly Subjects (MOSES) rates different areas of functioning (multidimensional), and this overcomes the difficulties of global ratings of impairment, which are sometimes regarded as being too broad. The MOSES was developed from a longitudinal research programme which included the development of the London Psychogeriatric Rating Scale (LPRS) (Hersch et al, 1978). The MOSES was developed by empirical factor analyses of earlier instruments identifying major areas of functioning, adding questions about depression and developing specific anchor points in the ratings. The final result was a 40-item test assessing five areas of functioning (eight items each): self-care functioning, disorientated behaviour, depressed/anxious mood, irritable behaviour and withdrawn behaviour (Helmes et al, 1985).

The original paper reports the results on 2542 individuals – inter-rater reliability was acceptable (e.g. intraclass correlation coefficients ranged from 0.50 to 0.99; internal consistency was around 0.8). Validity was tested by examining 12-month follow-up and comparisons with the Zung Depression Status Inventory (Zung, 1972) and the Robertson Short Status Questionnaire (Robertson et al, 1982), the Kingston Dementia Rating Scale (Lawson et al, 1977), the PAMIE Scale (page 248) (Gurel et al, 1972) and the London Psychogeriatric Rating Scale (Hersch et al, 1978). There were significant correlations between subscales of the MOSES and the other measures proving validity.

Additional references

Gurel L, Linn MW, Linn BS (1972) Physical and mental impairment-of-function evaluation in the aged: the PAMIE scale. *Journal of Gerontology* **27**: 83–90.

Helmes E, Csapo KG, Short JA (1985) *History, development and validation of a new rating scale for the institutionalized elderly: the Multidimensional Observation Scale for Elderly Subjects (MOSES) (Bulletin No 8501).* Dept of Psychiatry, University of Western Ontario, Canada.

Hersch EL, Kral VA, Palmer RB (1978) Clinical value of the London Psychogeriatric Rating Scale. *Journal of the American Geriatric Society* **26**: 348–54.

Lawson JS, Rodenburg M, Dykes JA (1977) A dementia rating scale for use with psychogeriatric patients. *Journal of Gerontology* **32**: 153–9.

Robertson D, Rockwood K, Stolee P (1982) A short mental status questionnaire. *Canadian Journal on Aging* **1**: 16–20.

Zung WWK (1972) The Depression Status Inventory: an adjunct to the Self-Rating Depression Scale. *Journal of Clinical Psychology* **28**: 539–43.

Address for correspondence

E Helmes
Psychology Department
London Psychiatric Hospital
Box 2532
Station A
London
Ontario N6A 4H1
Canada

Items covered in the Multidimensional Observation Scale for Elderly Subjects (MOSES)

1. Dressing
2. Bathing (Including baths and showers)
3. Grooming
4. Incontinence (Of either urine or feces)
5. Using the toilet
6. Physical mobility
7. Getting in and out of bed
8. Use of restraints
9. Understanding communication
10. Talking
11. Finding way around inside
12. Recognizing staff
13. Awareness of place
14. Awareness of time
15. Memory for recent events
16. Memory for important past events
17. Looking sad and depressed
18. Reporting sadness and depression
19. Sounding sad and depressed
20. Looking worried and anxious
21. Reporting worry and anxiety
22. Crying
23. Pessimism about the future
24. Self concern
25. Co-operation with nursing care
26. Following staff requests and instructions
27. Irritability
28. Reactions to frustration
29. Verbal abuse of staff
30. Verbal abuse of other residents
31. Physical abuse of others
32. Provoking arguments with other residents
33. Preferring solitude
34. Initiating social contacts
35. Responding to social contacts
36. Friendships with other residents
37. Interest in day-to-day events
38. Interest in outside events
39. Keeping occupied
40. Helping other residents

Cambridge Mental Disorders of the Elderly Examination (CAMDEX)

Reference: **Roth M, Tym E, Mountjoy CQ, Huppert FA, Hendrie H, Verma S, Goddard R (1986) CAMDEX. A standardised instrument for the diagnosis of mental disorder in the elderly with special reference to the early detection of dementia.** *British Journal of Psychiatry* **149: 698–709**

Time taken interview with subject approximately 60 minutes. Informant section approximately 20 minutes

Rating by interview

Main indications

An interview schedule for the diagnosis and measurement of dementia in the elderly.

Commentary

The Cambridge Mental Disorders of the Elderly Examination (CAMDEX) is a structured instrument comprising eight sections. The CAMDEX is designed to provide a formal diagnosis according to operational diagnostic criteria in one of 11 categories. Normally, four types of dementia are assessed: Alzheimer's disease, multi-infarct dementia, mixed Alzheimer's and multi-infarct dementia, and dementia due to other causes – delirium (with or without depression), depression, anxiety or phobic disorders, paranoid or paraphrenic illness, and other psychiatric disorders. A five-point scale allows severity of dementia and severity of depression to be rated. The original paper describes results on 92 patients. Inter-rater reliability ranged from a median of 0.83 for the observational parts of the CAMDEX up to 0.94 for the patient interview. With regard to clinical diagnoses of dementia, a cut-off of 79/80 on the CAMCOG (maximum = 106) yielded a result of 92% sensitivity and 96% specificity. A description of clinical diagnostic scales for Alzheimer's disease, multi-infarct dementia and depression is included.

Additional references

O'Connor D, Pollitt P, Hyde J et al (1990) The progression of mild idiopathic dementia in a community population. *Journal of the American Geriatrics Society* **39**: 246–51.

O'Connor D, Pollitt P, Hyde J et al (1990) Follow-up study of dementia diagnosed in the community using the CAMDEX. *Acta Psychiatrica Scandinavica* **81**: 78–82.

Address for correspondence

Felicia A Huppert
Department of Psychiatry
Level E4
Box 189
Addenbrooke's Hospital
Cambridge CB2 2QQ
UK

http://books.cambridge.org/0521462614.htm

The Cambridge Mental Disorders of the Elderly Examination (CAMDEX)

Section A
Particulars regarding present physical and mental state, past history, family history. It starts with 3 questions: name, age and date of bith. If the answers are obtained to 2 out of 3, section A is abandoned and Section B is completed.

Section B
This is the cognitive section which includes questions allowing the Mini-Mental State Examination to be completed as well as specific cognitive items in the CAMDEX and CAMCOG scales
orientation – time place
language – comprehension (motor response, verbal response, expression, naming, definitions, repetition, spontaneous speech, reading comprehension)
memory – recall (visual and verbal), recognition, retrieval of remote and recent information.
Registration – attention and concentration.
Praxis – copy and drawing, spontaneous writing, ideational praxis, writing to dictation, idea motor praxis.
Tactile perception – calculation, abstract thinking, visual perception (famous people), object, constancy, recognition of person/function.
Passage of time.

Section C
This consists of interviewer's observation on appearance, behaviour, mood, speech, mental slowing activity and thought process, bizarre behaviour and level of consciousness.

Section D
Simple physical examination.

Section E
Results of laboratory and radiological investigations.

Section F
Medication.

Section G
Additional information.

Section H
Interview with informant.
History of present difficulty (personality, memory, general mental function, functioning everyday activities, clouding/delirium, depressed mood, sleep, paranoid features, cerebro-vascular problems).

Questions pertaining to subject's past history.
Questions pertaining to family and past history.

Reproduced from the *British Journal of Psychiatry,* Roth M, Tym E, Mountjoy CQ, Huppert FA, Hendrie H, Verma S, Goddard R (1986) CAMDEX. A standardised instrument for the diagnosis of mental disorder in the elderly with special reference to the early detection of dementia, Vol. 149, pp. 698–709. © 1986 Royal College of Psychiatrists. Reproduced with permission.

Nurses' Observation Scale for Geriatric Patients (NOSGER)

Reference: **Spiegel R, Brunner C, Ermini-Fünfschilling D, Monsch A, Notter M, Puxty J, Tremmel L (1991) A new behavioural assessment scale for geriatric out- and in-patients: the NOSGER (Nurses' Observation Scale for Geriatric Patients).** *Journal of the American Geriatrics Society* **39: 339–47**

Time taken 20 minutes

Rating by nursing staff

Main indications

Assessment of behaviour and functioning in elderly patients.

Commentary

The Nurses' Observation Scale for Geriatric Patients (NOSGER) was developed from two existing scales: the Nurses' Observation Scale for Inpatient Evaluation (NOSIE; page 150) and the Geriatric Evaluation by Relative's Rating Instrument (GERRI; page 337). It was designed in view of the need to develop a useful instrument of longitudinal studies in psychogeriatrics, in particular fulfilling the requirements of the scale as follows:

(a) Applicable to institutionalized-community patients covering a wide range of behaviours.

(b) Easy to use for professionals and lay people.

(c) Covering a wide range of behaviours relevant to daily function independent of sex or social class.

The new scale was limited to 30 items, assigned on the basis of content to coincide with one of six areas of assessment: memory, instrumental activities of daily living, self-care, activities of daily living, mood, social behaviour and disturbing behaviour. Three validation studies have been carried out, which are referred to in the main paper. NOSGER items were selected specifically to avoid complicated and ambiguous expression and those which relatives might find offensive – delusions and hallucination were therefore omitted, as were questions with a negative formulation. Inter-rater reliability was found in the three validation studies to be 0.7, with the exception of mood and disturbing behaviour, where it were less than 0.6. The test/retest reliability yielded values between 0.8 and 0.9. Validity was assessed using a number of other scales, with generally good results.

Address for correspondence

R Spiegel
Clinical Research CNS Department
Sandoz Pharma Ltd
402 Basle
Switzerland

Nurses' Observation Scale for Geriatric Patients (NOSGER)

1.   Shaves or puts on makeup, combs hair without help.
2.   Follows favourite radio or TV programmes.
3.   Reports he/she feels sad.
4.   Is restless during the night.
5.   Is interested in what is going on around him/her.
6.   Tries to keep his/her room tidy.
7.   Is able to control bowels.
8.   Remembers a point in conversation after interruption.
9.   Goes shopping for small items (newspaper, groceries).
10. Reports feeling worthless.
11. Continues with some favourite hobby.
12. Repeats the same point in conversation over and over.
13. Appears sad or tearful.
14. Clean and tidy in appearance.
15. Runs aways.
16. Remembers names of close friends.
17. Helps others as far as physically able.
18. Goes out inappropriately dressed.
19. Is orientated when in usual surroundings.
20. When asked questions, seems quarrelsome and irritable.
21. Makes contact with people around.
22. Remembers where clothes and other things are placed.
23. Is aggressive (verbally or physically).
24. Is able to control bladder function (urine).
25. Appears to be cheerful.
26. Maintains contact with friends or family.
27. Confuses the identity of some people with others.
28. Enjoys certain events (visits, parties).
29. Appears friendly and positive in conversation with family members or friends.
30. Behaves stubbornly, does not follow instructions or rules.

Comments:

Answer with respect to last 2 weeks only
Score all as follows: All of the time
                        Most of the time
                        Often
                        Sometimes
                        Never

Reproduced with kind permission from Professor R Spiegel.

Comprehensive Assessment and Referral Evaluation (CARE)

Reference: **Gurland D, Kuriansky J, Sharpe L, Simon R, Stiller P, Birkett P (1977) The Comprehensive Assessment and Referral Evaluation (CARE): rationale, development and reliability.** *International Journal of Ageing and Human Development* **8: 9–42**

Time taken 45–90 minutes

Rating by trained interviewer

Main indications

A comprehensive measure of health and social problems of older people.

Commentary

The Comprehensive Assessment and Referral Evaluation (CARE) is an assessment technique intended to assimilate information on the health and social problems of older people. The CARE is essentially a semi-structured interview guide with an inventory of defined ratings. It is comprehensive in that it covers a whole range of problems – medical, psychiatric, nutritional, social and economic. It can be administered to all groups, and is therefore useful in deciding if a person should be referred, and its scope allows it to evaluate the effectiveness of a service. The CARE covers a number of different areas of functioning

outlined, and the original publication suggested (prior to a factor analysis being performed) the following dimensions: memory/disorientation; depression/anxiety; immobility/incapacity; physical/perceptual; isolation; and poor housing. The first two were indicative of psychiatric problems, the second two medical/physical problems and the last two socioeconomic problems. Reliability is presented for these dimensions in the form of intraclass correlations, and is generally good with the exception of the medical/physical ratings. Familiarity with the instrument was cited as the reason for the low scores.

Additional references

Copeland J (1976) A semi-structured clinical interview for the assessment of diagnosis and mental state in the elderly. *Psychological Medicine* **6**: 451–9.

Macdonald A, Mann A, Jenkins R et al (1982) An attempt to determine the impact of four types of care upon the elderly in London by the study of matched groups. *Psychological Medicine* **12**: 193–200.

Comprehensive Assessment and Referral Evaluation (CARE)

Identifying data/Dementia I: Census type data/Country of Origin/Race/Length of time spoken English

Dementia II: Error in length of residence/telephone number
General enquiries about main problems
Worry/depression/suicide/self-depreciation
Elation
Anxiety/fear of going out/infrequency of excursions
Referential and paranoid ideas
Household arrangement/loneliness
Family and friendly relationships/present and past Isolation index/closeness
Emergency assistance
Anger/family burden on subject
Obsessions/thought reading
Weight/appetite/digestion/difficulties in shopping and preparing food/dietary intake/alcohol intake
Sleep disturbance
Depersonalization

Dementia III: Subjective and objective difficulty with memory/tests or recall
Fits and faints/autonomic functions/bowel and bladder
Slowness and anergia/restlessness
Self-rating of health
Fractures and operations/medical and non-medical attention/examinations/medicines or drugs/drug addiction
Arthritis/aches and pains
Breathlessness/smoking/heart disease/hypertension/chest pain/cough/hoarseness/fevers
Limitation in mobility/care of feet/limitation of exertion/simple tests of motor function
Sores, growths, discharges/strokes/hospitalization and bed-rest
Hearing/auditory hallucinations
Vision/visual hallucinations
Hypochondriasis
Disfigurement/antisocial behavior
Loss of interests/activities list
History of depression
Organizations and religion/educational and occupational history
Work and related problems/retirement history
Income/health insurance/medical and other expenses/handling of finances/shortages
Housing facilities and related problems
Ability to dress/do chores/help needed or received
Neighborhood and crime
Overall self-rating of satisfaction/happiness/insight
Mute/stuporous/abnormalities of speech
Additional observations of subject and environment/communication difficulties

Reproduced from Gurland D, Kuriansky J, Sharpe L, Simon R, Stiller P, Birkett P (1977) The Comprehensive Assessment and Referral Evaluation (CARE): rationale, development and reliability. *International Journal of Ageing and Human Development* **8**: 9–42, published by Baywood Publishing Co.

The Philadelphia Geriatric Center Multilevel Assessment Instrument

Reference: **Lawton MP, Moss M, Fulcomer M, Kleban MH (1982) A research and service oriented multilevel assessment instrument.** *Journal of Gerontology.* **37: 91–9**

Time taken cannot be calculated

Rating by trained interviewer

Main indications

The instrument was developed to measure the well-being of older people in a number of significant domains, i.e. behavioural competence in the domains of health, activities of daily living, cognition, time use and social interactions, and in the sectors of psychological well-being and perceived environmental quality.

Commentary

The development of the MAI was stimulated by three main limitations of existing assessment measures: the inadequate representation of important classes of well-being, e.g. aspects of the environment, the incomplete use of psychometric scaling techniques in the production of the assessment package, and the fact that structural versatility is lacking in some instruments, for example debate as to the hazards of creating short forms of instruments, with trade-off regarding the amount of information that can be gleaned.

The main domains assessed were:

Physical health
a) Self-rated health 4 items
b) Health behaviour 3 items
c) Health conditions — A checklist asking people to report the presence or absence of 22 health conditions

Cognition
a) Mental status — The Mental Status Questionnaire of Khan et al (see page 75)
b) Cognitive symptoms — 4 questions constructed around memory problems, disorientation and confusion

Activities of daily living
a) Physical self-maintenance — Questions about toileting, ambulation, transfer, eating, bathing, dressing and grooming

Instrumental activities of daily living — This asks whether a person can perform a task. This avoids the problems associated with the sex-role or situation limited aspects

Time use — A 19-item checklist of non-instrumental ways of spending time (e.g. meetings, church, hobbies)

Social interaction — The final form included 2 subindices which had been defined by a principal components analysis of a larger battery of questions which yielded two factors, interaction with friends (5 items) and interaction with family (3 aggregated clusters). Another 8 items were retained

Personal adjustment
a) Morale — This was rated using the three highest-loaded items from each of the three factors of the revised Philadelphia Geriatric Center Morale Scale (Lawton, 1975; see page 357)
b) Psychiatric symptoms — These consisted of 10 common psychiatric symptoms, later reduced to five (sleeping, depression, nervousness, major fears, suicidal feelings)

Perceived environment
Housing quality 9 items
Neighbourhood quality 12 items
Personal security 3 items
Objective environment
Economic domain

Three groups were assessed, a sample of 590 people in total, 253 living independently at home and 173 tenants from 11 public housing sites; the second was a group receiving home services (99), and a further 65 people who were on the waiting list for institutions. Internal consistency was assessed using the alpha coefficient, and test/retest reliability was carried out after a 3-week gap. Validity was assessed in a variety of ways and was found to be satisfactory.

PRIME-MD

Reference: **Spitzer RL, Kroenke K, Williams JBW and the Patient Health Questionnaire Primary Care Study Group (1999) Validation and utility of a self-report version of PRIME-MD.** *Journal of the American Medical Association* **282: 1737–44**

Time taken 5 minutes (in 85% of cases a physician was able to interpret the score in less than 3 minutes)

Main indications

The Primary Care Indication of Mental Disorders (PRIME-MD) was developed as a screening instrument for the detection of psychiatric disorders. A clinician-administered version was rather limited in its clinical utility because of the time it took to give, and so a self-completing questionnaire was developed.

Commentary

The instrument was assessed in eight primary care centres in the USA, involving 3000 adult patients with a mean age of 46 but with a range of 18 to 99. Of these, 585 patients had an interview with a health professional shortly after completing the questionnaire. A diagnosis on the scale was present in 28% of the total sample and 29% of the smaller sample.

Address for correspondence

Dr Robert L Spitzer
Biometrics Research Department
New York State Psychiatric Institute
Unit 60 Riverside Drive
New York
NY 10032
USA
email: rls8@columbia.edu

Camberwell Assessment of Need for the Elderly (CANE)

Reference: Reynolds T, Thornicroft G, Abas M, Woods B, Hoe J, Leese M, Orrell M (2000) The Camberwell Assessment of Need for the Elderly (CANE); development, reliability and validity. *British Journal of Psychiatry* 176: 444–52

Time taken about 25 minutes

Rating by experienced interviewer

Main indications

A comprehensive assessment of needs for older people that allows ratings of patient, carer and staff views.

Commentary

The CANE is a comprehensive multi-agency needs assessment tool for older people developed from the Camberwell Assessment of Need. It defines whether needs are met or not met. It can be used to identify services and interventions required in a variety of settings including primary care, mental health services, and care homes. The CANE can be used by health and social care professionals; as an initial assessment, as a comprehensive review, as an outcome measure, for evaluation of services, to assess needs for service development, and for research. It has 24 areas of need covering psychological, physical, and social functioning and two areas for carer needs. It includes ratings for staff, user and carer views of needs. The older person can therefore have their own views of their needs rated separately and can express their level of satisfaction with services. It includes sections, to assess level of services received, and to take into account the individual's strengths, abilities and cultural context. The CANE is intended to model good clinical practice and the ratings are based upon expert professional assessment. The CANE has very good validity and reliability and a detailed manual is available. Training sessions can be arranged. It has been used widely in the UK and internationally and has been translated into several languages.

CANE items

1. Accommodation	2. Household activities
3. Food	4. Self care
5. Caring for another	6. Daytime activities
7. Memory	8. Eyesight/hearing/communication
9. Mobility	10. Continence
11. Physical health	12. Drugs
13. Psychotic symptoms	14. Psychological distress
15. Information	16. Deliberate self-harm
17. Accidental self-harm	18. Abuse/neglect
19. Behaviour	20. Alcohol
21. Company	22. Intimate relationships
23. Money	24. Benefits

Carer's items

A. Carer's need for information; B. Carer's psychological distress.

Additional references

Ashaye O, Livingston G, Orrell M (2003) Does standardised needs assessment improve the outcome of psychiatric day hospital care for older people? *Aging & Mental Health* 7(3): 195–9.

Martin M, Hancock G, Simmons P, Richardson B, Katona C, Mullan E, Orrell M (2002) An evaluation of needs in elderly continuing care settings. *International Psychogeriatrics* 14: 379–88.

Orrell M, Hancock G (2003) *Needs Assessment in Older People: the Camberwell Assessment of Need for the Elderly.* London: Gaskell.

Walters K, Iliffe S, Tai SS, Orrell M (2000) Assessing needs from the patient, carer and professional perspectives: the Camberwell Assessment of Need for the Elderly. *Age and Ageing* 29: 505–10.

Address for correspondence

Dr Martin Orrell
Reader in Psychiatry of Ageing
Department of Psychiatry
University College London
Wolfson Building, 48 Riding House St
London W1N 8AA, UK
Email: m.orrell@ucl.ac.uk
Website: www.thecane.co.uk

Easycare: Elderly Assessment System

Reference: **The EasyCare Development Group (2000) Sheffield Institute for Studies on Ageing (SISA). EasyCare. Elderly Assessment System. University of Sheffield 1999–2000**

Time taken varies for each subject

Main indications

EasyCare is a comprehensive assessment instrument looking at a variety of needs of older people. It is designed for the rapid assessment of an older person's physical, mental and social well-being and is focused on quality of life rather than disease, also recognizing the role of family members.

Commentary

EasyCare can be used in a number of different areas – initial contact, to assess changes in physical, mental health or social services, to act as part of screening or towards outcomes of care, as part of general surveys, and as part of an assessment of an older person prior to placement. A book is available from the authors at the Sheffield Institute for Studies on Ageing. It comprises 24 questions concerning disability, the four-item Geriatric Depression Scale and a six-item Cognitive Function Scale, originally described by Katzman (see p. 68). Questions at the end lay down goals that should be set.

1. Can you see? (with glasses if worn)
2. Can you hear? (with hearing aid if worn)
3. Do you have difficulty chewing food? (with dentures if worn)
4. Do you have difficulty making yourself understood because of problems with your speech?
5. In general, would you say your health is (excellent, very good, good, fair, poor)
6. Do you feel lonely?
7. In general, would you say your accommodation is (excellent, very good, good, fair, poor)
8. Can you do your housework?
9. Can you prepare your own meals?
10. Can you go shopping?
11. Can you handle your own money?
12. Can you use the telephone?
13. Can you take your own medicine?
14. Can you walk outside?
15. Can you get around indoors?
16. Can you manage stairs?
17. Can you move yourself from bed to chair, if next to each other?
18. Can you use the toilet (or commode)?
19. Can you use the bath or shower?
20. Can you keep up your personal appearance?
21. Can you dress yourself?
22. Can you feed yourself?
23. Do you have accidents with your bladder?
24. Do you have accidents with your bowels?

Geriatric Depression Scale (see page 2)
Katzman IMC test (see page 68)

Answered on ordinal scales giving rise to a maximum of 100 for most severe disability.

Address for correspondence

Professor Ian Philp
Sheffield Institute of Studies on Ageing
Community Sciences Centre
Northern General Hospital
Herrries Road
Sheffield S5 7AU
UK

easycare@sheffield.ac.uk

The MOS 36-Item Short-Form Health Survey (SF-36)

Reference: McHorney CA, Ware JE, Lu JFR, Sherbourne CD (1994) The MOS 36-item Short Form Health Survey (SF-36: III Tests of data quality, scaling assumptions and reliability across diverse patient groups). *Medical Care* 32: 40–66

Time taken estimated 10–15 minutes

Rater self-report measures. Little training required for the rater

Main indications

A standardized health survey. Constructed for use in health policy evaluations, general population surveys, clinical research and practice. For use in adults and older people.

Commentary

The MOS 36-Item Short Form Health Survey includes one multi-item scale measuring each of eight general health concepts: physical functioning; role limitations due to physical health problems; bodily pain; general health perceptions; vitality; social functioning; role limitations due to emotional problems; and mental health. All scales are linearly transformed on a scale from 0 to 100, with 100 indicating the most favourable health state and 0 the least favourable, the scores in between representing the percentage of the total possible score achieved. The total score provides a general index of favourable health. There is also a shortened form, the MOS SF-12. Analyses were conducted among 3445 patients and replicated across 24 subgroups, differing in sociodemographic characteristics, diagnosis and disease severity.

Additional reference

Ware JE Jr, Kosinski M, Keller SD (1996) A 12-item short-form health survey: construction of scales and preliminary tests of reliability and validity. *Medical Care* 34: 220–33.

Address for correspondence

Colleen A McHorney
The Health Institute
Box 345 New England Medical Center
750 Washington Street
Boston
MA 02111
USA

Health of the Nation Outcome Scales for Older People (HoNOS 65+)

Reference: **Burns A, Beever A, Lelliott P, Wing J, Blakey A, Orrell M, Mulinga J, Hadden S (1999) Health of the National Outcome Scales for Elderly People (HoNOS 65+).** *British Journal of Psychiatry* **174: 424–7**

Time taken 5–10 minutes (by a professional who knows the patient and once all the information is collected); 30 minutes in semi-structured interview

Rating by trained interviewer

Main indications

Global rating of mental and physical functioning and social circumstances of older people.

Commentary

The UK government's directive on health, enshrined in the *Health of the Nation* document, was a stimulus to the development of simple scales to measure mental health outcomes. A Health of the Nation Outcome scale for younger people with mental health problems (Wing et al, 1998) was developed, and there was clearly a need to adapt it for use in older adults. The work was coordinated by the Royal College of Psychiatrists Research Unit, and a series of multiprofessional focus groups was held to adapt the scale. Inter-rater reliability studies gave satisfactory levels of concordance in keeping with the general adult scale, and validity was assessed against the Mini-Mental State Examination (MMSE; page 36). The main amendments to the scale include specific ratings for agitation, restlessness and sleep disturbance, passive aspects of suicide ideation in the elderly, level of consciousness, and a

clear steer as to where incontinence should be scored. Ratings of sensory deficits were also included. It is important to note that the HoNOS 65+ is not a rating of the aetiology of problems, merely a description of their presence. HoNOS 65+ was able to distinguish between patients with organic functional illness in all the items except physical disability, hallucinations, living condition and relationships. The HoNOS 65+ is still subject to further field trials and amendments.

Additional references

Curtis R, Beevor A (1995) Health of the Nation Outcome Scales. In Wing JK, ed. *Measurement of mental health: contributions from the College Research Unit. College Research Unit Publication No. 2.* London: Royal College of Psychiatrists Research Unit, 33–46.

Wing JK, Beevor AS, Curtis RH et al (1998) Health of the Nation Outcome Scales (HoNOS): research and development. *British Journal of Psychiatry* **172**: 11–18.

Address for correspondence

Professor Alistair Burns
University of Manchester
School of Psychiatry and Behavioural Sciences
Education and Research Centre
Wythenshawe Hospital
Manchester M23 9LT, UK
e-mail: a_burns@man.ac.uk

Health of the Nation Outcome Scales for Older People (HoNOS 65+)

1. Aggression	5. Physical illness and disability	9. Relationships
2. Self-harm	6. Hallucinations and delusions	10. Activities of daily living
3. Drug and alcohol use	7. Depression	11. Residential environment
4. Cognitive problems	8. Other symptoms	12. Day-time activities

Rating:

Each item rated on a 5-point individualized rating from 0 (no problem) – 4 (serious problem).

1–3	= Behaviour
4–5	= Impairment
6–8	= Symptoms
9–12	= Social

Source: Reprinted with permission from Burns A *et al.* Br J Psychiatry 1999; **174**: 424–7.

Chapter 4

Physical examination

Cambridge Neurological Inventory

Reference: Chen EYH, Shapleske J, Luque R, McKenna PJ, Hodges JR, Calloway SP, Hymas NFS, Dening TR, Berrios GE (1995) The Cambridge Neurological Inventory: a clinical instrument for assessment of soft neurological signs in psychiatric patients. *Psychiatry Research* 56: 183–204

Time taken 20–40 minutes

Rating by trained examiner

Main indications

To identify soft neurological signs and other patterns of neurological impairment relevant to neurobiological localization and prognosis in schizophrenia and other psychiatric disorders.

Commentary

The Cambridge Neurological Inventory is a standardized inventory designed to complement the basic neurological examination. Items were drawn from other neurological scales (Quitkin et al, 1976; Walker, 1981; Tweedy et al, 1982; Buchanan and Heinrichs, 1988). The inventory required at least five practice trials before clinical use. The scale has a wider scope than others published, and is precise in using operational definitions for eliciting signs. Inter-rater reliability for most of the items is above 0.85, and was able to distinguish between patients with schizophrenia and controls.

Additional references

Buchanan RW, Heinrichs DW (1988) The Neurological Evaluation Scale (NES): a structured instrument for the assessment of neurological signs in schizophrenia. *Psychiatry Research* **27**: 335–50.

Quitkin F, Rifkin A, Klein DF (1976) Neurological soft signs in schizophrenia and character disorders. *Archives of General Psychiatry* **33**: 845–53.

Tweedy J, Reding M, Gracia C et al (1982) Significance of cortical disinhibition signs. *Neurology* **32**: 169–73.

Walker E (1981) Attentional and neuromotor functions of schizophrenic, schizoaffectives and patients with other affective disorders. *Archives of General Psychiatry* **38**: 1355–8.

Address for correspondence

Eric YH Chen
Department of Psychiatry
Univesity of Cambridge
Addenbrooke's Hospital
Cambridge CB2 2QQ
UK

Cambridge Neurological Inventory

PART 1

Speech assessment:	Articulation
	Aprosodic speech
	Unintelligible speech
Eye movement assessment:	Smooth pursuit – extent, smoothness, gaze impersistence
	Saccadia – smoothness, blink suppression, lateral head movement
Cranial nerve assessment:	Winlang (lateralization)
	Glabellar tap
	Rapid tongue movement

Extremity examinations:	Tone, strength, reflex

PART 2
Soft sign examinations
  i.e. primitive reflexes, repetitive movement, sensory integration, finger nose test, mirror movements, left–right orientation

PART 3
Posture and movement assessment – including catatonia, tardive dyskinesia, gait, balance

Rate as follows:
0 = Normal; 0.5 = Subthreshold; 1 = Definitely abnormal; 2 = Grossly abnormal;
9 = Missing/unable to test or lack of co-operation/comprehension

---

Webster Scale (and other Parkinson's Disease Scales)

Reference: **Webster DD (1988) Critical analysis of the disability in Parkinson's disease. *Modern Treatment* 5: 257–82**

Time taken 15–20 minutes (reviewer's estimate)

Rating by clinician

Main indications

Assessing the degree of disability in Parkinson's disease.

Commentary

The original paper is a model of clinical observation and clinical description and, while well supported by references, contains no empirical data about a patient population. The scale has been used in the assessment of dementia, e.g. Girling and Berrios (1990).

Other rating scales used in the assessment of Parkinson's disease include the Unified Parkinson's Disease Rating Scale (UPDRS) (England and Schwab, 1956; Fahn and Elton, 1987), a staging scale described by Hoehn and Yahr (1967), and the North Western University Disability Scale (Cantor et al, 1961). Other scales are available (for review, see Fahn and Elton, 1987).

Additional references

Cantor C, Torre R, Mier M (1961) A method of evaluating disability in patients with Parkinson's disease. *Journal of Nervous and Mental Disease* **133**: 143–7.

England A, Schwab R (1956) Post-operative evaluation of 26 selected patients with Parkinson's disease. *Journal of the American Geriatrics Society* **4**: 1219–32.

Fahn S, Elton R (1987) Unified Parkinson's Disease Rating Scale. In Fahn S, Marsden C, Goldstein M et al, eds. *Recent developments in Parkinson's disease*, Vol. 2. Macmillan Healthcare Information.

Girling D, Berrios G (1990) Extrapyramidal signs: primitive reflexes in frontal lobe function in senile dementia of the Alzheimer type. *British Journal of Psychiatry* **157**: 888–93.

Hoehn M, Yahr N (1967) Parkinsonism: onset, progression and mortality. *Neurology* **17**: 427–42.

Webster Scale

Bradykinesia of hands – including handwriting
0 No involvement.
1 Detectable slowing of the supination–pronation rate evidenced by beginning difficulty in handling tools, buttoning clothes, and with handwriting.
2 Moderate slowing of supination–pronation rate, one or both sides, evidenced by moderate impairment of hand function. handwriting is greatly impaired, micrographia present.
3 Severe slowing of supination–pronation rate. Unable to write or button clothes. Marked difficulty in handling utensils.
Rigidity
0 Non-detectable.
1 Detectable rigidity in neck and shoulders. Activation phenomenon is present. One or both arms show mild, negative, resting rigidity.
2 Moderate rigidity in neck and shoulders. Resting rigidity is positive when patient not on medication.
3 Severe rigidity in neck and shoulders. Resting rigidity cannot be reversed by medication.
Posture
0 Normal posture. Head flexed forward less than 4 inches.

1 Beginning poker spine. Head flexed forward up to 5 inches
2 Beginning arm flexion. Head flexed forward up to 6 inches. One or both arms raised but still below waist.
3 Onset of simian posture. Head flexed forward more than 6 inches. One or both hands elevated above the waist. Sharp flexion of hand, beginning interphalangeal extension. Beginning flexion of knees.
Upper extremity swing
0 Swings both arms well.
1 One arm definitely decreased in amount of swing.
2 One arm fails to swing.
3 Both arms fail to swing.
Gait
0 Steps out well with 18–30 inch stride. Turns about effortlessly.
1 Gait shortened to 12–18 inch stride. beginning to strike one heel. Turn around time slowing. Requires several steps.
2 Stride moderately shortened – now 6–12 inches. Both heels beginning to strike floor forcefully.

Scale continued opposite

3 Onset of shuffling gait, steps less than 3 inches. Occasional stuttering-type or blocking gait. Walks on toes – turns around very slowly.

Tremor

0 No detectable tremor found.

1 Less than one inch of peak-to-peak tremor movement observed in limbs or head at rest or in either hand while walking or during finger to nose testing.

2 Maximum tremor envelope fails to exceed 4 inches. Tremor is severe but not constant and patient retains some control of hands.

3 Tremor envelope exceeds 4 inches. Tremor is constant and severe. Patient cannot get free of tremor while awake unless it is a pure cerebellar type. Writing and feeding himself are impossible.

Facies

0 Normal. Full animation. No stare.

1 Detectable immobility. Mouth remains closed. Beginning features of anxiety or depression.

2 Moderate immobility. Emotion breaks through at markedly increased threshold. Lips parted some of the time. Moderate appearance of anxiety or depression. Drooling may be present.

3 Frozen facies. Mouth open ¼ inch or more. Drooling may be severe.

Seborrhea

0 None.

1 Increased perspiration, secretion remaining thin.

2 Obvious oiliness present. Secretion much thicker.

3 Marked seborrhea, entire face and head covered by thick secretion.

Speech

0 Clear, loud, resonant, clearly understood.

1 Beginning of hoarseness with loss of inflection and resonance. Good volume and still easily understood.

2 Moderate hoarseness and weakness. Constant monotone, unvaried pitch. Beginning of dysarthria, hesitancy, stuttering, difficult to understand.

3 Marked harshness and weakness. Very difficult to hear and to understand.

Self-care

0 No impairment.

1 Still provides full self-care but rate of dressing definitely impeded. Able to live alone and often still employable.

2 Requires help in certain critical areas, such as turning in bed, rising from chairs, etc. Very slow in performing most activities but manages by taking much time.

3 Continuously disabled. Unable to dress, feed himself, or walk alone.

Score as follows:

0 = No involvement/not detectable/not impaired

1 = Early disease

2 = Moderate disease

3 = Severe disease

Source: Webster DD (1968) Critical analysis of the disability in Parkinson's disease. *Modern Treatment* **5**: 257–82.

Tardive Dyskinesia Rating Scale (TDRS)

Reference: Simpson GM, Lee JH, Zoubok B, Gardos G (1979) A rating scale for tardive dyskinesia. *Psychopharmacology* 64: 171–9

Time taken 20–25 minutes (reviewer's estimate)

Rating by clinician

Main indications

For the assessment of the nature and severity of abnormal movements in psychiatric patients. Useful for studies in older people with schizophrenia.

Commentary

The Tardive Dyskinesia Rating Scale (TDRS) is a 43-item scale consisting of the standard assessment (from absent to very severe on a six-point scale) of neurological signs in the face, neck and trunk, and extremities, and changes affecting the whole body. Inter-rater reliability is generally high, ranging between 0.55 and 1.0 using Pearson's correlation. An abbreviated dyskinesia scale is also available consisting of 13 items with similar inter-rater reliability.

Additional reference

Simpson G (1988) Tardive dyskinesia rating scale. *Psychopharmacology Bulletin* **24**: 803–7.

Tardive Dyskinesia Rating Scale (TDRS)

Face

1. Blinking of eyes ___
2. Tremor of eyelids ___
3. Tremor of upper lip (rabbit syndrome) ___
4. Pouting of the (lower) lip ___
5. Puckering of lips ___
6. Sucking movements ___
7. Chewing movements ___
8. Smacking of lips ___
9. Bonbon sign ___
10. Tongue protrusion ___
11. Tongue tremor ___
12. Choreoathetoid movements of tongue ___
13. Facial tics ___
14. Grimacing ___
15. Other (describe) ___
16. Other (describe) ___

Neck and trunk

17. Head nodding ___
18. Retrocollis ___
19. Spasmodic torticollis ___
20. Torsion movements (trunk) ___
21. Axial hyperkinesia ___
22. Rocking movement ___
23. Other (describe) ___

24. Other (describe) ___

Extremities (upper)

25. Ballistic movements ___
26. Choreoathetoid movements – fingers ___
27. Choreoathetoid movements – wrists ___
28. Pill-rolling movements ___
29. Caressing or rubbing face and hair ___
30. Rubbing of thighs ___
31. Other (describe) ___
32. Other (describe) ___

Extremities (lower)

33. Rotation and/or flexion of ankles ___
34. Toe movements ___
35. Stamping movements – standing ___
36. Stamping movements – sitting ___
37. Restless legs ___
38. Crossing/uncrossing legs – sitting ___
39. Other (describe) ___
40. Other (describe) ___

Entire body

41. Holokinetic movements ___
42. Akathisia ___
43. Other (describe) ___

Score:

1 = Absent
2 = Questionable
3 = Mild
4 = Moderate
5 = Moderately severe
6 = Very severe

Neurological Evaluation Scale (NES)

Reference: **Buchanan RW, Heinrichs DW (1989) The Neurological Evaluation Scale (NES): a structured instrument for the assessment of neurological signs in schizophrenia.** *Psychiatry Research* **27: 335–50**

Time taken 30 minutes (reviewer's estimate)

Rating by clinician

Main indications

A structured neurological examination particularly focusing on areas of impairment found in schizophrenia.

Commentary

The Neurological Evaluation Scale (NES) was developed following an extensive search of systematic reviews and clinical studies of neurological abnormalities in patients with schizophrenia. Three functional areas were described: sensory dysfunction, motor and coordination, and impaired sequencing. A 28-item scale was described. Inter-rater reliability (intraclass correlations) was above 0.8 for the majority of items (reliability was also assessed by a

nurse, following training lasting approximately 20 hours) and reliability of above 0.72 was found. In 98 patients, validity was assessed by determining the ability of the scale to differentiate between patients and controls, and highly significant differences were found.

Additional reference

Heinrichs DW, Buchanan RW (1988) The significance and meaning of neurological signs in schizophrenia. *American Journal of Psychiatry* **145**: 11–18.

Address for correspondence

RW Buchanan
Department of Psychiatry
University of Maryland School of Medicine
Baltimore
MD 21228
USA

Neurological Evaluation Scale (NES)

1. Tandem walk
2. Romberg test
3. Adventitious overflow
4. Tremor
6. Cerebral dominance
7. Audio-visual integration
8. Stereognosis
9. Graphesthesia
10. Fist-ring test
11. Fist-edge-palm test
12. Ozeretski test
13. Memory
14. Rhythm tapping test
15. Rapid alternating movements
16. Finger-thumb opposition
17. Mirror movements
18. Extinction (face-hand test)
20. Right/left confusion
21. Synkinesis
22. Convergence
23. Gaze impersistence
24. Finger to nose test
25. Glabellar reflex
26. Snout reflex
27. Grasp reflex
28. Suck reflex

Assessments:
0 = Relatively normal
1 = Some disruption
2 = Major disruption

Quantification of Physical Illness in Psychiatric Research in the Elderly

Reference: **Burvill PW, Mowry B, Hall WD (1990) Quantification of physical illness in psychiatric research in the elderly.** *International Journal of Geriatric Psychiatry* 5: 161–70

Time taken 5 minutes

Rating by clinician

Main indications

The scale aims to allow for a rating of severity and disability of physical symptoms in different body systems: cardiovascular; CNS; endocrine; gastrointestinal; genitourinary; haematological; musculoskeletal; respiratory; other.

Commentary

One hundred and three patients, all with a DSM-III diagnosis of major depression were assessed for their physical health. Three types of data analysis were performed: a descriptive analysis of the basic data, the relationship between various measures and an analysis of the structure of these measures. An inter-rater test/retest reliability study was carried out which showed correlation coefficients of above 9 on all the measures. Distinct differences were seen on the comparison of body systems, suggesting that the scale could differentiate between them; the correlations between patients' own assessments and the psychiatric assessments were good, and a factor analysis revealed three factors that were independent of each other, one for acute illness, one for chronic illness, and one for the patient's own rating.

Criteria for rating severity and disability scores for each physical system:

Severity

Mild: An illness is present. Symptoms of the illness are absent or only mild. It either requires no treatment or is under good control with treatment.
Moderate: Symptoms of the chronic illness are of moderate severity. The illness is not under full control with treatment. There has not been any recent hospitalization. The illness is not life-threatening.
Severe: There are a number of severe symptoms. The illness requires substantial medical treatment with or without hospitalization, and/or the illness would be expected to reduce life expectancy in its present state.

Disability

Mild: The chronic illness causes the patient only relatively minor impairment of (a) physical, and/or (b) social functioning, and/or (c) in activities of daily living (ADL).
Moderate: The illness causes a moderate degree of impairment of (a) physical functioning, and/or (b) social functioning, and/or (c) in activities of daily living (ADL).
Severe: The illness causes marked impairments of (a) physical, and/or (b) social functioning, and/or (c) in activities of daily living (ADL).

London Handicap Scale

Reference: **Harwood RH, Gompertz P, Ebrahim S (1994) Handicap one year after stroke: validity of a new scale.** *Journal of Neurology, Neurosurgery and Psychiatry* **57: 825–9**

Time taken varies from subject to subject

Rating by self-rated questionnaire

Main indications

The aim was to determine the handicap experienced by people 1 year following stroke and to develop a handicap measurement scale.

Commentary

Three hundred and sixty-one people admitted to hospital with acute stroke were identified and outcomes at 12 months determined by a postal questionnaire comprising measures of disability with perceived health and life satisfaction. Construct validity of the scale was assessed using the correlation coefficients between other measures – the Barthel Index and the Nottingham Health Profile. Test/retest reliability was satisfactory.

Address for correspondence

Dr R Harwood
Department of Public Health and Primary Care
Royal Free Hospital School of Medicine
London NW3 2PF
UK

The London Handicap Scale

Your health and your life
This questionnaire asks six questions about your everyday life. Please answer each question. Tick the box next to the sentence which describes you best. Think about things you have done over the last week. Compare what you can do with what someone like you who is in good health can do.

Getting around (mobility)
Think about how you get from one place to another, using any help, aids of means of transport that you normally have available.
Does your health stop you from getting around?
1. Not at all: you go everywhere you want to, no matter how far away.
2. Very slightly: you go most places you want to, but not all.
3. Quite a lot: You get out of the house, but not far away from it.
4. Very much: you don't go outside, but you can move around from room to room indoors.
5. Almost completely: you are confined to a single room, but can move around in it.
6. Completely: you are confined to a bed or a chair. You cannot move around at all. There is no one to move you.

Looking after yourself (physical independence)
Think about things like housework, shopping, looking after money, cooking, laundry, getting dressed, washing, shaving and using the toilet.
Does your health stop you looking after yourself?
1. Not at all: you can do everything yourself.
2. Very slightly: now and again you need a little help.
3. Quite a lot: you need help with some tasks (such as heavy housework or shopping), but no more than once a day.
4. Very much: you can do some things but you need help more than once a day. You can be left alone safely for a few hours.
5. Almost completely: you need help to be available all the time. You cannot be left alone safely.
6. Completely: you need help with everything. You need constant attention, day and night.

Work and leisure (occupation)
Think about things like work (paid or not), housework, gardening, sports, hobbies, going out with friends, travelling, reading, looking after children, watching television and going on holiday.
Does your health limit your work or leisure activities?
1. Not at all: you can do everything you want to do
2. Very slightly: you can do almost all the things you want to do
3. Quite a lot: you find something to do almost all the time, but cannot do some things for as long as you would like.
4. Very much: you are unable to do a lot of things but can find something to do most of the time.
5. Almost completely: you are unable to do most things, but can find something to do some of the time.
6. Completely: you sit all day doing nothing. You cannot keep yourself busy or take part in any activities.

Getting on with people (social integration)
Think about family, friends and people you might meet during a normal day.
Does your health stop you getting on with people?
1. Not at all: you get on well with people, see everyone you want to see, and meet new people.
2. Very slightly: you get on well with people, but your social life is slightly limited.
3. Quite a lot: you are fine with people you know well, but you feel uncomfortable with strangers.

cont.

307

4. Very much: you are fine with people you know well, but you have few friends and little contact with neighbours. Dealing with strangers is very hard.
5. Almost completely: apart from the person who looks after you, you see no one. You have no friends and no visitors.
6. Completely: you don't get on with anyone, not even people who look after you.

Awareness of surroundings (orientation)
Think about taking in and understanding the world around you, and finding your way around in it.
Does your health stop you understanding the world around you?
1. Not at all: you fully understand the world around you. You see, hear, speak and think clearly, and your memory is good.
2. Very slightly: you have problems with hearing, speaking, seeing or your memory, but these do not stop you doing most things.
3. Quite a lot: you have problems with hearing, speaking, seeing or your memory which make life difficult a lot of the time, but you understand what is going on.
4. Very much: you have great difficulty understanding what is going on.
5. Almost completely: you are unable to tell where you are or what day it is. You cannot look after yourself at all.

6. Completely: you are unconscious, completely unaware of anything going on around you.

Affording the things you need (economic self-sufficiency)
Think about whether health problems have led to any extra expenses, or have caused you to earn less than you would if you were healthy.
Are you able to afford the things you need?
1. Yes, easily: you can afford everything you need. You have easily enough money to buy modern labour-saving devices and anything you may need because of ill-health.
2. Fairly easily: you have just about enough money. It is fairly easy to cope with expenses caused by ill-health.
3. Just about: you are less well-off than other people like you; however, with sacrifices you can get by without help.
4. Not really: you only have enough money to meet your basic needs. You are dependent on state benefits for any extra expenses you have because of ill-health.
5. No: you are dependent on state benefits or money from other people or charities. You cannot afford things you need.
6. Absolutely not: you have no money at all and no state benefits. You are totally dependent on charity for your most basic needs.

Source: Harwood RH *et al. J Neurol Neurosurg Psychiatry* 1994; **57**: 825–9. Reproduced by permission.

The General Medical Health Rating (GMHR)

Reference: **Lyketsos CG, Galik E, Steele C, Steinberg M, Rosenblatt A, Warren A, Sheppard JM, Baker A, Brandt J (1999) The General Medical Health Rating: a global rating of medical co-morbidity in patients with dementia.** *Journal of the American Geriatric Society* 47: 487–91

Time taken 10–15 minutes

Rating by clinician

Main indications

A rapid global rating scale of medical comorbidity in patients with dementia.

Commentary

The General Medical Health Rating (GMHR) was developed specifically for people with dementia to act as a bedside measure of general medical comorbidity (other scales being regarded as too cumbersome for general medical practice). In the study, 819 outpatients and 180 inpatients were included and the scale was found to be reliable (weighted kappa 0.91) across all stages and types of dementia

Address for correspondence

Dr CG Lyketsos
Osler 320
Johns Hopkins Hospital
Baltimore
MD 21287
USA

e-mail: Kostas@jhmi.edu

The General Medical Health Rating

Circle *one* of the numbers between 1 and 4 using the instructions next to each number *as a guide*. Please begin at the top and decide if the person meets each rating in sequence as written. If you are having trouble deciding between two adjacent ratings, rate the lower number.

4	EXCELLENT	no current unstable medical illness, may have up to two stable medical illnesses, is on very few (no more than two) medications, and appears healthy and in good condition
3	GOOD	may have one unstable medical illness that is being treated, or a few (up to four) stable medical illnesses, is on few (up to four) medications, and appears no more than mildly ill
2	FAIR	more than one (but no more than three) unstable medical illness, and/or several stable but chronic medical conditions, is on several medications, appears moderately ill
1	POOR	several unstable medical illnesses, multiple medications, appears quite ill, possibly in need of hospitalization

Simpson–Angus Scale (SAS)

References: **Simpson GM, Angus JWS (1970) A rating scale for extrapyramidal side-effects.** *Acta Psychiatrica Scandinavica* **212 (Suppl 44):11–19**

Simpson GM, Lee JH, Zoubok B, Gardos G (1979) A rating scale for tardive dyskinesia. *Psychopharmacology* **64: 171–9**

Time taken 10 minutes

Rating by physician

Main indications

A 10-item instrument used to measure drug-induced parkinsonism.

Commentary

The SAS consists of 10 items rated on a five-point scale (0 is complete absence of the condition, 4 is the presence of the condition in its extreme form). Seven of the 10 scale items measure rigidity. The remainder measure tremor and pooling of saliva in the mouth. The global score is a summation of all of the item ratings divided by the total number of items. Scores of up to 3 are considered within the normal range. The main disadvantage is the emphasis on rating rigidity and does not include ratings of akinesia or bradykinesia. It was validated in a double-blind study involving two dose levels of haloperidol and placebo. A modified version developed by Mindham in 1976 includes an item on lack of facial expression.

Additional references

Mindham RHS (1976) Assessment of drugs in schizophrenia: assessment of drug-induced extrapyramidal reactions and drugs given for their control. *British Journal of Clinical Pharmacology* **3** (Suppl 2): 395–400.

www.medafile.com/zyweb/SAMS.htm

Barnes Akathisia Rating Scale (BAS, BARS)

References: Barnes TRE (1989) A rating scale for drug-induced akathisia. *British Journal of Psychiatry* 154: 672–6

Barnes TRE (1992) Clinical assessment of the extrapyramidal side effects of antipsychotic drugs. *Journal of Psychopharmacology* 6: 214–21

Time taken 10–15 minutes

Rating by physician

Main indications

A scale to assess drug-induced akathisia.

Commentary

Developed in 1989, the Barnes Akathisia Rating Scale (BAS) assesses objective features of motor restlessness, subjective complaints of restlessness and associated distress. The scale incorporates diagnostic criteria for mild, moderate and severe akathisia, and includes an examination procedure that is recommended. Symptoms that have been observed in situations other than the interviewer examination may be included in the ratings. The final item is a clinical global assessment which may be used as an overall severity measure. The Hillside akathisia scale does not define the characteristic restless movements of akathisia and therefore the rater has to decide whether the movements qualify as manifestations of the condition or not. The BAS shows good inter-rater reliability. Its validity is derived from its basis in signs and symptoms identified in previous studies involving patients who received antipsychotic medication following acute psychiatric admissions, and schizophrenic patients on maintenance medication.

Additional references

Barnes TRE, Braude WM (1985) Akathisia variants and tardive dyskinesia. *Archives of General Psychiatry* 42: 874–8.

Fleischhacker W, Bergman KJ, Perovich R et al (1989) The Hillside akathisia scale: a new rating instrument for drug-induced akathisia, parkinsonism and hyperkinesias. *Acta Psychiatrica Scandinavica* 67: 178–87.

Address for correspondence

Professor Thomas Barnes
Division of Neuroscience and Psychological Medicine
Imperial College School of Medicine
Academic Centre, Ealing Hospital
St Bernard's Wing
Uxbridge Road
London UB1 3EU
UK

e-mail: t.r.barnes@ic.ac.uk
www.medafile.com/zyweb/Barnes.htm

Chapter 5

Delirium

Three scales purport to measure the symptoms of delirium. Two are firmly based on DSM criteria for the diagnosis of delirium: the Delirium Rating Scale (DRS; page 317) and the Confusion Assessment Method (CAM; page 315). The Delirium Symptom Interview (DSI; page 314) and CAM are devised to be completed by non-specialists. This is clearly an advantage considering the proportion of patients in non-specialist settings who may suffer from delirium.

Readers should also be aware of another two rating scales for delirium: The Delirium Assessment Scale (O'Keefe S, 1994, Rating the severity of delirium – The Delirium Assessment Scale. *International Journal of Geriatric Psychiatry* **9**: 551–6) and the Confusional State Evaluation (CSE) (Robertson B, Karlsson I. Styrud E, Gottfries C, 1997, Confusional state evaluation: an instrument for measuring severity of delirium in the elderly. *British Journal of Psychiatry* **170**: 565–70).

For information on the Delirium Index (DI), please see page 319.

Delirium Symptom Interview (DSI)

Reference: Albert MS, Levkoff SE, Reilly C, Liptzin B, Pilgrim D, Cleary PD, Evans D, Rowe JW (1992) The Delirium Symptom Interview: an interview for the detection of delirium symptoms in hospitalized patients. *Journal of Geriatric Psychiatry and Neurology* 5: 14–21

Time taken 10–15 minutes

Rating by lay interviewer

Main indications

To rate the symptoms of delirium.

Commentary

The Delirium Symptom Interview (DSI) was developed by an interdisciplinary group of investigators. One of the stimuli was the lack of easily administered instruments for delirium, which was impeding studies on the subject. The importance of ratings on a daily basis (in view of rapid changes seen in delirium) and the need therefore for ratings to be made by non-clinicians were emphasized.

Fifty patients on medical or surgical wards of an acute hospital were interviewed. Reliability for the various domains of the DSI range from 0.45 (sleep disturbance) to 0.80 (disturbance of consciousness), and ratings were made in the same interview. Reliability was 0.90 using a physicians' consensus. Sensitivity of the DSI in detecting delirium was 0.90, specificity 0.80, positive predictive value 0.87 and negative predictive value 0.84.

Address for correspondence

Marilyn S Albert
Department of Psychiatry and Neurology
Massachusetts General Hospital
Boston
MA
USA

Delirium Symptom Interview (DSI)

Symptom domains measured (from DSM III)
- Disorientation
- Sleep disturbance
- Perceptual disturbance
- Disturbance of consciousness
- Psychomotor activity
- General behaviour observations
- Fluctuating behaviour score

Domains assessed
Disorientation, disturbance of sleep, perceptual disturbance, disturbance of consciousness.

Observations
Disturbance of consciousness, incoherent speech, level of psychomotor activity, general behavioural observations, fluctuations in behaviour.

Score: or
1 = No
2 = Mild   1 = No
3 = Moderate   2 = Yes
4 = Severe   7 = Not applicable

A patient is defined as positive on the DSI if any one of the following is present: disorientation, disturbance of consciousness or perceptual disturbance.

Source: Albert MS, Levkoff SE, Reilly C, Liptzin B, Pilgrim D, Cleary P, Evans D, Rowe JW (1992) The Delirium Symptom Interview: an interview for the detection of delirium symptoms in hospitalized patients. *Journal of Geriatric Psychiatry and Neurology* **5**: 14–20.

Confusion Assessment Method (CAM)

Reference: Inouye SK, van Dyck CH, Alessi CA, Balkin S, Siegal AP, Horwitz RI (1990) Clarifying confusion: the Confusion Assessment Method. *Annals of Internal Medicine* 113: 941–8

Time taken 5 minutes

Rating by clinician

Main indications

For the non-psychiatric clinician to detect delirium. Some training required.

Commentary

The Confusion Assessment Method (CAM) instrument consists of nine operationalized criteria from DSM-III-R including the four cardinal features of acute onset and fluctuation, inattention, disorganized thinking and altered level of consciousness. Both the first and second feature, and either the third or fourth, are required. Face and content validity, concurrent validation, inter-rater reliability and convergent validity were all assessed. The results were validated against a psychiatric diagnosis and for cognitive tests. Sensitivity was 94% and 100% (in two study sites), with specificity 90% and 95% respectively. There was a good correlation with ratings on cognitive tests, and inter-rater reliability was around 0.81. Test/retest reliability was not carried out because of fluctuations in the clinical condition of the patients. Individual clinical features of the CAM include acute onset and fluctuating course, inattention and disorganized thinking, altered level of consciousness, disorientation, memory impairment, perceptional disturbance, abnormal psychomotor activity and altered sleeping cycle.

Address for correspondence

Sharon K Inouye
Yale–New Haven Hospital
20 York Street
Tomkins Basement 15
New Haven
CT 06504
USA

Confusion Assessment Method (CAM)

Acute onset

1. Is there evidence of an acute change in mental status from the patient's baseline?

Inattention*

2. A. Did the patient have difficulty focusing attention, for example, being easily distractible, or having difficulty keeping track of what was being said?

   Not present at any time during interview.
   Present at some time during interview, but in mild form.
   Present at some time during interview, in marked form.
   Uncertain.

   B. (If present or abnormal) Did this behavior fluctuate during the interview, that is, tend to come and go or increase and decrease in severity?

   Yes.
   No.
   Uncertain.
   Not applicable.

   C. (If present or abnormal) Please describe this behavior:

Disorganized thinking

3. Was the patient's thinking disorganized or incoherent, such as rambling or irrelevant conversation, unclear or illogical flow of ideas, or unpredictable switching from subject to subject?

Altered level of consciousness

4. Overall, how would you rate this patient's level of consciousness?

   Alert (normal).
   Vigilant (hyperalert, overly sensitive to environmental stimuli, startled very easily).
   Lethargic (drowsy, easily aroused).
   Stupor (difficult to arouse).
   Coma (unrousable).
   Uncertain.

Disorientation

5. Was the patient disoriented at any time during the interview, such as thinking that he or she was somewhere other than the hospital, using the wrong bed, or misjudging the time of day?

Memory impairment

6. Did the patient demonstrate any memory problems during the interview, such as inability to remember events in the hospital or difficulty remembering instructions?

Perceptual disturbances

7. Did the patient have any evidence of perceptual distrubances, for example, hallucinations, illusions, or misinterpretations (such as thinking something was moving when it was not)?

Psychomotor agitation

8. Part 1.
   At any time during the interview, did the patient have an unusually increased level of motor activity, such as restlessness, picking at bedclothes, tapping fingers, or making frequent sudden changes of position?

Psychomotor retardation

8. Part 2.
   At any time during the interview, did the patient have an unusually decreased level of motor activity, such as sluggishness, staring into space, staying in one position for a long time, or moving very slowly?

Altered sleep–wake cycle

9. Did the patient have evidence of disturbance of the sleep–wake cycle, such as excessive daytime sleepiness with insomnia at night?

*The questions listed under this topic are repeated for each topic where applicable.

Source: *Annals of Internal Medicine*, 113, 941–948, 1990. Copyright 1990, the American College of Physicians. Reprinted by permission.

Delirium Rating Scale (DRS)

Reference: **Trzepacz PT, Baker RW, Greenhouse J (1988) A symptom rating scale for delirium. *Psychiatry Research* 23: 89–97**

Time taken 5–10 minutes

Rating by clinician

Main indications

Assessment of symptoms of delirium.

Commentary

The Delirium Rating Scale (DRS) consists of ten items based on DSM-III criteria for delirium. Twenty patients with delirium were compared against nine with chronic schizophrenia, nine with dementia and nine medically ill subjects. Other ratings included the Mini-Mental State Examination (MMSE; page 36), the Trail Making Test and the Brief Psychiatric Rating Scale (BPRS; page 272). Inter-rater reliability was 0.97. Ratings on the DRS were significantly higher for the delirium group compared with the other three groups. It is suggested that the test can be used in conjunction with the electroencephalogram and cognitive tests to measure delirium.

Address for correspondence

PT Trzepacz
Allegheny General Hospital
320 E North Avenue
Pittsburgh
PA 15213
USA

Delirium Rating Scale (DRS)

Item 1: Temporal onset of symptoms

0. No significant change from longstanding behavior, essentially a chronic or chronic-recurrent disorder.
1. Gradual onset of symptoms, occurring within a 6-month period.
2. Acute change in behavior or personality occurring over a month.
3. Abrupt change in behavior, usually occurring over a 1- to 3-day period.

Item 2: Perceptual disturbances

0. None evident by history or observation.
1. Feelings of depersonalization or derealization.
2. Visual illusions or misperceptions including macropsia, micropsia, e.g. may urinate in wastebasket or mistake bedclothes for something else.
3. Evidence that the patient is markedly confused about external reality, not discriminating between dreams and reality.

Item 3: Hallucination type

0. Hallucinations not present.
1. Auditory hallucinations only.
2. Visual hallucinations present by patient's history or inferred by observation, with or without auditory hallucinations.
3. Tactile, olfactory, or gustatory hallucinations present with or without visual or auditory hallucinations.

Item 4: Delusions

0. Not present.
1. Delusion are systematized, i.e. well-organized and persistent.
2. Delusions are new and not part of a preexisting primary psychiatric disorder.
3. Delusions are not well circumscribed; are transient, poorly organized, and mostly in response to misperceived environmental cues; e.g. are paranoid and involve persons who are in reality caregivers, loved ones, hospital staff, etc.

Item 5: Psychomotor behavior

0. No significant retardation or agitation.
1. Mild restlessness, tremulousness, or anxiety evident by observation and a change from patient's usual behavior.
2. Moderate agitation with pacing, removing i.v.s etc.
3. Severe agitation, needs to be restrained, may be combative; or has significant withdrawal from the environment, but not due to major depression or schizophrenic catatonia.

Item 6: Cognitive status during formal testing

0. No cognitive deficits, or deficits which can be alternatively explained by lack of education or prior mental retardation.
1. Very mild cognitive deficits which might be attributed to

inattention due to acute pain, fatigue, depression, or anxiety associated with having a medical illness.
2. Cognitive deficit largely in one major area tested, e.g. memory, but otherwise intact.
3. Significant cognitive deficits which are diffuse, i.e. affecting many different areas tested; must include periods of disorientation to time or place at least once each 24-hr period; registration and/or recall are abnormal; concentration is reduced.
4. Severe cognitive deficits, including motor or verbal perseverations, confabulations, disorientation to person, remote and recent memory deficits, and inability to cooperate with formal mental status testing.

Item 7: Physical disorder

0. None present or active
1. Presence of any physical disorder which might affect mental state.
2. Specific drug, infection, metabolic, central nervous system lesion, or other medical problem which can be temporally implicated in causing the altered behavior or mental status.

Item 8: Sleep-wake cycle disturbance

0. Not present, awake and alert during the day, and sleeps without significant disruption at night.
1. Occasional drowsiness during day and mild sleep continuity disturbances at night; may have nightmares but can readily distinguish from reality.
2. Frequent napping and unable to sleep at night, constituting a significant disruption of or a reversal of the usual sleep-wake cycle.
3. Drowsiness prominent, difficulty staying alert during interview, loss of self-control over alertness and somnolence.
4. Drifts into stuporous or comatose periods.

Item 9: Lability of mood

0. Not present; mood stable.
1. Affect/mood somewhat altered and changes over the course of hours; patient states that mood changes are not under self-control.
2. Significant mood changes which are inappropriate to situation, including fear, anger, or tearfulness; rapid shifts of emotion, even over several minutes.
3. Severe disinhibition of emotions, including temper outbursts, uncontrolled inappropriate laughter, or crying.

Item 10: Variability of symptoms

0. Symptoms stable and mostly present during daytime.
2. Symptoms worsen at night.
4. Fluctuating intensity of symptoms, such that they wax and wane during a 24-hr period.

Reprinted from *Psychiatry Research*, 23, Trzepacz PI, Baker RW, Greenhouse J, pp. 89–97. Copyright (1988), with permission from Elsevier Science.

The Delirium Index (DI)

Reference: **McCusker J, Cole M, Bellavance F, Primeau F (1998) Reliability and validity of a new measure of severity of delirium.** *International Psychogeriatrics* 10: 421–33

Time taken 5–10 minutes

Rating by trained observer

Main indication

To rate the severity of delirium.

Commentary

The Delirium Index (DI) was designed from the Confusion Assessment Method (CAM; see page 315) and DSM-III-R Criteria for Delirium.

The final instrument is a seven symptom rating scale, each scored on a 3 point measure, increased from an original 2 point scale, with a view to increasing sensitivity.

The scale was assessed in three studies looking at inter-rater reliability, and construct and criterion validity. Inter-rater reliability between a research assistant and psychiatrist ranged between 0.77 and 0.93. Criterion validity was assessed against the Delirium Rating Scale (Trzepacz et al 1998, page 317) and correlation with that instrument was high. Correlations with the Mini-Mental State Examination (page 36) and the Barthel Index (page 190) were 0.7 and 0.6 respectively. The DI is a measure of the severity of delirium, allowing standardized measurements of changes over time to be undertaken.

Address for Correspondence

Dr Jane McCusker
Department of Clinical Epidemiology and Community Studies
St Mary's Hospital Center, Room 2508
3830 Lacombe Avenue
Montreal
Quebec H3T 1M5
Canada

The Delirium Index (DI)

The DI is an instrument for the measurement of severity of symptoms of delirium that is based solely upon observation of the individual patient, without additional information from family members, nursing staff, or the patient medical chart. The DI was designed to be used in conjunction with the MMSE: At least the first five questions of the MMSE comprise the basis of observation. Additional questions may be necessary for scoring certain symptoms as noted.

I. Attention
  0   Attentive
  I   Generally attentive but makes at least one error in spelling 'World' backwards.
  2   Questions can generally be answered but subject is distractible and at times has difficulty in keeping track of questions. May have some difficulty in shifting attention to new questions or questions may have to be repeated several times.
  3   Either unresponsive or totally unable to keep track of or answer questions. Has great difficulty in focusing attention and is often distracted by irrelevant stimuli.
  9   Cannot assess.

2. Disorganized Thinking
  0   Responses are logical, coherent, and relevant.
  I   Responses are vague or unclear.
  2   Thought is occasionally illogical, incoherent, or irrelevant.
  3   Either unresponsive or thought is fragmented, illogical, incoherent, and irrelevant.
  9   Cannot assess.

3. Level of Consciousness
  0   Normal.
  I   Hypervigilant or hypovigilant (glassy eyed, decreased reaction to questions).
  2   Drowsy/sleepy. Responds only to simple, loud questions.
  3   Unresponsive or comatose.

4   Disorientation (Additional questions on age, birthdate, and birthplace may be used.)
  0   Knows today's date (± I day) and the name of the hospital.
  I   Either does not know today's date (±I day) or does not know the name of the hospital.
  2   Either does not know the month or year or does not know that he is in hospital.
  3   Either unresponsive or or does not know name or birthdate.
  9   Cannot assess.

5   Memory (Additional questions may be asked on how long patient has been in hospital, circumstances of admission.)
  0   Recalls 3 words and details of hospitalization.
  I   Either cannot recall I of the words or has difficulty recalling details of the hospitalization.
  2   Either cannot recall 2 of the 3 words or recalls very few details of the hospitalization.
  3   Either unresponsive or cannot recall any of the 3 words or cannot recall any details of the hospitalization.
  9   Cannot assess.

6   Perceptual Disturbance (Patient is asked whether he has had any unusual experiences and has seen or heard things that other people do not see or hear. If yes, he is asked whether these occur during the daytime or at night and how frequently. Patient is also observed for any evidence of disordered perception.)
  0   Either unresponsive or no perceptual disturbance observed or cannot assess.
  I   Misinterprets stimuli (for example, interpreting a door closing as a gunshot).
  2   Occasional nonthreatening hallucinations.
  3   Frequent, threatening hallucinations.

7. Motor Activity
  0   Normal.
  I   Responds well to questions but either moves frequently or is lethargic/sluggish.
  2   Moves continuously (and may be restrained) or very slow with little spontaneous movement.
  3   Agitated, difficult to control (restraints are required) or no voluntary movement.

Scoring

I Total score is sum of 7 item scores.

2 If questions I, 2 4 or 5 are checked '9' (e.g. patient refuses to answer questions), replace 9 by the score of Item 3.

Source: McCusker J, Cole M, Bellavance F, Primeau F (1998) Reliability and validity of a new measure of severity of delirium. *International Psychogeriatrics* 10(4): 421–33. © 1998 Springer Publishing Company, Inc., New York 10012, used by permission.

Chapter 6

Caregiver assessments

This is an ever expanding field with much current interest in the views and experiences of carers. Psychological distress is best measured using the General Health Questionnaire (GHQ; page 334) – the gold standard in terms of the rating of psychological distress. Lists of the number of problems exist, and other scales cover activity, intimacy and hassles in more detail. The gold standard remains Gilleard's Problem Checklist and Strain Scale (page 322). Other inventories include the Screen for Caregiver Burden (SCB; page 326), the Caregiving Hassles Scale (page 328), the Revised Memory and Behavior Problems Checklist (page 332), the TRIMS Behavioral Problem Checklist (BPC; page 336) and the Geriatric Evaluation by Relative's Rating Instrument (GERRI; page 337). More detailed information, looking at the mechanisms of strain, is dealt with by the Marital Intimacy Scale (page 330) and the Ways of Coping Checklist (page 324). The Caregiver Activity Survey (CAS; page 333) measures time spent, while the Zung Self-Rating Depression Scale (page 339) and GHQ are included as they are commonly used assessments of psychological disturbance and depression in relatives.

Problem Checklist and Strain Scale

Reference: **Gilleard CJ (1984)** *Living with dementia: community care of the elderly mental infirm.* **Beckenham: Croom Helm**

Time taken 20 minutes (reviewer's estimate)

Rating by interviewer

Main indications

Problem Checklist: assessment of problems experienced by carers of patients with dementia. Strain Scale: assessment of strain.

Commentary

The Problem Checklist was derived from three main studies on day patients, largely in the Edinburgh region of Scotland (Gilleard and Watt, 1982). The 34-item Problem Checklist is rated on a three-point scale: not present, occasionally occurring and frequently/continually occurring, with those items rated as occasionally or frequently further rated as no problem, a small problem or a great problem. The Strain Scale is derived from Machin (1980) and contains 12 items.

Additional references

Gilleard CJ, Watt G (1982) The impact of psychogeriatric day care on the primary supporter of the elderly mentally infirm. In Taylor R, Gilmore A, eds. *Current trends in British gerontology.* Aldershot: Gower Publishing, 139–47.

Machin E (1980) A survey of the behaviour of the elderly and their supporters at home. Unpublished MSc thesis, University of Birmingham.

Address for correspondence

CJ Gilleard
Director of Psychology
Department of Psychology
Springfield Hospital
61 Glenburnie Road
Tooting
London SW17 7DJ
UK

Problem Checklist and Strain Scale

Problem Checklist

1. Unable to dress without help
2. Demands attention
3. Unable to get in and out of a chair without help
4. Uses bad language
5. Unable to get in and out of bed without help
6. Disrupts personal and social life
7. Unable to wash without help
8. Physically aggressive
9. Needs help at mealtimes
10. Vulgar habits (e.g. spitting, table manners)
11. Incontinent – soiling
12. Creates personality clashes
13. Forgets things that have happened
14. Temper outbursts
15. Falling
16. Rude to visitors
17. Unable to manage stairs
18. Not safe if outside the house alone
19. Cannot be left alone for even one hour
20. Wanders about the house at night
21. Careless about own appearance
22. Unable to walk outside house
23. Unable to hold a sensible conversation
24. Noisy, shouting
25. Incontinent – wetting
26. Shows no concern for personal hygiene
27. Unsteady on feet
28. Always asking questions
29. Unable to take part in family conversations
30. Unable to read newspapers, magazines, etc.
31. Sits around doing nothing
32. Shows no interest in news about friends and relatives
33. Unable to watch and follow television (or radio)
34. Unable to occupy himself/herself doing useful things

Strain Scale

Dangers
1. Do you fear accidents or dangers concerning the elderly person (e.g. fire, gas, falling over, etc.)?

Embarrassment
2. Do you ever feel embarrassed by the elderly person in any way?

Sleep
3. Is your sleep ever interrupted by the elderly person?

Coping
4. How often do you feel it is difficult to cope with the situation you are in and in particular with the elderly person?

Depression
5. Do you ever get depressed about the situation?

Worry
6. How much do you worry about the elderly person?

Household routine
7. Has your household routine been upset in caring for the elderly relative?

Frustration
8. Do you feel frustrated with your situation?

Enjoyment of role
9. Do you get any pleasure from caring for the elderly person?

Holidays
10. Do the problems of caring prevent you from getting away on holiday?

Finance
11. Has your standard of living been affected in any way due to the necessity of caring for your elderly relative?

Health
12. Would you say that your health had suffered from looking after your relative?

Attention
13. Do you find the demand for companionship and attention from the elderly person gets too much for you?

Scoring system:
Problem checklist:

0 = Not present
1 = Occasionally occurring
2 = Frequently/continually occurring

Strain scale:

5 = A great deal of the time
4 = Sometimes
3 = Never

Scoring for item 9 is reversed

Reproduced with permission of Dr Christopher J Gilleard.

Ways of Coping Checklist: Revision and Psychometric Properties

Reference: **Vitaliano PP, Russo J, Carr JE, Maiuro RD, Becker J (1985) The Ways of Coping Checklist: revision and psychometric properties.** *Multivariate Behavioral Research* **20: 3–26**

Time taken estimated 30 minutes

Rating by trained psychologist

Main indications

A measure of an individual's ability to cope based on Lazarus's transactional model of stress.

Commentary

Originally derived from Lazarus's transactional model of stress, whereby an event is considered stressful when a person appraises it as potentially dangerous to his or her psychological well-being. Four psychometric properties were examined, including the reproducibility of the factor structure of the original scales, internal consistency reliabilities and intercorrelations of the original and revised scales, the construct and concurrent validity of the scales, and their relationship to demographic factors. These properties were studied on three distress samples, psychiatric outpatients, spouses of patients with Alzheimer's disease, and medical students. The revised scales were shown to be more reliable and to share substantially less variance than the original scales across all samples.

Additional references

Folkman S, Lazarus RS (1980) An analysis of coping in a middle-aged community sample. *Journal of Health and Social Behavior* **21**: 219–39.

Lazarus RS, Launier R (1978) Stress related transactions between the person and environment. In: Pervin LA, Lewis M, eds. *Perspective in interactional psychology*. New York: Plenum.

Address for correspondence

PP Vitaliano
Department of Psychiatry and Behavioral Sciences
University of Washington
Washington, DC
USA

Ways of Coping Checklist

	Revised scale	*Original item source*

Problem-focused

1. Bargained or compromised to get something positive from the situation. — P
2. Concentrated on something good that could come out of the whole thing. — P
3. Tried not to burn my bridges behind me, but left things open somewhat. — W
4. Changed or grew as a person in a good way. — G
5. Made a plan of action and followed it. — P
6. Accepted the next best thing to what I wanted. — W
7. Came out of the experience better than when I went in. — G
8. Tried not to act too hastily or follow my own hunch. — W
9. Changed something so things would turn out all right. — P
10. Just took things one step at a time. — P
11. I know what had to be done, so I doubled my efforts and tried harder to make things work. — P
12. Came up with a couple of different solutions to the problem. — P
13. Accepted my strong feelings, but didn't let them interfere with other things too much. — W
14. Changed something about myself so I could deal with the situation better. — G
15. Stood my ground and fought for what I wanted. — P

Seeks social support

1. Talked to someone to find out about the situation. — M
2. Accepted sympathy and understanding from someone. — S
3. Got professional help and did what they recommended. — M
4. Talked to someone who could do something about the problem. — P
5. Asked someone I respected for advice and followed it. — M
6. Talked to someone about how I was feeling. — S

Blamed self

1. Blamed yourself. — B
2. Criticized or lectured yourself. — B
3. Realized you brought the problem on yourself. — B

Wishful thinking

1. Hoped a miracle would happen. — W
2. Wished I was a stronger person – more optimistic and forceful. — W
3. Wished that I could change what had happened. — W
4. Wished I could change the way that I felt. — W
5. Daydreamed or imagined a better time or place than the one I was in. — W
6. Had fantasies or wishes about how things might turn out. — W
7. Thought about fantastic or unreal things (like perfect revenge or finding a million dollars) that made me feel better. — M
8. Wished the situation would go away or somehow be finished. — W

Avoidance

1. Went on as if nothing had happened. — Min
2. Felt bad that I couldn't avoid the problem. — W
3. Kept my feelings to myself. — W
4. Slept more than usual. — M
5. Got mad at the people or things that caused the problem. — M
6. Tried to forget the whole thing. — Min
7. Tried to make myself feel better by eating, drinking, smoking, taking medications. — M
8. Avoided being with people in general. — M
9. Kept others from knowing how bad things were. — W
10. Refused to believe it had happened. — M

Abbreviations for scales are:
P, Problem-focused; W, Wishful thinking; G, Growth; M, Mixed; Min, Minimized; B, Blamed self; S, Seeks social support

Source: *Multivariate Behavioral Research* (pp. 11–13), by PP Vitaliano, J Russo, JE Carr, RD Maiuro, J Becker, 1985, New Jersey, USA: Lawrence Erlbaum Associates. Copyright 1985 by Lawrence Erlbaum Associates. Reprinted with permission.

Screen for Caregiver Burden (SCB)

Reference: **Vitaliano PP, Russo J, Young HM, Becker J, Maiuro RD (1991) The Screen for Caregiver Burden.** *Gerontologist* **31: 76–83**

Time taken 20 minutes (reviewer's estimate)

Rating by interview

Main indications

The assessment of perceived burden of caring for a person with Alzheimer's disease.

Commentary

The Screen for Caregiver Burden (SCB) is a 25-item scale providing scores for objective and subjective burden. The former refers to the number of caregiver experiences occurring independently of their distress and the latter evaluates overall distress. Internal consistency of the two scales was above 0.85 and test/retest reliability between 0.64 and 0.70. Construct validity was examined with an explanatory model of distress previously described by the authors (Vitaliano et al, 1987). Convergent and divergent validity were examined in relation to measures taken of the patient's clinical condition and measures of anxiety and depression in the carers. The scale was also shown to be sensitive to changes over time, and correlate with changes in the same measures of the patient's functioning and ratings of the carer's mood.

Additional reference

Vitaliano PP, Maiuro RD, Bolton PA et al (1987) A psychoepidemiologic approach to the study of disaster. *Journal of Community Psychology* 15: 99–122.

Address for correspondence

PP Vitaliano
Department of Psychiatry and Behavioral Sciences
University of Washington
Washington, DC
USA

Screen for Caregiver Burden (SCB)

1. My spouse continues to drive when he/she shouldn't.
2. I have little control over my spouse's illness.
3. I have little control over my spouse's behavior.
4. My spouse is constantly asking the same questions over and over.
5. I have to do too many jobs/chores (feeding, shopping, paying bills) that my spouse used to perform.
6. I am upset that I cannot communicate with my spouse.
7. I am totally responsible for keeping our household in order.
8. My spouse doesn't cooperate with the rest of our family.
9. I have had to seek public assistance to pay for my spouse's medical bills.
10. Seeking public assistance in demeaning and degrading.
11. My spouse doesn't recognize me all the time.
12. My spouse has struck me on various occasions.
13. My spouse has gotten lost in the grocery store.
14. My spouse has been wetting the bed.
15. My spouse throws fits and has threatened me.
16. I have to constantly clean up after my spouse eats.
17. I have to cover up for my spouse's mistakes.
18. I am fearful when spouse gets angry.
19. It is exhausting having to groom and dress my spouse every day.
20. I try so hard to help my spouse but he/she is ungrateful.
21. It is frustrating trying to find things that my spouse hides.
22. I worry that my spouse will leave the house and get lost.
23. My spouse has assaulted others in addition to me.
24. I feel so alone – as if I have the world on my shoulders.
25. I am embarrassed to take my spouse out for fear that he/she will do something.

Burden Interview

Reference: **Zarit SH, Reever KE, Bach-Peterson J (1980) Relatives of the impaired elderly: correlates of feeling of burden.** *The Gerontologist* **20: 649–55**

Time taken 25 minutes (reviewer's estimate)

Rating by self-report during an assessment interview

Main indications

Assessment of the feelings of burden of caregivers in caring for an older person with dementia.

Commentary

Twenty-nine patients with senile dementia and their caregivers were interviewed, and the Burden Interview was compared with measures of cognitive function (Khan Mental Status Questionnaire; Khan et al, 1960), a measure of mental state (Jacobs et al, 1977), a measure of the Memory and Problems Checklist and activities of daily living as assessed by scales described by Lawton (1971). The amount of burden assessed was found to be less when more visits were made by carers to the patient with dementia, and severity of behavioural problems was not associated with higher levels of burden. The paper was one of the earlier studies to underscore the importance of providing support to caregivers in the community care of older people with dementia.

Additional references

Jacobs JW, Bernhard JR, Delgado A et al (1977) Screening for organic mental syndromes in the medically ill. *Annals of Internal Medicine* **86**: 40–6.

Khan RL, Goldfarb AI, Pollack J et al (1960) A brief objective measure for the determination of mental status of the aged. *American Journal of Psychiatry* **117**: 326–8.

Lawton MP (1971) The functional assessment of elderly people. *Journal of the American Geriatrics Society* **19**: 465–80.

Address for correspondence

Steve Zarit
Gerontology Center
College of Health and Human Development
Pennsylvania State University
105 Henderson Building South
University Park
PA 16802-6500
USA
e-mail: Z67@psu.edu

Burden Interview

1. I feel resentful of other relatives who could but who do not do things for my spouse.
2. I feel that my spouse makes requests which I perceive to be over and above what s/he needs.
3. Because of my involvement with my spouse, I don't have enough time for myself.
4. I feel stressed between trying to give to my spouse as well as to other family responsibilities, job, etc.
5. I feel embarrassed over my spouse's behavior.
6. I feel guilty about my interactions with my spouse.
7. I feel that I don't do as much for my spouse as I could or should.
8. I feel angry about my interactions with my spouse.
9. I feel that in the past, I haven't done as much for my spouse as I could have or should have.
10. I feel nervous or depressed about my interactions with my spouse.
11. I feel that my spouse currently affects my relationships with other family members and friends in a negative way.
12. I feel resentful about my interactions with my spouse.
13. I am afraid of what the future holds for my spouse.
14. I feel pleased about my interactions with my spouse.
15. It's painful to watch my spouse age.
16. I feel useful in my interactions with my spouse.
17. I feel my spouse is dependent.
18. I feel strained in my interactions with my spouse.
19. I feel that my health has suffered because of my involvement with my spouse.
20. I feel that I am contributing to the well-being of my spouse.
21. I feel that the present situation with my spouse doesn't allow me as much privacy as I'd like.
22. I feel that my social life has suffered because of my involvement with my spouse.
23. I wish that my spouse and I had a better relationship.
24. I feel that my spouse doesn't appreciate what I do for him/her as much as I would like.
25. I feel uncomfortable when I have friends over.
26. I feel that my spouse tries to manipulate me.
27. I feel that my spouse seems to expect me to take care of him/her as if I were the only one s/her could depend on.
28. I feel that I don't have enough money to support my spouse in addition to the rest of our expenses.
29. I feel that I would like to be able to provide more money to support my spouse than I am able to now.

Caregiving Hassles Scale

Reference: **Kinney JM, Stephens MAP (1989) Caregiving Hassles Scale: assessing the daily hassles of caring for a family member with dementia.** *Gerontologist* **29: 328–32**

Time taken 25 minutes (reviewer's estimate)

Rating by caregivers

Main indications

To examine the daily burden of caring for a patient with Alzheimer's disease.

Commentary

The Caregiving Hassles Scale was developed specifically to assess minor events of the day-to-day experience of caregiving rather than longer-term events or wider caregiver responsibilities. The development of the scale was based on the work of Lazarus and Folkman (1984), which regards stress as a measure of minor irritation of daily living. Sixty caregivers of patients with Alzheimer's disease were interviewed with measures of construct validity. Test/retest reliability and internal consistency were also measured. Originally, 110 items were considered (Kinney and Stephens, 1987). Statistically this was reduced to 42 items, and each was coded according to its relevance to a number of constructs: basic activities of daily living, instrumental activities of daily living, patient's cognitive status and behaviour and the caregiver's support network. Test/retest reliability was 0.83 and internal consistency 0.91. There were significant correlations with other measures of the impact of caregivers: the Caregiver's Impact Scale (Poulshock and Deimling, 1984), the SCL-90-R (an inventory to measure psychological distress: Derogatis, 1983) and the London Psychogeriatric Rating Scale.

Additional references

Derogatis LR (1983) *The SCL-90-R: administration, scoring and procedures manual II.* Baltimore, MD: Clinical Psychometric Research Unit, Johns Hopkins University.

Kinney JM, Stephens MAP (1987) *The Caregiving Hassles Scale: administration, reliability and validity.* Kent, OH: Psychology Department, The State University.

Lazarus RS, Folkman S (1984) *Stress, appraisal and coping.* New York: Springer.

Poulshock SW, Deimling GT (1984) Families caring for elders: issues in the measurement of burden. *Journal of Gerontology* 39: 230–9.

Caregiving Hassles Scale

1.	BEH	Care-recipient criticizing complaining.
2.	COG	Care-recipient declining mentally.
3.	BADL	Assisting care-recipient with walking.
4.	IADL	Extra expenses due to caregiving.
5.	SN	Friends not showing understanding about caregiving.
6.	BEH	Care-recipient losing things.
7.	COG	Undesirable changes in care-recipient's personality.
8.	BADL	Assisting with care-recipient's toileting.
9.	IADL	Transporting care-recipient to doctor/other places.
10.	BEH	Conflicts between care-recipient and family.
11.	COG	Care-recipient not showing interest in things.
12.	BADL	Bathing care-recipient.
13.	SN	Family not showing understanding about caregiving.
14.	BEH	Care-recipient yelling/swearing.
15.	BEH	Care-recipient's not cooperating.
16.	COG	Care-recipient's forgetfulness.
17.	BADL	Assisting care-recipient with exercise/therapy.
18.	IADL	Doing care-recipient's laundry.
19.	BEH	Care-recipient leaving tasks uncompleted.
20.	COG	Care-recipient being confused/not making sense.
21.	BADL	Lifting or transferring care-recipient.
22.	SN	Not receiving caregiving help from friends.
23.	BEH	Care-recipient frowning/scowling.
24.	COG	Care-recipient living in past.
25.	BADL	Helping care-recipient eat.
26.	IADL	Picking up after care-recipient.
27.	BEH	Care-recipient verbally inconsiderate; not respecting others' feelings.
28.	BEH	Being in care-recipient's presence.
29.	COG	Care-recipient talking about/seeing things that aren't real.
30.	BADL	Dressing care-recipient.
31.	SN	Not receiving caregiving help from family.
32.	BEH	Care-recipient asking repetitive questions.
33.	COG	Care-recipient not recognizing familiar people.
34.	BADL	Giving medications to care-recipient.
35.	IADL	Preparing meals for care-recipient.
36.	BEH	Care-recipient wandering off.
37.	COG	Care-recipient's agitation.
38.	BADL	Assisting care-recipient with health aids (e.g. dentures, braces)
39.	IADL	Care-recipient requiring day supervision.
40.	SN	Leaving care-recipient with others at home.
41.	BEH	Care-recipient hiding things.
42.	IADL	Care-recipient requiring night supervision.

BADL	=	Hassle assisting with basic ADL.
IADL	=	Hassle assisting with instrumental ADL.
COG	=	Hassle with care-recipient's cognitive status.
BEH	=	Hassle with care-recipient's behavior.
SN	=	Hassle with caregiver's support network.

Reproduced from the *Gerontologist,* Vol. 29, no. 3, pp. 328–32, 1989. Copyright © The Gerontological Society of America.

Marital Intimacy Scale

Reference: **Morris LW, Morris RG, Britton PG (1988) The relationship between marital intimacy, perceived strain and depression in spouse caregivers of dementia sufferers.** *British Journal of Medical Psychology* 61: 231–6

Time taken 20 minutes (reviewer's estimate)

Rating essentially self-report but with guidance from interviewer

Main indications

This scale aims to assess the relationship between marital intimacy and that of strain and depression in spouse carers of individuals suffering from dementia.

Commentary

The Marital Intimacy Scale was adapted by Morris and his colleagues from the Waring Intimacy Questionnaire (Waring and Reddon, 1983; Waring and Patten, 1984). Nine areas were assessed: conflict resolution, affection, cohesion, sexuality, identity, compatibility, autonomy, expressiveness and desirability. Morris et al (1988) administered the 24-item questionnaire twice: once to obtain a measure of present intimacy with statements being rated as they applied at the time, and again to assess past intimacy where the caregivers were asked to rate the statements as they applied before the partner became ill. Essentially the questionnaire consists of a number of statements, with the person circling one of five choices: strongly agree, agree, undecided, disagree, strongly disagree. Twenty spouse caregivers were interviewed. A

measure of subjective burden was assessed using a screen scale devised for the study: a seven-point bipolar rating scale anchored at each end by statements 'I feel more strain because of the way my partner is nowadays' (1) to 'I feel severe strain because of the way my partner is nowadays' (7). The Beck Depression Inventory (BDI; page 7) and the Problem Checklist and Strain Scale (page 322) were also administered to the carers. Higher levels of perceived strain and depression were found in carers who experienced lower levels of marital intimacy, the decline in intimacy being estimated from the difference between the levels of past and present intimacy.

The scale has been used in studies of dementia to assess the relationship between marital intimacy and behavioural problems in dementia (Fearon et al, 1998).

Additional references

Fearon M, Donaldson C, Burns A, Tarrier N (1998) Intimacy as a determinant of expressed emotion in carers of people with Alzheimer's disease. *Psychological Medicine* **28**: 1085–90.

Waring E, Reddon J (1983) Waring Intimacy Questionnaire. *Journal of Clinical Psychology* **39**: 53–7.

Waring E, Patton D (1984) Marital intimacy in depression. *British Journal of Psychiatry* **145**: 641–4.

Marital Intimacy Scale

Introduction to rating of present intimacy

Please say whether you strongly agree, agree, are undecided, disagree or strongly disagree with each of the following statements as they apply to you AT PRESENT. It is best not to spend too long thinking about your answers. Please circle the letter that corresponds to your answer.

Introduction to rating of past intimacy

Please think back to the time before you suspected that your partner was ill. Please say whether you strongly agreed, agreed, have been undecided, disagreed or strongly disagreed with each of the following statements AT THAT TIME. Please try to remember as accurately as you can but it is best not to spend too long on each question. Circle the letter that corresponds to each answer.

		Strongly agree	Agree	Unde-cided	Disagree	Strongly disagree
1.	The feelings I have for my partner are warm and affectionate.	A	B	C	D	E
2.	My partner and I find it difficult to agree when making important decisions.	A	B	C	D	E
3.	I am very committed to my partner.	A	B	C	D	E
4.	My partner makes unreasonable demands on my spare time.	A	B	C	D	E
5.	All my partner's habits are good and desirable ones.	A	B	C	D	E
6.	I enjoy pleasant conversations with my partner.	A	B	C	D	E
7.	I wish my partner was more loving and affectionate to me.	A	B	C	D	E
8.	My partner has helped me to feel that I am a worthwhile person.	A	B	C	D	E
9.	I am unable to tell my partner in words that I love him/her.	A	B	C	D	E
10.	On occasion, I have told a small lie to my partner.	A	B	C	D	E
11.	My partner is liked and accepted by my relatives.	A	B	C	D	E
12.	I look outside my marriage for things that make life worthwhile and interesting.	A	B	C	D	E
13.	When I am unhappy about some aspect of our relationship I am able to tell my partner about it.	A	B	C	D	E
14.	My marriage has 'smothered' my personality.	A	B	C	D	E
15.	I sometimes have thoughts and ideas I would not like to tell my partner.	A	B	C	D	E
16.	I am happy with the physical relationship in my marriage.	A	B	C	D	E
17.	My partner does not understand the way I feel.	A	B	C	D	E
18.	My relationship with my partner is the most important and meaningful relationship I have.	A	B	C	D	E
19.	I wish my partner worked harder to make our relationship more satisfying for us both.	A	B	C	D	E
20.	I have never had an argument with my partner.	A	B	C	D	E
21.	My partner confides his/her innermost thoughts and beliefs to me.	A	B	C	D	E
22.	I have become angry, upset or irritable because of things that occur in my marriage.	A	B	C	D	E
23.	My partner and I enjoy several mutually satisfying outside interests together.	A	B	C	D	E
24.	I am unable to say to my partner all that I would like.	A	B	C	D	E
25.	I sometimes boast in front of my partner.	A	B	C	D	E
26.	My partner and I share views on what is right and proper conduct.	A	B	C	D	E
27.	My partner is critical of decisions I make.	A	B	C	D	E
28.	My marriage helps me to achieve the goals I have set myself in life.	A	B	C	D	E
29.	My marriage suffers from disagreement concerning matters of leisure and recreation.	A	B	C	D	E
30.	Once in a while, I lose my temper and get angry with my partner.	A	B	C	D	E

Thank you for answering these questions.

Reproduced with kind permission from R Morris.

Revised Memory and Behavior Problems Checklist

Reference: **Teri L, Truax P, Logsdon R, Uomoto J, Zarit S, Vitaliano PP (1992) Assessment of behavioral problems in dementia: the Revised Memory and Behavior Problems Checklist. *Psychology and Aging* 7: 622–31**

Time taken 15–20 minutes (reviewer's estimate)

Rating from caregiver reports

Main indications

Assessment of behavioural problems in patients with dementia.

Commentary

The Revised Memory and Behavior Problems Checklist is a 24-item checklist which provides one total score and three subscores for the following problems: memory related, depression and disruptive behaviours. It assesses both the frequency of behaviours and caregiver reactions. Some 64 items were gathered from the original Memory and Problems Checklist (Zarit and Zarit, 1983) plus additional items. Validity was assessed by the Mini-Mental State Examination (MMSE; page 36), the Hamilton Depression Scale (page 6),

the Center for Epidemiological Studies – Depression Scale (CES-D; page 13) and the Caregiver Hassles Scale (page 328), and it was found to be good. Internal consistency was 0.75 for the frequency estimates and 0.87 for caregiver reactions. Some 201 subjects and their carers were examined.

Additional reference

Zarit SH, Zarit JM (1983) Cognitive impairment. In Lewinsohn PM, Teri L, eds. *Clinical geropsychology.* Elmsford, NY: Pergamon Press, 38–81.

Address for correspondence

Linda Teri
Department of Psychiatry and Behavioral Sciences
University of Washington Medical Center
RP-10 Seattle
WA 98195, USA
e-mail: lteri@u.washington.edu

Revised Memory and Behavior Problems Checklist

1. Asking the same question over and over.
2. Trouble remembering recent events (e.g. items in the newspaper or on TV).
3. Trouble remembering significant past events.
4. Losing or misplacing things.
5. Forgetting what day it is.
6. Starting, but not finishing, things.
7. Difficulty concentrating on a task.
8. Destroying property.
9. Doing things that embarrass you.
10. Waking you or other family members up at night.
11. Talking loudly and rapidly.
12. Appears anxious or worried.
13. Engaging in behavior that is potentially dangerous to self or others.
14. Threats to hurt oneself.
15. Threats to hurt others.
16. Aggressive to others verbally.
17. Appears sad or depressed.
18. Expressing feelings of hopelessness or sadness about the future (e.g. 'Nothing worthwhile ever happens,' 'I never do anything right').
19. Crying and tearfulness.
20. Commenting about death of self or others (e.g. 'Life isn't worth living,' 'I'd be better off dead').
21. Talking about feeling lonely.
22. Comments about feeling worthless or being a burden to others.
23. Comments about feeling like a failure or about not having any worthwhile accomplishments in life.
24. Arguing, irritability, and/or complaining.

Rate both frequency and reaction as follows:

Frequency:
0 = Never occurred
1 = Not in past week
2 = 1–2 times in past week
3 = 3–6 times in past week
4 = Daily or more often
9 = Do not know/not applicable

Reaction:
0 = Not at all
1 = A Little
2 = Moderately
3 = Very much
4 = Extremely
9 = Do not know/not applicable

Reproduced with kind permission from Dr L Teri.

Caregiver Activity Survey (CAS)

Reference: **Davis KL, Marin DB, Kane R, Patrick D, Peskind ER, Raskind MA, Puder KL (1997) The Caregiver Activity Survey (CAS): development and validation of a new measure for caregivers of persons with Alzheimer's disease.** *International Journal of Geriatric Psychiatry* **12: 978–88**

Time taken 5 minutes

Rating by self-report

Main indications

A measure of time spent with the carer and caregiver burden.

Commentary

The Caregiver Activity Survey (CAS) was developed to assess the amount of time caregivers were spending looking after patients with Alzheimer's disease. Forty-two patients with Alzheimer's disease and their carers were studied with measures of test/retest reliability over a 3-week period and validity assessed by comparison with the Alzheimer's Disease Assessment Scale – Cognitive Section (ADAS-CoG; page 48) and the Mini-Mental State Examination (MMSE; page 36). The final version of the CAS consisted of six items. There was high test/retest reliability, intra-class correlation was 0.88 and conversion validity was high in comparison with the three scales. In the final scale, the inclusion of a dimension reflecting caregiver burden was not successful.

Address for correspondence

Dr KL Davis
Mount Sinai School of Medicine
One Gustave L Levy Place
Box 1230
New York NY 10029-6574
USA

e-mail: Kenneth.davis@mssm.edu

Caregiver Activity Survey (CAS)

Areas assessed:

I	– Communication	III	– Dressing
II	– Using transportation	IV	– Eating
		V	– Looking after self-appearance
		VI	– Supervision necessary

Scoring is by the amount of time spent in the last 24 hours doing those activities assessed

General Health Questionnaire (GHQ)

Reference: **Goldberg DP, Williams P (1988)** *A User's Guide to the General Health Questionnaire.* **Windsor: NFER-NELSON**

Time taken depends on version (e.g. 5 minutes for 12-item GHQ)

Rating by self-rating

Main indications

A self-administered screening test in detecting psychiatric disorders in community settings and non-psychiatric clinical settings.

Commentary

The General Health Questionnaire (GHQ) is the most widely used self-rating instrument for the detection of psychiatric disorder and psychological morbidity. It is not used primarily in older people, but it is included here as it is used as a measure of psychological distress and psychiatric morbidity in carers of patients. For details, the rater is referred to the *User's Guide to the General Health Questionnaire*, and the 12-item questionnaire (GHQ-12), which is reproduced here. Essentially, four versions are available: 12-, 28-, 30- and 60-item questionnaires. Where scaled subscores are required, the GHQ-28 should be used. For more intensive examination, with literate subjects with plenty of time the GHQ-60 is the best, but the GHQ-12 still does a good job with regard to sensitivity and specificity (e.g. GHQ-12, 89% sensitivity, 80% specificity; GHQ-28, 84% and 82% respectively; GHQ-30, 74% and 82% respectively; and GHQ-60, 78% and 87% respectively). These sensitivity and specificity measurements are in relation to the ability of the questionnaire to discriminate between cases and non-cases.

Address for correspondence

NFER Nelson
Freepost
Windsor
Berks SL4 1BU
UK

General Health Questionnaire (GHQ-12)

Sample only

Please read this carefully:
We should like to know if you have had any medical complaints, and how your health has been in general, over the past few weeks. Please answer ALL the questions simply by underlining the answer which you think most nearly applies to you. Remember that we want to know about present and recent complaints, not those you had in the past. It is important that you try to answer ALL the questions.

Thank you very much for your co-operation.

HAVE YOU RECENTLY:

1	–	been able to concentrate on whatever you're doing?	Better than usual	Same as usual	Less than usual	Much less than usual
2	–	lost much sleep over worry?	Not at all	No more than usual	Rather more than usual	Much more than usual
3	–	felt that you are playing a useful part in things?	More so than usual	Same as usual	Less useful than usual	Much less useful
4	–	felt capable of making decisions about things?	More so than usual	Same as usual	Less so than usual	Much less capable
5	–	felt constantly under strain?	Not at all	No more than usual	Rather more than usual	Much more than usual
6	–	felt you couldn't overcome your difficulties?	Not at all	No more than usual	Rather more than usual	Much more than usual
7	–	been able to enjoy your normal day-to-day activities?	More so than usual	Same as usual	Less so than usual	Much less than usual
8	–	been able to face up to your problems?	More so than usual	Same as usual	Less able than usual	Much less able
9	–	been feeling unhappy and depressed?	Not at all	No more than usual	Rather more than usual	Much more than usual
10	–	been losing confidence in yourself?	Not at all	No more than usual	Rather more than usual	Much more than usual
11	–	been thinking of yourself as a worthless person?	Not at all	No more than usual	Rather more than usual	Much more than usual
12	–	been feeling reasonably happy, all things considered?	More so than usual	About same as usual	Less so than usual	Much less than usual

Source: GHQ-12 © David Goldberg, 1978. Reproduced by permission of the Publishers, NFER-NELSON, Darville House, 2 Oxford Road East, Windsor SL4 1DF, England. All rights reserved.

TRIMS Behavioral Problem Checklist (BPC)

Reference: **Niederehe G (1988) TRIMS Behavioral Problem Checklist (BPC).**
Psychopharmacology Bulletin 24: 771–8

Time taken 25 minutes (reviewer's estimate)

Rating by carers

Main indications

The Texas Research Institute of Mental Science (TRIMS) Behavioral Problem Checklist (BPC) was developed for the assessment of the range of behavioural problems of patients with dementia and their effect on carers.

Commentary

Six subgroups were described as part of the BPC scale: cognitive symptoms, self-care deficits, instrumental activities of daily living deficits, dysphoric mood, acting-out behaviour and inactivity/withdrawal. The scales were all intercorrelated. Cronbach's alpha showed excellent internal consistency (0.93), and symptoms correlated with the measures of activities of daily living and AOLS.

Additional reference

Zarit SH, Reever KE, Bach-Peterson J (1980) Relatives of the impaired elderly: correlates of feelings of burden. *Gerontologist* **20**: 649–55.

Address for correspondence

George Niederehe
Mental Disorders of the Aging Research Branch
National Institute of Mental Health
Room 11C-03
5600 Fishers Lane
Rockville
MD 20857
USA

TRIMS Behavioral Problem Checklist (BPC)

Cognitive symptoms	Dysphoric mood
Self-care deficits	Acting-out behaviour
Instrumental activities of daily living deficits	Inactivity/withdrawal

---

Frequency: How often does your relative show the problem?
0 = Never happens (If behavior never happens, go on to next question)
1 = Has happened but not in the past week
2 = 1 to 2 times in past week
3 = 3 to 6 times in past week
4 = Happens daily or more often

Duration: When did the problem begin?
0 = Never happens
1 = Recently (1–6 months ago)
2 = Within the past year (7–12 months ago)
3 = Within the previous year (13–24 months ago)
4 = Over 2 years ago (2+ years ago)

Reaction: How much does this problem bother or upset you?
0 = Not at all
1 = A little
2 = A moderate amount
3 = Quite a lot
4 = Very much, extremely

Reproduced from Niederehe G (1988) TRIMS Behavioral Problem Checklist (BPC). *Psychopharmacology Bulletin* **24**: 771–8.

Geriatric Evaluation by Relative's Rating Instrument (GERRI)

Reference: **Schwartz GE (1988) Geriatric Evaluation by Relative's Rating Instrument (GERRI).** *Psychopharmacology Bulletin* **24:** 713–16

Time taken 20 minutes (reviewer's estimate)

Rating by carer

Main indications

Assessment of a number of behaviours in elderly people.

Commentary

The Geriatric Evaluation by Relative's Rating Instrument (GERRI) consists of 49 short phrases covering behavioural disturbances and problems with cognitive function, social functioning and mood. Ratings are on a five-point frequency scale from 'almost all the time' to 'almost never'. The scale assesses behaviour over the last 2 weeks and can be repeated at this time interval. High inter-rater reliability and high internal consistency have been demonstrated (Schwartz, 1983), and it has been validated against the London Psychogeriatric Rating Scale, the Mini-Mental State Examination (MMSE; page 36) and an activities of daily living index (Sheikh et al, 1979).

Additional references

Schwartz GE (1983) Development and validation of the Geriatric Evaluation by Relative's Rating Instrument (GERRI). *Psychological Reports* **53**: 479–88.

Sheikh K, Smith D, Meade T et al (1979) Repeatability and validity of a modified activities of daily living (ADL) index in studies of chronic disability. *Internal Rehabilitation Medicine* **1**: 51–8.

Address for correspondence

Gerri E Schwartz
Janssen Research Foundation
40 Kingsbridge Road
Piscataway
NJ 08855-3998
USA

Geriatric Evaluation by Relative's Rating Instrument (GERRI)

1.	Remembers name of spouse/children living with him/her.	C
2.	Shaves or puts on makeup, combs hair without help.	S
3.	Prepares coffee, tea, or simple meals for self when necessary.	S
4.	Remembers where small items, such as keys, jewelry, or wallets are placed.	C
5.	Reports he/she feels sad.	M
6.	Appears restless and fidgety.	M
7.	Pays bills with checks.	S
8.	Remembers familiar phone numbers.	C
9.	Grasps point of newspaper articles, news broadcasts, etc.	C
10.	Reports feeling of hopelessness about the future.	M
11.	Forgets names of common objects.	C
12.	Handles incoming calls.	S
13.	Gets lost – leaves house and does not know where he/she lives.	C
14.	Remembers point in conversation after interruption.	C
15.	Handles money shopping for simple grocery items or newspaper or cigarettes.	S
16.	Reports feeling worthless.	M
17.	Continues to work on some favorite hobby.	S
18.	Does not recognize familiar people.	C
19.	Repeats same point in conversation over and over.	C
20.	Appears tearful.	M
21.	Leaves clothes soiled.	S
22.	Physically dirty or sloppy in appearance.	S
23.	Mood changes from day to day, happy one day, sad the other.	M
24.	Forgets the day of the week.	C
25.	Goes out inappropriately dressed.	S
26.	Embarrassing behavior.	S
27.	Forgets what he/she is looking for in the house.	C
28.	Forgets appointments.	C
29.	Remembers names of close friends.	C
30.	Acts childish.	S
31.	Continues to watch or 'follow' favorite TV or radio program.	C
32.	When asked questions, seems quarrelsome and irritable.	M
33.	Does not pursue every day activities.	S
34.	Overquick or 'jumpy' reaction to sudden noises or sights.	M
35.	Has difficulty concentrating or paying attention.	C
36.	Does not socialize with friends.	S
37.	Has fluctuations in memory – good one day, bad the next.	C
38.	Remembers where clothes are placed.	C
39.	Wants to have things his/her own way.	S
40.	Irregular eating habits, misses meals or eats meals consecutively.	S
41.	Remembers to lock door when leaving the house.	C
42.	Initiates phone contacts with friends.	S
43.	Appears to be easily annoyed or angered.	M
44.	Remembers to take medication.	C
45.	Reports feeling optimistic about future.	M
46.	Appears to be cheerful.	M
47.	Forgets to turn off stove.	C
48.	Appears friendly and positive in conversations with family members.	S
49.	Behaves stubbornly, such as refuses to take medication.	S

C = Cognitive functioning
S = Social functioning
M = Mood

Score:
1 = Almost all the time
2 = Most of the time
3 = Often
4 = Sometimes
5 = Almost never
6 = Does not apply

Reproduced with permission of author and publisher from: Schwartz, G.E. 'Development and validation of the Geriatric Evaluation by Relatives Rating Instrument (GERRI).' *Psychological Reports*, 1983, **53**, 479–488. © Psychological Reports 1983.

Zung Self-Rating Depression Scale

Reference: **Zung WWK (1965) A Self-Rating Depression Scale.** *Archives of General Psychiatry* **12: 63–70**

Time taken 3 minutes

Rating by self-rating

Main indications

Self-rating of depression.

Commentary

The 20-item Zung Self-Rating Depression Scale has been used extensively for the assessment of mood in older people, and has excellent reliability and internal consistency. It has been validated both as a screening instrument and as one sensitive to change (Zung, 1983). Like the Beck Depression Inventory (BDI; page 7), it has been used to assess depression in carers of patients with dementia. The scale was originally assessed on 56 patients, and validity was shown by its ability to discriminate between those with depressive disorders and those with other psychiatric conditions.

Additional reference

Zung W (1983) Self-rating scales for psychopathology. In Crook T, Ferris S, Bartus R, eds. *Assessment in geriatric psychopharmacology.* New Canaan: Mark Powley Associates.

www.fpnotebook.com/PSY85.htm

Zung Self-Rating Depression Scale

1. I feel down-hearted and blue.*
2. Morning is when I feel the best.
3. I have crying spells or feel like it.*
4. I have trouble sleeping at night.*
5. I eat as much as I used to.
6. I still enjoy sex.
7. I notice that I am losing weight.*
8. I have trouble with constipation.*
9. My heart beats faster than usual.*
10. I get tired for no reason.*
11. My mind is as clear as it used to be.
12. I find it easy to do the things I used to.
13. I am restless and can't keep still.*
14. I feel hopeful about the future.
15. I am more irritable than usual.*
16. I find it easy to make decisions.
17. I feel that I am useful and needed.
18. My life is pretty full.
19. I feel that others would be better off if I were dead.*
20. I still enjoy the things I used to do.

Rating:
1=A little of the time
2=Some of the time
3=Good part of the time
4=Most of the time

Each is graded on a 4-point scale (1–4), there being 10 positive and 10 negative items, so that a global score out of a maximum of 80 gives a measure of the severity of depression. Converted to a percentage, >50% is suggested to indicate depression.

*rated 1–4
Others rated 4–1

Reproduced (with the permission of the American Medical Association) from Zung WWK (1965) A Self-Rating Depression Scale. *Archives of General Psychiatry* **12**: 63–70.

Behavioural and Mood Disturbance Scale (BMDS)

Reference: **Greene JG, Smith R, Gardiner M, Timbury GC (1982) Measuring behavioural disturbance of elderly demented patients in the community and its effect on relatives: a factor analytic study.** *Age and Ageing* **11: 121–6**

Time taken 15–20 minutes

Rating by interview

Main indications

Assessment of behaviour and mood of a patient by a relative.

Commentary

The Behavioural and Mood Disturbance Scale (BMDS) aims to enable relatives to make a standard assessment of mood and behaviour disturbance shown by older people with dementia living at home. The scale grew out of existing literature such as the PAMIE Scale (page 248), the Stockton Geriatric Rating Scale (page 250), the Clifton Assessment Procedures for the Elderly (CAPE; page 56) and the Psychogeriatric Dependency Rating Scales (PGDRS; page 243). Thirty-eight day patients with dementia and their carers were interviewed. The items (as below) were rated, with a 0–4 severity scale. Three factors were extracted: apathetic/withdrawn behaviour, active/disturbed behaviour, and mood disturbance. Validation was by means of factor analysis, and a test/retest study achieved satisfactory results.

Additional reference

Greene JG, Timbury GC (1979) A geriatric psychiatry day hospital service: a five-year review. *Age and Ageing* 8: 49–53.

Behavioural and Mood Disturbance Scale (BMDS)

Does he/she . . . .

*1. Play or talk with the children?	21. Ever seem lost in a world of his/her own?
*2. Watch and follow television?	22. Ever get lost in the house?
*3. Read newspapers, magazines etc.?	23. Ever fail to recognize familiar people?
*4. Keep his/herself busy doing useful things?	24. Ever get mixed up about the day, year, etc.?
*5. Help out with domestic chores?	25. Get mixed up about where he/she is?
6. Sit around doing nothing?	26. Ever moan and complain?
*7. Take part in family conversations?	27. Ever talk out loud to him/herself?
8. Ever talk nonsense?	28. Ever mutter to him or herself?
*9. Understand what is said to him/her?	29. Ever get up unusually early in the morning?
*10. Ever start and maintain a sensible conversation?	30. Ever go on and on about certain things?
*11. Respond sensibly when spoken to?	31. Wander outside the house at night?
12. Ever wander off the subject?	32. Wander outside the house and get lost?
*13. Show an interest in news about friends and relatives?	33. Have to be prevented from wandering outside the house?
14. Ever cry for no obvious reason?	34. Ever accuse people of things?
15. Ever become angry and threatening?	35. Ever hoard useless things?
16. Ever appear unhappy and depressed?	36. Ever endanger him/herself?
17. Ever appear restless and agitated?	37. Ever pace up and down wringing his or her hands?
18. Ever look frightened and anxious?	38. Talk all the time?
19. Ever become irritable and easily upset?	39. Ever shout at the children?
20. Mood ever change for no apparent reason?	40. Attempt to help with the housework but prove more of a hindrance than help?

Score: 0 = Never; 1 = Rarely, now and again; 2 = Sometimes, in between; 3 = Frequently, most of the time, quite a bit; 4 = Always, all the time; * = Scoring reversed.

The Pleasant Events Schedule – AD

Reference: **Teri L, Logsdon RG (1991) Identifying pleasant activities for Alzheimer's disease patients: The Pleasant Events Schedule – AD.** *Gerontologist* **31: 124–27**

Time taken less than 30 minutes

Rating by caregiver

Main indications

To help caregivers identify appropriate and pleasant activities for patients with Alzheimer's disease.

Commentary

The Pleasant Events Schedule – AD was developed from two earlier schedules: Lewinshon and Talkington (1979) and one modified for the elderly by Teri and Lewinshon (1982). The amendments consist of the deleting of items not relevant to patients with Alzheimer's disease. The 53 items are each rated three times: the number of times the event occurred in the last month is rated on a 3-point scale (not at all, a few times, and often); each item is rated according to the availability or opportunities the patient has had to engage in the activity on the same 3-point scale; and a 2-point scale rates enjoyability (now enjoys and enjoyed in the past). The psychometric properties of the previous scales are documented (Cronbach's alpha 0.98).

Logston and Teri (1977) describe a short 20-item version validated on 42 patients with Alzheimer's disease. Items are rated with regard to their frequency and availability during the last month on a 3-point scale (not at all, a few times (1–6 times) and often (7 or more times)). The rating is also made as to whether the patient enjoys the activity now and whether the activity was enjoyed in the past. An overall summary score of frequency of enjoyable activities is a cross product of current enjoyment with frequency, and is calculated for each item. Each item therefore receives a score of 0 (either does not enjoy or has not done in the past month), 1 (enjoys and has done a few times) and 2 (enjoys and has done often). The sum of these items' scores represents the frequency of pleasant activities during the last month and is called the ENJOY. Internal consistency and split half reliability of the scales were excellent. The 20-item version was obtained by excluding 33 items – three were judged by the author to be difficult to rate, eight were enjoyed by fewer than 30% of the subjects and so eliminated, and items with item total correlations below 0.35 were also eliminated (22).

Additional references

Lewinshon PM, Talkington J (1979) Studies on the measurement of unpleasant events and relations with depression. *Applied Psychological Measurement* **3**: 83–101.

Logston R, Teri L (1977) The Pleasant Event Schedule – AD. *Gerontologist* **37**: 40–5.

Teri L, Lewinshon PM (1982) Modification of pleasant and unpleasant events schedules for use with the elderly. *Journal of Consulting and Clinical Psychology* **50**: 444–5.

Address for correspondence

Linda Teri
University of Washington
Department of Psychiatry and Behavioral Science
1959 NE Pacific St
Seattle
WA 98195
USA

e-mail: lteri@u.washington.edu

	Frequency			Availability			Enjoyability	
	Not at all	A few times	Often	Not at all	A few times	Often	Now enjoys	Enjoyed in the past

*1.   Being outside (sitting outside, being in the country)
2.   Meeting someone new or making new friends
3.   Planning trips or vacations, looking at travel brochures, traveling
*4.   Shopping, buying things (for self or others)
5.   Being at the beach
*6.   Reading or listening to stories, novels, plays, or poems
*7.   Listening to music (radio, stereo)
*8.   Watching TV
9.   Camping
10.   Thinking about something good in the future
11.   Completing a difficult task
*12. Laughing
13.   Doing jigsaw puzzles, crosswords, and word games
*14. Having meals with friends or family (at home or out, special occasions)
15.   Taking a shower or bath
16.   Being with animals or pets
17.   Listening to nonmusic radio programs (talk shows)
*18. Making or eating snacks
*19. Helping others, helping around the house, dusting, cleaning, setting the table, cooking
20.   Combing or brushing my hair
21.   Taking a nap
*22. Being with my family (children, grandchildren. siblings, others)
23.   Watching animals or birds (in a zoo or in the yard)
*24. Wearing certain clothes (such as new, informal, formal, or favorite clothes)
*25. Listening to the sounds of nature (birdsong, wind, surf)
26.   Having friends come to visit
*27. Getting/sending letters, cards, notes
28.   Watching the clouds, sky, or a storm
*29. Going on outings (to the park, a picnic, a barbeque, etc.)
30.   Reading, watching, or listening to the news
31.   Watching people
*32. Having coffee, tea, a soda, etc. with friends
*33. Being complimented or told I have done something well
34.   Being told I am loved
35.   Having family members or friends tell me something that makes me proud of them
36.   Seeing or speaking with old friends (in person or on the telephone)
37.   Looking at the stars or moon
38.   Playing cards or games
39.   Doing handwork (crocheting, woodworking, crafts, knitting, painting, drawing, ceramics, clay work, other)
*40. Exercising (walking, aerobics, swimming, dancing, other)
41.   Indoor gardening or related activities (tending plants)
42.   Outdoor gardening or related activities (mowing lawn, raking leaves, watering plants, doing yard work)
43.   Going to museums, art exhibits, or related cultural activities
44.   Looking at photo albums and photos
45.   Stamp collecting, or other collections
46.   Sorting out drawers or closets
*47. Going for a ride in the car
48.   Going to church, attending religious ceremonies
49.   Singing
*50. Grooming self (wearing makeup, having hair done)
51.   Going to the movies
*52. Recalling and discussing past events
53.   Participating or watching sports (golf, baseball, football, etc.)

Caregiver Time Use

Reference: **Clipp EC, Moore MJ (1995) Caregiver time use: an outcome measure in clinical trial research on Alzheimer's disease.** *Clinical Pharmacology and Therapeutics* **58: 228–236**

Time taken 15 minutes (reviewer's estimate)

Rating by informant who knows the patient

Main indications

To assess the time spent caring for a person with dementia.

Commentary

A direct relationship was found between improvement in cognitive function (as affected by velnacrine) and reduced unpaid caregiving time: at the highest dose of the drug it was an equivalent to 3.3 hours per day.

Address for correspondence

Dr Elizabeth E Clipp
Veterans Affairs Medical Center
508 Fulton Street
Durham
NC 27705
USA

Caregiver Activities Time Survey (CATS)

CARE BY PAID PROFESSIONALS

☐ NONE

Description of Caregiver (check all that apply)	Number of Visits* in Last 2 Weeks	Average Number of Hours and Minutes per Visit*	
		Hours	Minutes
☐ VISITING NURSE	_|_	_|_	_|_
☐ HOME HEALTH AIDE	_|_	_|_	_|_
☐ ATTENDANT	_|_	_|_	_|_
☐ HOUSEKEEPER	_|_	_|_	_|_
☐ MEALS ON WHEELS	_|_	_|_	_|_
☐ DAY CARE PROGRAM	_|_	_|_	_|_
☐ TRANSPORTATION	_|_	_|_	_|_
☐ OTHER	_|_	_|_	_|_

*Includes attendance at day care program.

UNPAID CARE BY FAMILY OR FRIENDS

☐ NONE

Type of Care Provided (check all that apply)	Number of Hours & Minutes Spent in a Typical Day	
	Hours	Minutes
☐ FEEDING	_|_	_|_
☐ TOILETING	_|_	_|_
☐ BATHING	_|_	_|_
☐ DRESSING	_|_	_|_
☐ ADMINISTERING MEDICATION	_|_	_|_
☐ SUPERVISION	_|_	_|_
☐ HOUSEKEEPING	_|_	_|_
☐ TRANSPORTATION	_|_	_|_
☐ OTHER _____	_|_	_|_

Multidimensional Caregiver Burden Inventory

Reference: **Novak M, Guest C (1989) Application of a multidimensional caregiver burden inventory.** *The Gerontologist* 29: 798–803

Time taken 10 minutes

Rater a trained interviewer

Main indications

A diverse multidimensional instrument that measures the impact of burden on caregivers.

Commentary

The sample for the study consisted of 107 caregivers (28 male, 79 female), the care receivers having a diagnosis of Alzheimer's disease, senile dementia or organic brain syndrome. The scale consists of a 24-item, five subscale caregiver burden inventory and looks specifically at time dependence, development burden, physical burden, social burden and emotional burden. Depending on CBI scores a caregiver burden profile can be constructed which enables the scores to be graphically displayed and can compare the burden score among subscales.

Additional reference

Novak M, Guest C (1989) Caregiver response to Alzheimer's disease. *International Journal of Aging and Human Development* **28**: 67–79.

Address for correspondence

Dr Mark Novak
Continuing Education Division
University of Manitoba
Winnipeg
Manitoba
Canada
R3T 2N2

Caregiver Burden Inventory (CBI) (Mean = 22.14; SD = 16.30)

Factor	Factor loading	Factor	Factor loading
Factor 1: Time-Dependence Burden (Mean = 6.98; SD = 5.89)		2. My health has suffered	.73
1. My care receiver needs my help to perform many daily tasks	.88	3. Caregiving has made me physically sick	.70
2. My care receiver is dependent on me	.77	4. I'm physically tired	.69
3. I have to watch my care receiver constantly	.77	*Factor 4: Social Burden (Mean = 2.54; SD = 3.54)*	
4. I have to help my care receiver with many basic functions	.71	1. I don't get along with other family members as well as I used to	.81
5. I don't have a minute's break from my caregiving chores	.66	2. My caregiving efforts aren't appreciated by others in my family	.79
Factor 2: Developmental Burden (Mean = 7.08; SD = 5.89)		3. I've had problems with my marriage	.73
1. I feel that I am missing out on life	.78	4. I don't do as good a job at work as I used to	.61
2. I wish I could escape from this situation	.78	5. I feel resentful of other relatives who could but do not help	.60
3. My social life has suffered	.71	*Factor 5: Emotional Burden (Mean = 2.02; SD = 3.04)*	
4. I feel emotionally drained due to caring for my care receiver	.65	1. I feel embarrassed over my care receiver's behavior	.81
5. I expected that things would be different at this point in my life	.63	2. I feel ashamed of my care receiver	.74
Factor 3: Physical Burden (Mean = 5.47; SD = 5.9)		3. I resent my care receiver	.64
1. I'm not getting enough sleep	.73	4. I feel uncomfortable when I have friends over	.64
		5. I feel angry about my interactions with my care receiver	.53

Source: Reproduced with permission from Novak M, Guest C. *Gerontologist* 1989; **29**: 798–803.

Chapter 7

Memory functioning

Cognitive Failures Questionnaire (CFQ)

Reference: Broadbent DE, Cooper PF, FitzGerald P, Parkes KR (1982) Cognitive Failures Questionnaire (CFQ) and its correlates. *British Journal of Clinical Psychology* 21: 1–16

Time taken 10 minutes

Rating self-rating

Main indications

A measure of self-reported failures in perception, memory and motor function.

Commentary

The Cognitive Failures Questionnaire (CFQ) is only weakly correlated with indices of social desirability set or of neuroticism, but is significantly correlated with ratings of the respondent by his or her spouse. The score has been found to be reasonably stable over long periods; however, it does correlate with the number of current psychiatric symptoms. Responses relate to the last six months. Validity was assessed by correlations with the Short Inventory of Memory Experiences (Herrmann and Neisser, 1978) and a number of neuropsychological tests. The use of the CFQ in memory clinics may highlight areas of concern for the clinician.

Additional reference

Herrmann D, Neisser U (1978) An inventory of everyday memory experiences. In Gruneberg MM, Morris PE, Sykes RN, eds. *Practical aspects of memory*. London: Academic Press.

Cognitive Failures Questionnaire (CFQ)

The following questions are about minor mistakes which everyone makes from time to time, but some of which happen more than others. We want to know how often these things have happened to you in the last six months. Please circle the appropriate number.

		Very often	Quite often	Occasionally	Very rarely	Never
1	Do you read something and find you haven't been thinking about it and must read it again?	4	3	2	1	0
2	Do you find you forget why you went from one part of the house to the other?	4	3	2	1	0
3	Do you fail to notice signposts on the road?	4	3	2	1	0
4	Do you find you confuse right and left when giving directions?	4	3	2	1	0
5	Do you bump into people?	4	3	2	1	0
6	Do you find you forget whether you've turned off a light or a fire or locked the door?	4	3	2	1	0
7	Do you fail to listen to people's names when you are meeting them?	4	3	2	1	0
8	Do you say something and realize afterwards that it might be taken as insulting?	4	3	2	1	0
9	Do you fail to hear people speaking to you when you are doing something else?	4	3	2	1	0
10	Do you lose your temper and regret it?	4	3	2	1	0
11	Do you leave important letters unanswered for days?	4	3	2	1	0
12	Do you find you forget which way to turn on a road you know well but rarely use?	4	3	2	1	0
13	Do you fail to see what you want in a supermarket (although it's there)?	4	3	2	1	0
14	Do you find yourself suddenly wondering whether you've used a word correctly?	4	3	2	1	0
15	Do you have trouble making up your mind?	4	3	2	1	0
16	Do you find you forget appointments?	4	3	2	1	0
17	Do you forget where you put something like a newspaper or a book?	4	3	2	1	0
18	Do you find you accidentally throw away the thing you want and keep what you meant to throw away – as in the example of throwing away the matchbox and putting the used match in your pocket?	4	3	2	1	0
19	Do you daydream when you ought to be listening to something?	4	3	2	1	0
20	Do you find you forget people's names?	4	3	2	1	0
21	Do you start doing one thing at home and get distracted into doing something else (unintentionally)?	4	3	2	1	0
22	Do you find you can't quite remember something although it's on the tip of your tongue?	4	3	2	1	0
23	Do you find you forget what you came to the shops to buy?	4	3	2	1	0
24	Do you drop things?	4	3	2	1	0
25	Do you find you can't think of anything to say?	4	3	2	1	0

Reprinted with kind permission of the *British Journal of Clinical Psychology*.

Informant Questionnaire on Cognitive Decline in the Elderly (IQCODE)

References: Jorm AF, Jacomb PA (1989) An Informant Questionnaire on Cognitive Decline in the Elderly (IQCODE): socio-demographic correlates, reliability, validity and some norms. *Psychological Medicine* 19: 1015–22.

Jorm AF, Scott R, Jacomb PA (1989) Assessment of cognitive decline in dementia by informant questionnaire. *International Journal of Geriatric Psychiatry* 4: 35–9

Time taken 10–15 minutes (reviewer's estimate)

Rating by interviewer

Main indications

The Informant Questionnaire on Cognitive Decline in the Elderly (IQCODE) is a questionnaire administered to an informant about changes in the everyday cognitive function of an elderly person and aims to assess cognitive decline independent of premorbid ability.

Commentary

These two companion papers outline the rationale behind the development of the IQCODE, emphasizing the three methods of assessing cognitive decline: comparison with estimated premorbid ability, self-reported questionnaires and a third informant's report (n = 362). Jorm analysed returns from a postal questionnaire, as well as a smaller and more direct validity exercise, on 31 volunteers from hostels and nursing homes in Canberra.

The internal consistency of the IQCODE was 0.93 and the validity measured against the Mini-Mental State Examination (MMSE; page 36) showed a correlation of 0.78.

Jorm and Jacomb (1989) provided some additional data showing test/retest reliability and a correlation of 0.75; patients with worse scores did move into institutional care at follow-up.

Further studies have shown that the IQCODE is as good as the MMSE in the diagnosis of dementia (Jorm et al, 1991, 1996). A 16-item version has been described and found to perform as well as the long version (Jorm, 1994). Validity has been affirmed by showing that ratings of moderate or severe decline have greater changes than quantitative tests over time (Jorm et al, 1996). The scale has also been successfully translated into French (Mulligan et al, 1996). A retrospective version is available (26 items) for analysis after a patient has died.

Additional references

Jorm AF (1994) A short form of the Informal Questionnaire on Cognitive Decline in the Elderly (IQCODE): development and cross-validation. *Psychological Medicine* 24: 145–53.

Jorm AF, Scott R, Cullen JS, Mackinnon AJ (1991) Performance of the Informant Questionnaire on Cognitive Decline in the Elderly (IQCODE) as a screening test for dementia. *Psychological Medicine* 21: 785–90.

Jorm AF, Broe GA, Creasey H et al (1996) Further data on the validity of the Informant Questionnaire on Cognitive Decline in the Elderly (IQCODE). *International Journal of Geriatric Psychiatry* 11: 131–9.

Mulligan R, Mackinnon A, Jorm AF (1996) A comparison of alternative methods of screening for dementia in clinical settings. *Archives of Neurology* 53: 532–6.

Address for correspondence

AF Jorm
NH & MRC Social Psychiatry Research Unit
The Australian National University
Canberra 0200
Australia

http://www.anu.edu.au/iqcode/

Informant Questionnaire on Cognitive Decline in the Elderly (IQCODE) (short form)

Now we want you to remember what your friend or relative was like 10 years ago and to compare it with what he/she is like now. 10 years ago was in 19___. Below are situations where this person has to use his/her memory or intelligence and we want you to indicate whether this has improved, stayed the same or got worse in that situation over the past 10 years. Note the importance of comparing his/her present performance with 10 years ago. So if 10 years ago this person always forgot where he/she had left things, and he/she still does, then this would be considered 'Hasn't changed much'. Please indicate the changes you have observed by circling the appropriate answer.

Compared with 10 years ago how is the person at:

	1	2	3	4	5
1. Remembering things about family and friends e.g. occupations, birthdays, addresses	Much improved	A bit improved	Not much change	A bit worse	Much worse
2. Remembering things that have happened recently	Much improved	A bit improved	Not much change	A bit worse	Much worse
3. Recalling conversations a few days later	Much improved	A bit improved	Not much change	A bit worse	Much worse
4. Remembering his/her address and telephone number	Much improved	A bit improved	Not much change	A bit worse	Much worse
5. Remembering what day and month it is	Much improved	A bit improved	Not much change	A bit worse	Much worse
6. Remembering where things are usually kept	Much improved	A bit improved	Not much change	A bit worse	Much worse
7. Remembering where to find things which have been put in a different place from usual	Much improved	A bit improved	Not much change	A bit worse	Much worse
8. Knowing how to work familiar machines around the house	Much improved	A bit improved	Not much change	A bit worse	Much worse
9. Learning to use a new gadget or machine around the house	Much improved	A bit improved	Not much change	A bit worse	Much worse
10. Learning new things in general	Much improved	A bit improved	Not much change	A bit worse	Much worse
11. Following a story in a book or on TV	Much improved	A bit improved	Not much change	A bit worse	Much worse
12. Making decisions on everyday matters	Much improved	A bit improved	Not much change	A bit worse	Much worse
13. Handling money for shopping	Much improved	A bit improved	Not much change	A bit worse	Much worse
14. Handling financial matters e.g. the pension, dealing with the bank	Much improved	A bit improved	Not much change	A bit worse	Much worse
15. Handling other every day arithmetic problems e.g. knowing how much food to buy, knowing how long between visits from family or friends	Much improved	A bit improved	Not much change	A bit worse	Much worse
16. Using his/her intelligence to understand what's going on and to reason things through	Much improved	A bit improved	Not much change	A bit worse	Much worse

Sources: Jorm AF, Jacomb PA (1989) An Informant Questionnaire on Cognitive Decline in the Elderly (IQCODE): socio-demographic correlates, reliability, validity and some norms. *Psychological Medicine* **19**: 1015–22. Reproduced with kind permission from Cambridge University Press. Also Jorm AF, Scott R, Jacomb PA (1989) Assessment of cognitive decline in dementia by informant questionnaire. *International Journal of Geriatric Psychiatry* **4**: 35–9. Copyright John Wiley & Sons Limited. Reproduced with permission.

Metamemory in Adulthood (MIA) Questionnaire

Reference: **Dixon RA, Hultsch DF, Hertzog C (1988) The Metamemory in Adulthood (MIA) Questionnaire.** *Psychopharmacology Bulletin* 24: 671–88

Time taken 30 minutes (reviewer's estimate)

Rating self-rating

Main indications

Self-rating of memory function.

Commentary

The Metamemory in Adulthood (MIA) Questionnaire consists of 108 items divided into seven scales: strategy (knowledge and reported use of memory strategies), task (knowledge of basic memory process), capacity (beliefs regarding one's own memory), change (change in the ability to remember), anxiety (perceptions of the relationship between anxiety and memory performance), achievement (perception of one's own motivation to perform well in memory tasks) and locus (sense of control over memory skills). An eighth scale, activity (regularity of activities supportive of memory), has also been described, adding 12 items. A number of samples have been described in ages ranging from 18 to 84, and validation against personality,

depression and other scales has been carried out (Hultsch et al, 1988). Internal consistency as assessed by Cronbach's alpha is high, and discriminant validity demonstrates that MIA constructs are not easily accounted for by other psychological indices such as depression or anxiety. While not meant as a device for measuring actual memory problems, it can measure knowledge, beliefs and affect about memory.

Additional reference

Hultsch DF, Hertzog C, Dixon RA et al (1988) Memory, self-knowledge and self-efficacy in the aged. In Howe ML, Brainerd CJ, eds. *Cognitive development in adulthood: progress in cognitive developmental research.* New York: Springer-Verlag, 65–92.

Address for correspondence

Roger A Dixon
Department of Psychology
University of Victoria
Victoria BC
V8W 2Y2
Canada

Metamemory in Adulthood (MIA) Questionnaire

Main items:

Strategy	Anxiety
Task	Achievement
Capacity	Locus
Change	Activity

Memory Functioning Questionnaire (MFQ)

Reference: **Gilewski MJ, Zelinski EM (1988) Memory Functioning Questionnaire (MFQ).**
***Psychopharmacology Bulletin* 24: 665–70**

Time taken 25 minutes (reviewer's estimate)

Rating self-rating

Main indications

Detection of memory complaints in elderly people.

Commentary

The Memory Functioning Questionnaire (MFQ) is a 64-item instrument with seven scales: general rating of memory, retrospective functioning, frequency of forgetting, frequency of forgetting when reading, remembering past events, seriousness of forgetting, and mnemonics usage. It is a revision of an earlier scale which had an additional 28 questions in nine scales (Zelinski et al, 1980). A principal components analysis of a larger scale in a population of some 800 adults revealed three factors: general frequency of forgetting, seriousness, and retrospective functioning/mnemonics. The parent questionnaire has been shown to correlate significantly with formal tests of cognitive function (Zelinski et al, 1980).

Additional reference

Zelinski EM, Gilewski MJ, Thompson LW (1980) Do laboratory tests relate to self-assessment of memory ability in the young and old? In Poon LW, Fozard JL, Cermak LS et al, eds. *New directions in memory and ageing: proceedings of the George A Talland Memorial Conference.* Hillsdaee, NJ: Erlbaum, 519–44.

Address for correspondence

Elizabeth M Zelinski
Leonard Davis School of Gerontology
University of Southern California
Los Angeles
CA 90089-0191
USA

Memory Functioning Questionnaire (MFQ)

Main items:	Frequency of forgetting when reading
Memory rating	Remembering past events
Retrospective functioning	Seriousness of forgetting
Frequency of forgetting	Mnemonics usage

Reproduced from Gilewski MJ, Zelinski EM (1988) Memory Functioning Questionnaire (MFQ). *Psychopharmacology Bulletin* **24**: 665–70.

The Knowledge of Memory Aging Questionnaire

Reference: **Cherry KE, West RL, Reese CM, Yassuda M (2000) The Knowledge of Memory Aging Questionnaire.** *Educational Gerontology* **26: 195–219**

Time taken 10 minutes

Rating by questionnaire

Main indications

To assess the general knowledge of normal and pathological memory ageing. It can be used with students, older adults, and service providers who work with the elderly

Commentary

The questionnaire consists of 28 true/false items covering a broad range of aspects of memory that would be either normal age-related memory changes or abnormal memory deficits due to dementia. From an educational point of view the KMAQ can assess the baseline level of ageing knowledge so that it may be increased. From a research perspective the instrument can be used to examine the relationship between knowledge of memory ageing, self-reported appraisals of memory, and objective memory performance.

Address for correspondence

Katie E Cherry
Department of Psychology
Louisiana State University
Baton Rouge
Louisiana 70803-5501
USA
pskatie@lsu.edu

Knowledge of Memory Aging Questionnaire

1. 'A picture is worth a thousand words' in that it is easier for both younger and older people to remember pictures than remember words. (N-true)
2. Older people tend to have more trouble concentrating than younger people. That is, older people are more likely to be distracted by background noises and other happenings around them. (N-true)
3. Regardless of how memory is tested, younger adults will remember far more material than older adults. (N-false)
4. Confusion and memory lapses in older people can sometimes be due to physical conditions that doctors can treat so that these symptoms go away over time. (P-true)
5. Becoming disoriented (such as getting lost or losing track of what day it is) happens to persons with Alzheimer's disease, but only in the later stages of the disease. (P-false)
6. Older people remember to do future planned activities (such as returning a book to the library) better than they remember past actions that they have already completed. (N-true)
7. Medications that are prescribed by doctors for heart and circulation problems do *not* affect memory in older adults. (P-false)
8. Sometimes the effects of intense grief over the loss of a loved one may be mistaken for early Alzheimer's disease in older adults. (P-true)
9. A complete physical exam by a doctor is routinely recommended if a diagnosis of Alzheimer's disease is suspected. (P-true)
10. Older people tend to remember specific past events in their daily life better than they remember the meanings of words (vocabulary) and general facts (such as the capital of the United States). (N-false)
11. Frequent complaining about memory problems is an early sign of Alzheimer's disease. (P-false)
12. The only way to tell for sure if an individual has Alzheimer's disease is to do an autopsy after that person has died. (P-true)
13. If an older adult is unable to recall a specific fact (e.g. remembering a person's name), then providing a cue to prompt or jog the memory is unlikely to help. (N-false)
14. When older people are trying to memorize new information, the way they study it does *not* affect how much they will remember later. (N-false)
15. If one has lived to be 85 years old and shows no signs of Alzheimer's disease, then the chances are very high that this person will live out the rest of his or her life without developing the disease. (P-false)
16. For older adults, the ability to remember something is unrelated to the number of other thoughts or issues on their mind when trying to recall this information. (N-false)
17. Memory for how to do well-learned things, such as reading a map or riding a bike, does *not* change very much, if at all, in later adulthood. (N-true)
18. Signs and symptoms of Alzheimer's disease show up gradually and become more noticeable to family members and close friends over time. (P-true)
19. When an older adult comes in for a checkup, doctors and psychologists can now clearly tell the difference between the symptoms of mental health problems and the symptoms of physical illness. (P-false)
20. Immediate memory (such as repeating a telephone number) is about the same for younger and older people, but an older person's memory for things that happened days, weeks, or months ago is typically worse than that of a younger person. (N-true)
21. If an older person has gone into another room and cannot remember what he or she had intended to do there, going back to the place where the thought first came to mind will often help one recall what he or she had intended to do. (N-true)
22. Alzheimer's disease is the only illness that leads to confusion and memory problems in older adults. (P-false)
23. For older people, education, occupation, and verbal skills tend to have little influence on their memory. (N-false)
24. Modern-day memory improvement methods that are based on organization (e.g. grouping similar items together) and association (e.g. linking new information to what is already known) can actually be traced back to the ancient Greek scholars, such as Aristotle and Plato. (N-true)
25. Healthy older adults have trouble remembering how to use familiar gadgets (like a key chain) and appliances (like a can opener). (P-false)
26. Dramatic changes in personality and relationships with others may be seen in persons who have Alzheimer's disease. (P-true)
27. Memory training programs are *not* helpful for older persons, because the memory problems that occur in old age cannot be improved by educational methods. (N-false)
28. Lifelong alcoholism may result in severe memory problems in old age. (P-true)

N = normal; P = pathological

Source: Cherry KE *et al. Educ Gerontol* 2000; **26**: 195–219. Reproduced by permission.

Chapter 8

Other scales

Multiphasic Environmental Assessment Procedure (MEAP)

Reference: **Moos RH, Lemke S (1992)** *Multiphasic Environmental Assessment Procedure user's guide.* **Palo Alto, CA: Center for Health Care Evaluation, Department of Veterans' Affairs and Stanford University Medical Centers.**

Time taken variable

Rating various

Main indications

The Multiphasic Environmental Assessment Procedure (MEAP) is a five-part procedure for making a comprehensive evaluation of the physical and social environments in group residential facilities for older people.

Commentary

The MEAP comprises five separate instruments corresponding to four conceptual domains as summarized below. A detailed analysis is beyond the scope of this book. The rater is referred to the user's guide and appropriate references.

Overview of the Multiphasic Environmental Assessment Procedure (MEAP) instruments

Instrument	Aspect of environment assessed	Source
Resident and Staff Information Form (RESIF)	Suprapersonal factors, such as the average background and personal characteristics of people living or working the facility (6 subscales)	Records, interviews, and staff reports
Physical and Architectural Features Checklist (PAF)	Physical features, covering location, features inside and outside the facility, and space allowances (8 subscales)	Direct observation
Policy and Program Information Form (POLIF)	Facility policies, including types of rooms available, how the facility is organized, and what services are provided (9 subscales)	Facility administrator and staff reports
Sheltered Care Environment Scale (SCES)	Social milieu, including relationships, personal growth and system maintenance and change (7 subscales)	Resident and staff reports
Rating Scale	Physical environment and resident and staff functioning (4 subscales)	Direct observation

Source: Moos RH, Lemke S, Multiphasic Environmental Assessment Procedure user's guide. Reprinted by permission of Sage Publications.

Philadelphia Geriatric Center Morale Scale

Reference: **Lawton MP (1975) Philadelphia Geriatric Center Morale Scale: a revision.** *Journal of Gerontology* 30: 85–9

Time taken rating as one part of a 60-minute interview

Rating by interview

Main indications

Assessment of morale in elderly people.

Commentary

The original paper describes a principal components analysis of the scale on over 1000 elderly people. The work builds on the original description scale (Lawton, 1972) and a companion paper (Morris and Sherwood, 1975). Three consistently reproducible factors emerged: agitation, attitude towards own ageing and lonely dissatisfaction. Using 17 of the original items, internal consistency as determined by Cronbach's alpha statistics was 0.85, 0.81 and 0.85 respectively. The 17 items were designated as the revised Philadelphia Geriatric Center Morale Scale.

Additional references

Lawton MP (1972) The dimensions of morale. In Kent D, Kastenbaum R, Sherwood S, eds. *Research, planning and action for the elderly.* New York: Behavioral Publications.

Morris JN, Sherwood S (1975) A retesting and modification of the Philadelphia Geriatric Centre Morale Scale. *Journal of Gerontology* 15: 77–84.

	YES	NO

Agitation

* Little things bother me more this year (no)	—	—
* I sometimes worry so much that I can't sleep (no)	—	—
I have a lot to be sad about (no)	—	—
* I am afraid of a lot of things (no)	—	—
* I get mad more than I used to (no)	—	—
Life is hard for me most of the time (no)	—	—
* I take things hard (no)	—	—
* I get upset easily (no)	—	—

Attitude toward own aging

* Things keep getting worse as I get older (no)	—	—
* I have as much pep as I had last year (yes)	—	—
Little things bother me more this year (no)	—	—
* As you get older you are less useful (no)	—	—
* As I get older, things are better/worse than I thought they would be (better)	—	—
I sometimes feel that life isn't worth living (no)	—	—
* I am as happy now as when I was younger (yes)	—	—

Lonely dissatisfaction

* How much do you feel lonely? (not much)	—	—
* I see enough of my friends and relatives (yes)	—	—
* I sometimes feel that life isn't worth living (no)	—	—
* Life is hard for much of the time (no)	—	—
* How satisfied are you with your life today? (satisfied)	—	—
* I Have a lot to be sad about (no)	—	—
People had it better in the old days (no)	—	—
A person has to live for today and not about tomorrow (yes)	—	—

High morale responses are indicated in parentheses

(*) Items selected as best representative of the factor

Cumulative Illness Rating Scale (CIRS)

Reference: **ConwellY, Forbes NT, Cox C, Caine ED (1993) Validation of a measure of physical illness burden at autopsy: the Cumulative Illness Rating Scale.** *Journal of the American Geriatrics Society* **41: 38–41**

Time taken 20 minutes (reviewer's estimate)

Rating by trained examiners to complete medical examination and health history

Main indications

An objective measure of physical illness burden.

Commentary

The Cumulative Illness Rating Scale (CIRS) is useful in several scenarios – for example in predicting outcome in longitudinal studies of late-life affective illness, and as an outcome variable in studies of social factors or health behaviour on overall physical wellbeing. The CIRS is a measure of physical illness in which a cumulative score is derived from ratings of severity of impairment in each of 13 organ systems. Using information from physicians, interview and review of medical records, the CIRS was correlated with post-mortem ratings made independently at tissue autopsy on victims of suicide. Inter-rater reliability is about 0.83. CIRS ratings made by examination of tissue at autopsy were highly predictive of analogous ratings based on historical data, accounting for 75% of the variance in CIRS scores.

Additional reference

Linn MW, Linn BS, Gurel L (1967) Physical resistance in the aged. *Geriatrics* **22**: 134–8.

Address for correspondence

Yeates Conwell
University of Rochester
300 Crittenden Blvd
Rochester
NY 14642
USA

e-mail: Yeates.conwell@urmc.rochester.edu

Cumulative Illness Rating Scale (CIRS)

		Rating
	Cardiovascular–Respiratory System	
1.	Cardiac (heart only)	___
2.	Vascular (blood, blood vessels and cells, marrow, spleen, lymphatics)	___
3.	Respiratory (lungs, bronchi, trachea below larynx)	___
4.	EENT (eye, ear, nose, throat, larynx)	___
	Gastrointestinal System	
5.	Upper GI (esophagus, stomach, duodenum, biliary and pancreatic trees)	___
6.	Lower GI (intestines, hernias)	___
7.	Hepatic (liver only)	___
	Genitourinary System	
8.	Renal (kidneys only)	___
9.	Other GU (ureters, bladder, urethra, prostate, genitals)	___
	Musculo-Skeletal-Integumentary System	
10.	MSI (muscles, bone, skin)	___
	Neuropsychiatric System	
11.	Neurologic (brain, spinal cord, nerves)	___
12.	Psychiatric (mental)	___
	General System	
13.	Endocrine-Metabolic (includes diffuse infections, poisonings)	___
	Total	___

Rate as follows for each system:
0 = No impairment to organ/system
1 = Mild impairment
    No interference normal activity
    Treatment required
    Prognosis excellent

2 = Moderate impairment
    Interference with normal activity
    Treatment required
    Prognosis is good
3 = Severe impairment
    Disability

    Urgent treatment required
    Prognosis guarded
4 = Extrememly severe impairment
    Life threatening
    Treatment is emergent or of no avail
    Grave prognosis

Measurement of Morale in the Elderly

Reference: **Pierce RC, Clarke MM (1973) Measurement of morale in the elderly.**
International Journal of Aging and Human Development **4: 83–101**

Time taken 20–25 minutes (reviewer's estimate)

Rating by clinical interviewer

Main indications

Designed to assess level of morale amongst older people with mental health problems.

Commentary

The Measurement of Morale in the Elderly scale was developed using original items and ones taken from previous studies (Thompson et al, 1960; Srole et al, 1962). There were eight identifiable factors for factor analysis: depression/satisfaction, will to live, equanimity (all referring to morale), positive or negative attitudes to ageing, social alienation (representing attitudes to ageing), physical health and sociability. The study was able to discriminate between two groups of ageing subjects; those with possible mental health problems and normal controls. A 1978

research version is also available, which has 35 items rated on a 4/5 point scale (agree strongly/never – disagree strongly/often).

Additional references

Srole L, Langner TS, Michael ST et al (1962) *Mental health in the metropolis: the midtown Manhattan study.* Vol. 1. New York: McGraw-Hill.

Thompson WE, Streib GF, Kosa J (1960) The effect of retirement on personal adjustment: a panel analysis. *Journal of Gerontology* **15**: 165–9.

Address for correspondence

Robert C Pierce
99 Golden Hind Blvd
San Rafael
CA 94903
USA

Measurement of Morale in the Elderly

1.   How is your appetite? (Poor.)
2.   How has you general health been this past year? (Extremely poor.)
3.   Do you find you are less interested lately in things like your personal appearance and table manners and things like that? (No.)
4.   Do you have as much energy as you did a year ago? (Less.)
5.   Interviewer's rating of the subject's reaction to interview. (Any 'abnormal' reaction.)
6.   Interviewer's rating of the subject's affectivity. (Any 'Abnormal' rating; e.g., tense, irritable, overly cheerful, tearful, etc.)
7.   Interviewer's rating of the subject's cooperativeness. (Uncooperative.)
8.   Do you often feel irritable and impatient? (No.)
9.   Have you been worried during the past year for no reason? (No.)
10. Do you often feel moody and blue? (No.)
11. Have you felt lately that life is not worth living? (No.)
12. All in all, how much happiness would you say you find in life today? (Almost none.)
13. In general, how would you say you feel most of the time, in good spirits or in low spirits? (Usually low.)
14. On the whole, how satisfied would you say you are with your life today? (Not very satisfied.)
15. How often do you get the feeling that your life today is not very useful? (Hardly ever.)
16. How often do you find yourself feeling blue? (Hardly ever.)
17. How often do you get upset by the things that happen in your day-to-day life? (Hardly ever.)
18. These days I find myself giving up hope of trying to improve myself. (Disagree.)
19. Almost eveything these days is a racket. (Disagree.)
20. How much do you plan ahead the things that you will be doing the next week or week after? (Almost no plans.)
21. There's little use in writing to public officials because often they aren't interested in the problems of the average man. (Disagree.)
22. Nowadays a person has to live pretty much for today and let tomorow take care of itself. (Disagree.)
23. In spite of what some people say, the lot of the average man is getting worse, not better. (Disagree.)
24. It's hardly fair to bring children into the world with the way things look for the future. (Disagree.)
25. These days a person doesn't know who he can count on. (Disagree.)
26. Young people underestimate the capabilities of older people. (Disagree.)
27. When you are old there's not much use in going to a lot of trouble to look nice. (Disagree.)
28. I'd rather die than grow older. (Disagree.)
29. Old people can generally solve problems better because they have more experience. (Disagree.)
30. I'd like to live another 20 years. (Disagree.)
31. Life doesn't really begin until 60. (Disagree.)
32. I feel sorry for old people. (Disagree.)
33. Sometimes I wish I were 25 or 30 again. (Disagree.)
34. Everybody takes advantage of older people. (Disagree.)
35. The main problem in old age is money. (Disagree.)
36. When you get old you begin to forget things. (Disagree.)
37. I have more friends now than I did when I was 50. (Disagree.)
38. Young people don't realize that old folks have problems. (Disagree.)
39. Lots of old people don't seem to care about keeping themselves neat and clean. (Disagree.)
40. When you're older you appreciate the world more. (Disagree.)
41. When you get old, more people go out of their way to be nice to you. (Disagree.)
42. When you're old you take longer to make up your mind. (Disagree.)
43. The only good things about being older is that you are near the end of your suffering. (Disagree.)
44. When you get old your thinking is not as good as it used to be. (Disagree.)
45. I can't think of any problems that older people have. (Disagree.)

Scale continued overleaf

1978 Research Version

For each of the following items, please circle the number of the alternative that you feel applies best to you.

1. Do you ever feel moody?
   4_____ Never
   3_____ Once in a while
   2_____ Fairly often
   1_____ Often

2. I'd rather die than grow very old
   1_____ Agree strongly
   2_____ Agree moderately
   3_____ Undecided
   4_____ Disagree moderately
   5_____ Disagree strongly

3. I'd like to live at least another twenty years
   1_____ Disagree strongly
   2_____ Disagree moderately
   3_____ Undecided
   4_____ Agree moderately
   5_____ Agree strongly

4. I look forward to life in the next several years
   5_____ Agree strongly
   4_____ Agree moderately
   3_____ Undecided
   2_____ Disagree moderately
   1_____ Disagree strongly

5. All in all, how much happiness would you say you find in life today?
   1_____ Almost none
   2_____ Some, but not much
   3_____ A good deal

6. On the whole, how satisfied would you say you are with your way of life today?
   3_____ Very satisfied
   2_____ Fairly satisfied
   1_____ Not very satisfied

7. Loud noises make me jump
   5_____ Disagree strongly
   4_____ Disagree moderately
   3_____ Undecided
   2_____ Agree moderately
   1_____ Agree strongly

8. I've been feeling a lot of stress and strain recently
   5_____ Agree strongly
   4_____ Agree moderately
   3_____ Undecided
   2_____ Disagree moderately
   1_____ Disagree strongly

9. In general, how would you say you feel most of the time, in good spirits or in low spirits?
   1_____ Usually in low spirits
   2_____ Sometimes in good, sometimes in low
   3_____ Usually in good spirits

10. I've been feeling awfully jumpy lately
    5_____ Disagree strongly
    4_____ Disagree moderately
    3_____ Undecided
    2_____ Agree moderately
    1_____ Agree strongly

11. Do you sometimes find yourself feeling impatient?
    1_____ Often
    2_____ Fairly often
    3_____ Once in a while
    4_____ Never

12. I think my life in the next few years will be better than ever
    5_____ Agree strongly
    4_____ Agree moderately
    3_____ Undecided
    2_____ Disagree moderately
    1_____ Disagree strongly

13. I'd like to live to a ripe old age
    1_____ Disagree strongly
    2_____ Disagree moderately
    3_____ Undecided
    4_____ Agree moderately
    5_____ Agree strongly

14. How often do you find yourself feeling blue?
    4_____ Never
    3_____ Once in a while
    2_____ Fairly often
    1_____ Often

15. I seem to get nervous very easily nowadays
    5_____ Disagree strongly
    4_____ Disagree moderately
    3_____ Undecided
    2_____ Agree moderately
    1_____ Agree strongly

16. Do you get upset by the things that happen in your day-to-day life?
    1_____ Often
    2_____ Fairly often
    3_____ Once in a while
    4_____ Never

17. If things get any worse I think I'll kill myself
    1_____ Agree strongly
    2_____ Agree moderately
    3_____ Undecided
    4_____ Disagree moderately
    5_____ Disagree strongly

18. I think I am a very calm person
    5_____ Agree strongly
    4_____ Agree moderately
    3_____ Undecided
    2_____ Disagree moderately
    1_____ Disagree strongly

19. I hate it when things go wrong
    5_____ Disagree strongly
    4_____ Disagree moderately
    3_____ Undecided
    2_____ Agree moderately
    1_____ Agree strongly

20. I'm generally pretty easygoing
    5_____ Disagree strongly
    4_____ Disagree moderately
    3_____ Undecided
    2_____ Agree moderately
    1_____ Agree strongly

21. How often do you feel grouchy for no particular reason?
    4_____ Never
    3_____ Once in a while

cont.

| 2 _____ | Fairly often |
| 1 _____ | Often |

22. How often do you feel irritable?

1 _____	Often
2 _____	Fairly often
3 _____	Once in a while
4 _____	Never

23. How often do you get the feeling that your life today is not very useful?

4 _____	Never
3 _____	Once in a while
2 _____	Fairly often
1 _____	Often

24. Have you been worried during the past year for no reason?

1 _____	Often
2 _____	Fairly often
3 _____	Once in a while
4 _____	Never

25. Do you fly off the handle easy?

4 _____	Never
3 _____	Once in a while
2 _____	Fairly often
1 _____	Often

26. I'd like to take it easy, but circumstances won't allow me

5 _____	Disagree strongly
4 _____	Disagree moderately
3 _____	Undecided
2 _____	Agree moderately
1 _____	Agree strongly

27. I'm not as enthusiastic about things as I used to be

1 _____	Disagree strongly
2 _____	Disagree moderately
3 _____	Undecided
4 _____	Agree moderately
5 _____	Agree strongly

28. I'm contented with what I've done in life

5 _____	Agree strongly
4 _____	Agree moderately
3 _____	Undecided
2 _____	Disagree moderately
1 _____	Disagree strongly

29. I'm tired a lot

1 _____	Disagree strongly
2 _____	Disagree moderately
3 _____	Undecided
4 _____	Agree moderately
5 _____	Agree strongly

30. I feel discouraged

5 _____	Agree strongly
4 _____	Agree moderately
3 _____	Undecided
2 _____	Disagree moderately
1 _____	Disagree strongly

31. I've been having a hard time getting started lately

1 _____	Disagree strongly
2 _____	Disagree moderately
3 _____	Undecided
4 _____	Agree moderately
5 _____	Agree strongly

32. I'm generally satisfied with the way I am

5 _____	Agree strongly
4 _____	Agree moderately
3 _____	Undecided
2 _____	Disagree moderately
1 _____	Disagree strongly

33. Sometimes I just don't like myself

1 _____	Disagree strongly
2 _____	Disagree moderately
3 _____	Undecided
4 _____	Agree moderately
5 _____	Agree strongly

34. I have some bad qualities

5 _____	Agree strongly
4 _____	Agree moderately
3 _____	Undecided
2 _____	Disagree moderately
1 _____	Disagree strongly

35. Life has been pretty good to me

1 _____	Disagree strongly
2 _____	Disagree moderately
3 _____	Undecided
4 _____	Agree moderately
5 _____	Agree strongly

Scoring:

The individual taking the inventory should circle the number of the most appropriate alternative for each question.

To score the inventory, add the number of the alternative for the items composing the scales Satisfaction, Will-to-live, and Equanimity, as follows:

Satisfaction	Equanimity	Will-to-live
1	7	2
5	8	3
6	10	4
9	11	12
14	15	13
23	16	17
27	19	
28	20	
29	21	
30	22	
31	24	
32	25	
33	26	
34		
35		

Reproduced from Pierce RC, Clarke MM (1973) Measurement of morale in the elderly. *International Journal of Aging and Human Development* **4**: 83–101, published by Baywood Publishing Co.

Retrospective Postmortem Dementia Assessment (RCD-1)

Reference: **Davis PB, White H, Price JL, McKeel D, Robins LN (1991) Retrospective Postmortem Dementia Assessment: validation of a new clinical interview to assist neuropathologic study.** *Archives of Neurology* **48: 613–17**

Time taken 40 minutes

Rating retrospective structured telephone interview

Main indications

Retrospective gathering of information about a patient after his or her death.

Commentary

The Retrospective Postmortem Dementia Assessment (RCD-1) is a screening interview for use after the death of a patient to enable retrospective information to be gathered so that a clinical diagnosis of the type of dementia can be achieved. It is particularly useful in studies looking at clinicopathological correlations where one may not have had the opportunity to collect information prospectively. A number of different topics are included, including demographic data, family history, physical functioning, physical condition, drug and alcohol intake, hearing and vision, memory and orientation, neuropsychiatric features and particular signs such as aphasia. Extracts from existing scales include the Blessed Dementia Scale (page 46) and the Clinical Dementia Rating (CDR; page 238). Agreement between RCD-1 interview and post-mortem diagnosis was 91%, and between RCD-1 interview and medical records 100%.

Additional reference

Regier DA, Meyers JK, Kramer M et al (1984) The NIMH Epidemologic Catchment Area Program. *Archives of General Psychiatry* **41**: 934–40.

Address for correspondence

Paula Bonino
Senior Associate Geriatrician
Geriatric Care Services/Lutheran Affiliated Services
500 Wittenberg Way
Box 928
Mars
PA 16046–0928
USA

Retrospective Postmortem Dementia Assessment (RCD-1)

The assessment encompasses the following areas

Demographics	Medications
Family history – siblings, parents	Hearing
Health status/physical functioning	Vision
Physical conditions	Problems related to memory and orientation
	Behaviour/changes in personality
	Social support/functioning

Quality of Interactions Schedule (QUIS)

Reference: **Dean R, Proudfoot R, Lindesay J (1993) The Quality of Interactions Schedule (QUIS): development, reliability and use in the evaluation of two domus units.** *International Journal of Geriatric Psychiatry* **8: 819–26**

Time taken observation period can be varied

Rating by trained observer

Main indications

An observer-rated measure of interactions between residents and care staff.

Commentary

In some situations, direct observations of interactions between staff and residents are valuable in evaluating and planning services. Event-sampling strategies have been devised (Godlove et al, 1982) and shorter versions validated (Macdonald et al, 1985). The Quality of Interactions Schedule (QUIS) was developed to assess the number and quality of interactions as part of a prospective evaluation of two residential units for elderly people with mental illness. The number and quality of interaction are estimated on the basis of a series of ten 15-minute observation times across the working day, over a period of approximately two weeks. Interactions are coded in one of five categories: positive social, positive care, neutral, negative protective and negative restrictive, based on the work of Clark and Bowling (1989).

Observation and coding consistently produce kappa reliability statistics of above 0.75, with a range of 0.60–0.91.

Additional references

Clark P, Bowling A (1989) Observational study of quality of life in nursing homes and a long stay ward for the elderly. *Ageing Soc* **9**: 123–48.

Godlove C, Richard L, Rodwell G (1982) *Time for action. An observational study of elderly people in four different care environments.* Social Services Monographs, Research in Practice. Sheffield: Community Care, University of Sheffield, Joint Unit for Social Services Research.

Macdonald AJD, Craig TKJ, Warner LAR (1985) The development of short observation method for the study of activity and contacts of old people in residential settings. *Psychological Medicine* **15**: 167–72.

Address for correspondence

James Lindesay
Leicester General Hospital
Gwendolen Road
Leicester LE5 4PW, UK
e-mail: Jeb1@le.ac.uk

Quality of Interactions Schedule (QUIS): guidelines and examples for coding interactions

Positive social
Interaction principally involving 'good, constructive, beneficial' conversation and companionship.

Positive care
Interactions during the appropriate delivery of physical care.

Neutral
Brief, indifferent interactions not meeting the definitions of the other categories.

Negative protective
Providing care, keeping safe or removing from danger, but in a restrictive manner, without explanation or reassurance.

Negative restrictive
Interactions that oppose or resist residents' freedom of action without good reason, or which ignore resident as a person.

INSIGHT

Reference: **Verhey FRJ, Rozendaal N, Ponds RWHM, Jolles J (1993) Dementia, awareness and depression.** *International Journal of Geriatric Psychiatry* **8: 851–6**

Time taken 5 minutes

Rating by interview

Main indications

Assessment of awareness of cognitive decline.

Commentary

Awareness of cognitive decline in dementia is an important area, and the terms 'unawareness of deficit', 'lack of insight' and 'anosognosia' are usually used interdependently. Generally, insight tends to decrease with increasing severity of dementia (McGlynn and Schachter, 1989). The authors of the original paper on INSIGHT rated insight in 170 patients, the majority of whom had Alzheimer's disease. Standard guidelines were used to rate the awareness of cognitive decline, the final rating being made on a four-point scale. Level of awareness was significantly related to the severity of dementia but not depression.

Additional reference

McGlynn SM, Schachter DL (1989) Unawareness of deficits in neuropsychological syndromes. *Journal of Experimental Neuropsychology* 1: 143–205.

Address for correspondence

FRJ Verhey
Department of Psychiatry
University Hospital of Maastricht
PO Box 5800
6202 AZ Maastricht
The Netherlands

e-mail: f.verhey@np.unimaas.nl

INSIGHT

Please tell me about the problems you are here for. Why did Dr . . . send you to this clinic?

When the patient has other complaints not directly related to dementia:

Do you have any other complaints?

When the patient has no spontaneous complaints about his cognitive functions:

How is your memory functioning? Do you think you have a poor memory?

When the patient denies deficits of memory or other cognitive functions:

So, there are no memory problems at all? Is everything going all right for you?

Complaints are then discussed and the same question adopted to ask the caregiver.

Scoring:
4 = Adequate
3 = Mildly disturbed
2 = Moderately disturbed
1 = Severely disturbed

Ischaemic Score

Reference: Hackinski VC, Iliff LD, Zilka E et al (1975) Cerebral blood flow in dementia. *Archives of Neurology* 32: 632–7

Time taken 2 minutes (once all the information is gathered)

Rating by clinician

Main indications

Assessment of vascular contribution to the aetiology of dementia.

Commentary

On the basis of the Ischaemic Score, the concept of multi-infarct dementia was introduced based on the assumption that in many patients dementia was as a result of single or multiple large infarctions. The Ischaemic Score was validated using functional brain imaging to divide patients with dementia into those with vascular disease and those with primary degenerative dementia. The average age of the group was 63, and there seems to be a bimodal distribution of the scores in relation to the appearances on the scan, reflecting cerebral blood flow. A score of 4 or below was indicative of a primary degenerative dementia and 7 or above of vascular dementia. A number of authors have commented on the scale and adaptations have been suggested. The most obvious omission is the lack of evidence from brain imaging to show vascular changes in the brain. Hachinski

(1983) confirmed that the scale is designed to identify strokes and so is considered by many to be more of an infarct than an ischaemic scale. Validity studies with amended versions of the scale have been published (e.g. Rosen et al, 1980; Loeb and Godolfo, 1983; Fischer et al, 1991). Grasel et al (1990) found the best discriminating factors to be fluctuation course, stepwise deterioration, abrupt onset, history of strokes, and the presence of focal neurological signs and symptoms.

Additional references

Fischer P et al (1991) Neuropathological validation of the Hachinski scale *Journal of Neural Transmission* 1: 57.

Grasel E et al (1990) What contribution can the Hachinski ischaemic scale make to the differential diagnosis between multi-infarct dementia and primary degenerative dementia? *Archives of Gerontology and Geriatrics* 11: 63–75.

Hachinski C (1983) Multifocal dementia. *Neurologic Clinics* 1: 27–36.

Loeb C, Godolfo C (1983) Diagnostic evaluation of degenerative and vascular dementia. *Stroke* 14: 399–401.

Rosen WG et al (1980) Pathological verification of ischaemic score in dementias. *Annals of Neurology* 7: 486–8.

Ischaemic Score			
Abrupt onset	2	Emotional incontinence	1
Stepwise deterioration	1	History of hypertension	1
Fluctuating course	2	History of strokes	2
Nocturnal confusion	1	Generalized atherosclerosis	1
Relative preservation of personality	1	Focal neurological symtoms	2
Depression	1	Focal neurological signs	2
Somatic complaints	1		

The CAGE Questionnaire

Reference: **Ewing J (1984) Detecting alcoholism: the CAGE questionnaire.** *Journal of the American Medical Association* **252: 1905–7**

Time taken 1 minute

Rating by nurse or clinician

Main indications

To screen for alcohol use disorders.

Commentary

The CAGE is the oldest and most widely used alcohol screening questionnaire. It consists of four questions and the acronym CAGE is based on the first letter of the key word of each item in the questionnaire.

The CAGE was originally developed for use in young adult populations but has also been used in elderly patient populations. The utility of various cut-off scores on the CAGE alcohol use disorders has been computed in younger adult and elderly populations. The sensitivity and specificity of a cut-off score of ≥2 varies between 48–70% for sensitivity and 56–100% for specificity. The CAGE has been used in a number of different settings including medical outpatients, nursing homes and individuals who are housebound. The CAGE has good test accuracy in older people and is superior to both the MAST-G and AUDIT in this population.

Additional reference

Mayfield D, McCleod D, G Jall P (1974) A validation of a new alcohol screening instrument. *American Journal of Psychiatry* **131**: 1121–3.

Morton JL, Jones TV, Manganaro MA (1996) Performance of alcoholism screening questionnaires in elderly veterans. *American Journal of Medicine* **101**: 153.

Address for correspondence

Dr John A Ewing
Center for Alcohol Studies
Wing B Medical School
207-H UNC-CH Chapel Hill
NC 27514
USA

The CAGE questions

Have you ever felt the need to **C**ut down drinking?
Have you ever felt **A**nnoyed by criticism of drinking?
Have you ever had **G**uilty feelings about drinking?
Have you ever taken a morning **E**ye-opener?

MAST-G

Reference: Blow F (1991) Michigan Alcoholism Screening Test – Geriatric Version (MAST-G). Ann Arbour: University of Michigan Alcohol Research Centre

Rating by self-administered questionnaire

Main indications

To screen for alcohol use disorders.

Commentary

This is an elderly specific alcohol screening instrument. It consists of 24 items in a Yes/No format. Scores range from 0–24 and the optimal cut-off for alcohol dependence is ≥5. The MAST-G has been used in nursing home patients, geriatric outpatients and has shown high sensitivity, varying between 91–93% and good specificity varying between 65–84%.

MAST-G

Directions: The following is a list of questions about your past and present drinking habits. Please answer yes or no to each question by marking the line next to the question. When you are finished answering the questions, please add up how many 'yes' responses you checked and put that number in the space provided at the end.

		YES (1)	NO (2)
1.	After drinking have you ever noticed an increase in your heart rate or beating in your chest?	1. _____	_____
2.	When talking with others, do you ever underestimate how much you actually drink?	2. _____	_____
3.	Does alcohol make you sleepy so that you often fall asleep in your chair?	3. _____	_____
4.	After a few drinks, have you sometimes not eaten or been able to skip a meal because you didn't feel hungry?	4. _____	_____
5.	Does having a few drinks help decrease your shakiness or tremors?	5. _____	_____
6.	Does alcohol sometimes make it hard for you to remember parts of the day or night?	6. _____	_____
7.	Do you have rules for yourself that you won't drink before a certain time of day?	7. _____	_____
8.	Have you lost interest in hobbies or activities you used to enjoy?	8. _____	_____
9.	When you wake up in the morning, do you ever have trouble remembering part of the night before?	9. _____	_____
10.	Does having a drink help you sleep?	10. _____	_____
11.	Do you hide your alcohol bottles from family members?	11. _____	_____
12.	After a social gathering, have you ever felt embarrassed because you drank too much?	12. _____	_____
13.	Have you ever been concerned that drinking might be harmful to your health?	13. _____	_____
14.	Do you like to end an evening with a night cap?	14. _____	_____
15.	Did you find your drinking increased after someone close to you died?	15. _____	_____
16.	In general, would you prefer to have a few drinks at home rather than go out to social events?	16. _____	_____
17.	Are you drinking more now than in the past?	17. _____	_____
18.	Do you usually take a drink to relax or calm your nerves?	18. _____	_____
19.	Do you drink to take your mind off your problems?	19. _____	_____
20.	Have you ever increased your drinking after experiencing a loss in your life?	20. _____	_____
21.	Do you sometimes drive when you have had too much to drink?	21. _____	_____
22.	Has a doctor or nurse ever said they were worried or concerned about your drinking?	22. _____	_____
23.	Have you ever made rules to manage your drinking?	23. _____	_____
24.	When you feel lonely does having a drink help?	24. _____	_____

TOTAL 'YES' response _____

Scoring: 5 or more 'yes' responses is indicative of alcohol problem.

Source: Reproduced with permission from Blow (1991).

AUDIT

Reference: **Saunders JB, Aasland OG, Babor TF et al (1993) Development of the Alcohol Use Disorders Identification Test (AUDIT): WHO Collaborative Project on Early Detection of Persons with Harmful Alcohol Consumption–II.** *Addiction* 88: 791–804

Rating by self-administered questionnaire

Main indications

To screen for alcohol use disorders.

Commentary

This instrument was originally developed for WHO International Studies on problem drinking in General Practice. It was designed with young populations in mind and on the detection of current drinking problems. It is a 10-item screening questionnaire. It ranges in score from 0 to 41, with 0 indicating no levels of alcoholism and 41 indicating a very high likelihood of alcoholism. The conventional cut-off for alcohol abuse disorders is ≥8.

AUDIT has been compared to both the CAGE and the MAST-G in elderly populations and has been shown to be inferior to both MAST-G and CAGE in terms of detecting alcohol abuse.

The AUDIT Core Questionnaire

1. How often do you have a drink containing alcohol?
   (0) Never   (1) Less than monthly   (2) Monthly   (3) Weekly   (4) Daily or almost daily

2. How many drinks containing alcohol do you have on a typical day when you are drinking?
   (0) None   (1) 1 or 2   (2) 3 or 4   (3) 5 or 6   (4) 7 to 9   (5) 10 or more

3. How often do you have six or more drinks on one occasion?
   (0) Never   (1) Less than monthly   (2) Monthly   (3) Weekly   (4) Daily or almost daily

4. How often during the last year have you found that you were not able to stop drinking once you had started?
   (0) Never   (1) Less than monthly   (2) Monthly   (3) Weekly   (4) Daily or almost daily

5. How often during the last year have you failed to do what was normally expected from you because of drinking?
   (0) Never   (1) Less than monthly   (2) Monthly   (3) Weekly   (4) Daily or almost daily

6. How often during the last year have you needed a first drink in the morning to get yourself going after a heavy drinking session?
   (0) Never   (1) Less than monthly   (2) Monthly   (3) Weekly   (4) Daily or almost daily

7. How often during the last year have you had a feeling of guilt or remorse after drinking?
   (0) Never   (1) Less than monthly   (2) Monthly   (3) Weekly   (4) Daily or almost daily

8. How often during the last year have you been unable to remember what happened the night before because you had been drinking?
   (0) Never   (1) Less than monthly   (2) Monthly   (3) Weekly   (4) Daily or almost daily

9. Have you or someone else been injured as a result of your drinking?
   (0) No   (2) Yes, but not in the last year   (4) Yes, during the last year

10. Has a relative or friend or a doctor or other health worker been concerned about you drinking or suggested you cut down?
    (0) No   (2) Yes, but not in the last year   (4) Yes, during the last year

Numbers in parentheses are scoring weights. AUDIT Core Questionnaire total score is the sum of the scoring weights.

Source: Reproduced with permission from Saunders JB *et al. Addiction* 1993; **88**: 791–804.

Mini Nutritional Assessment

Reference: **Guigoz Y, Vellas B, Garry PJ (1994) Mini Nutritional Assessment: a practical assessment tool for grading the nutritional state of elderly patients.** *Facts and Research in Gerontology* **Suppl 2: 15–59**

Time taken 20 minutes

Rating by trained rater

Main indications

A nutritional assessment to evaluate the risk of malnutrition.

Commentary

The Mini Nutritional Assessment (MNA) test has five components:

1. Anthropometric measurements
2. Global assessment
3. Dietary questionnaire
4. Subjective assessments
5. Biological markers.
   The biological markers included a maximum score of 30 points, broken down into:

(a) normal (adequate nutrition)
(b) borderline (at risk of malnutrition)
(c) undernutrition.

The MNA has been developed and cross-validated in elderly populations from the very frail to the healthy.

Additional reference

Destky AS, Smalley PS, Chang J (1994) Is this patient malnourished? *Journal of the American Medical Association* **271**: 54–8.

Address for correspondence

Y Guigoz
Nestlé Research Centre
Nestec Ltd
Vers-chez-les Blanc
1000 Lausanne 26
Switzerland

The Resource Utilization in Dementia (RUD) Instrument

Reference: **Wimo A, Nordberg G, Jansson W, Grafstrom M (2000) Assessment of informal services to demented people with the RUD instrument.** *International Journal of Geriatric Psychiatry* **15: 969–71**

Time taken Between 5 and 40 minutes, depending on resource use

Rating by experienced interviewer

Main indications

This instrument was designed to assess resource utilization in people with dementia.

Commentary

Information on resource utilization is obtained by doing a structured interview with the caregiver. The RUD can be administered by nurses, clinicians or specialists. There are two parts to the questionnaire: Part A constitutes the baseline assessments. Information on the primary caregiver and their relationship with the patient, the amount of time given to assisting the patient with ADL, their current employment status, work loss through caring for the patient, the amount of hospitalization, physician time, and medications consumed by the caregiver are assessed.

The living accommodation, home services and the amount of hospitalization, physician time, and medications consumed by the patient are also assessed.

Part B is similar to the first but is for use in follow-up visits (see below).

Additional reference

Evaluation of the Healthcare Resource Utilization and Caregiver Time in Anti-Dementia Drug Trials – A quantitative battery. In: Wimo A, Jansson W, Karlsson G et al. (eds). *Health Economics of Dementia.* Oxford: Wiley, 1998.

Address for correspondence

Professor A Wimo
HC Bergsjo
Box 16
S-82070
Sweden

e-mail: anders.wimo@neurotec.ki.se

Follow-up questionnaire (Part B)

B1 caregiver
 Caregiver time
 Work status
 Health care resource utilization

B2 Patient
 Accommodation
 Health care resource utilization

The Alzheimer's Disease Knowledge Test

Reference: **Dieckmann L, Zarit S, Zarit JM, Gatz M (1988) The Alzheimer's Disease Knowledge Test.** *The Gerontologist* **28: 402–7**

Time taken 10 minutes

Rating by self-administered questionnaire

Main indications

To assess the level of knowledge of Alzheimer's disease in caregivers, professionals and other personnel involved in the care of Alzheimer's patients.

Commentary

The instrument consists of 20 multiple-choice questions with five response alternatives, consisting of the correct response, three distractors and an 'I do not know' alternative.

The test appears to be useful in providing the kind of information about the overall level of knowledge, information and misinformation that is needed to plan educational programmes for those involved with Alzheimer disease patients.

Address for correspondence

Lisa Dieckmann
Department of Psychology
Seely G Mudd Building
University of Southern California
Los Angeles
CA 90089-1061
USA

Alzheimer's Disease Knowledge Test

Question

1. The percentage of people over 65[a] who have severe dementia caused by Alzheimer's disease or a related disorder is estimated to be
   +1 A. less than 2%
     0 B. about 5%
   −1 C. about 10%
   −1 D. 20–25%
        E. I don't know
2. The prevalance of Alzheimer's disease in the general population of the United States is expected to
   +1 A. decrease slightly
   +1 B. remain approximately the same
     0 C. increase in proportion to the number of people over 65
   −1 D. nearly triple by the year 2000
        E. I don't know
3. The cause of Alzheimer's disease is
        A. old age
        B. hardening of the arteries
        C. senility
     0 D. unknown
        E. I don't know
4. Preliminary research concerning the role of heredity in Alzheimer's disease suggests that
     0 A. persons with a close relative with Alzheimer's disease have an increased risk of becoming afflicted
   −1 B. Alzheimer's disease is always transmitted genetically
   −1 C. Alzheimer's disease is only inherited if both parents are carriers of the disease
   +1 D. Alzheimer's disease is never inherited
        E. I don't know

cont.

5. Larger than normal amounts of aluminum have been found in the brains of some people with Alzheimer's disease. Studies investigating the role of aluminum in causing Alzheimer's disease
    A. have determined that it is the major cause
    B. have established that it plays a role in the onset of the disease
  0 C. are inconclusive
    D. have proven that it is not a cause
    E. I don't know

6. A person suspected of having Alzheimer's disease should be evaluated as soon as possible because
  +1 A. prompt treatment of Alzheimer's disease may prevent worsening of symptoms
  +1 B. prompt treatment of Alzheimer's disease may reverse symptoms
   0 C. it is important to rule out and treat reversible disorders
  −1 D. it is best to institutionalize an Alzheimer's disease patient early in the course of the disease
    E. I don't know

7. Which of the following procedures is required to confirm that symptoms are due to Alzheimer's disease?
    A. Mental status testing
  0 B. Autopsy
    C. CT scan
    D. Blood test
    E. I don't know

8. Which of the following conditions sometimes resembles Alzheimer's disease?
    A. Depression
    B. Delirium
    C. Stroke
  0 D. All of the above
    E. I don't know

9. Which of the following is always present in Alzheimer's disease?
   0 A. Loss of memory
  −1 B. Loss of memory, incontinence
  −1 C. Loss of memory, incontinence, hallucinations
  −1 D. None of the above
    E. I don't know

10. Although the rate of progression of Alzheimer's disease is variable, the average life expectancy after onset is
    A. 6 months–1 year
    B. 1–5 years
  0 C. 6–12 years
    D. 15–20 years
    E. I don't know

11. Most researchers investigating the use of lecithin as a treatment for Alzheimer's disease have concluded that it
  +1 A. reverses symptoms
  +1 B. prevents further decline
  −1 C. reverses symptoms and prevents further decline
   0 D. has no effect on the disease
    E. I don't know

12. Which of the following statements describes a reaction Alzheimer's disease patients may have to their illness?
    A. They are unaware of their symptoms
    B. They are depressed
    C. They deny their symptoms
  0 D. All of the above
    E. I don't know

13. Sometimes Alzheimer's disease patients wander away from home. caregivers can best manage this problem by
  +1 A. reasoning with the patient about the potential dangers of wandering
  +1 B. sharing feelings of concern with the patient in a calm and reassuring manner
   0 C. making use of practical solutions such as locked doors
  −1 D. remaining with the patient at all times to prevent the behavior
    E. I don't know

14. Which statement is true concerning treatment of Alzheimer's disease patients who are depressed?
  −1 A. It is usually useless to treat them for depression because feelings of sadness and inadequacy are part of the disease process
   0 B. Treatment of depression may be effective in alleviating depressive symptoms
  −1 C. Anti-depressant medication should not be prescribed
  +1 D. Proper medication may alleviate symptoms of depression and prevent further intellectual decline
    E. I don't know

cont.

15. What is the role of nutrition in Alzheimer's disease?
    +1 A. Proper nutrition can prevent Alzheimer's disease
    +1 B. Proper nutrition can reverse the symptoms of Alzheimer's disease
     0 C. Poor nutrition can make the symptoms of Alzheimer's disease worse
    −1 D. Nutrition plays no role in Alzheimer's disease
       E. I don't know

16. What is the effect of orienting information (i.e. reminders of the date and place) on Alzheimer's disease patients?
    +1 A. It produces permanent gains in memory
    +1 B. It will slow down the course of the disease
    −1 C. It increases confusion in approximately 50% of patients
     0 D. It has no lasting effect on the memory of patients
       E. I don't know

17. People sometimes write notes to themselves as reminders. How effective is this technique for Alzheimer's disease patients?
    −1 A. It can never be used because reading and comprehension are too severely impaired
     0 B. It may be useful for the mildly demented patient
    −1 C. It is a crutch which may contribute to further decline
    +1 D. It may produce permanent gains in memory
       E. I don't know

18. When an Alzheimer's disease patient begins to have difficulty performing self-care activities, many mental health professionals recommend that the caregiver
    +1 A. allow the patient to perform the activities regardless of the outcome
     0 B. assist with the activities so that the patient can remain as independent as possible
    −1 C. take over the activities right away to prevent accidents
    −1 D. make plans to have the patient moved to a nursing home
       E. I don't know

19. Medicare will pay for which of the following for Alzheimer's disease patients?
     0 A. A physician's diagnostic evaluation of the patient
       B. Nursing home care expenses
       C. Homecare expenses
       D. All of the above
       E. I don't know

20. Which of the following is a primary function of the Alzheimer's Disease and Related Disorders Association (ADRDA)?
       A. Conducting research
       B. providing medical advice
     0 C. Family support and education
       D. Providing day care for Alzheimer's disease patients
       E. I don't know

Note: The correct answer is indicated by 0. Positive and negative bias are indicated by +1 and −1, respectively.
[a]The age specification was inadvertently omitted from item 1 for analyses on the final 20 items.

Source: Reproduced by permission from Dieckmann L *et al. The Gerontologist* 1988; **28**: 402–7.

Appendix

What to use and when

Clinical or research issue	Suggested scales	Page No.
Depression		
Screening for depression:		
General practice	GDS	2
	BASDEC	10
	SELFCARE (D)	11
	EBAS-DEP	31
Medical/geriatric	GDS	2
Inpatients	BASDEC	10
Community surveys	CES-D	13
	GMSS	279
	Canberra Interview for the Elderly (CIE)	280
	CAMDEX	286
In nursing/residential homes	GDS	2
	BASDEC	10
	Geriatric Depression Scale (Residential)	4
	SELFCARE (D)	11
With cognitive impairment	Cornell Scale for Depression in Dementia	9
	DSS	15
	NIMH Dementia Mood Assessment Scale (DMAS)	23
Post-stroke	Emotionalism and Mood Disorders after Stroke	26
Rating severity of depression	Hamilton Depression Rating Scale	6
Symptom profile in depression	Hamilton Depression Rating Scale	6
Self-rating scales	GDS	2
	BDI	7
	Zung Self-Rating Depression Scale	339
Monitoring change	MADRS	8
	Hamilton Depression Rating Scale	6

Clinical or research issue	Suggested scales	Page No.
Cognitive impairment		
Screening for cognitive impairment:		
General practice	MMSE	36
	MTS/AMTS	44
	Clock Drawing Test	51
	SKT	69
	7 Minute Neurocognitive Screening Battery	77
Nursing/residential homes	MMSE	36
Medical/geriatric inpatients	MMSE	36
	Clock Drawing Test	51
In depressed patients	MMSE	36
	Clock Drawing Test	51
Community surveys	SIDAM	275
	GMSS	279
	Canberra Interview for the Elderly (CIE)	280
	CAMDEX	286
Global ratings of psychiatric symptomatology	Psychogeriatric Assessment Scales	278
Dementia		
Detailed profile of cognitive deficits		
Early/mild	ADAS-Cog	48
	MMSE	36
Severe	Severe Impairment Battery	69
	SMMSE	38
Global ratings	GDS	236
	CDR	238
Staging of disease	GDS	236
	CDR	238
Measuring therapeutic effects:		
Cognitive function	MMSE	36
	ADAS-Cog	48
Global changes	CIBIC and variants	240
	ADCS-CGIC	256
Activities of daily living	IDDD	188
	The Bristol Scale	195
	DAD	219
Psychiatric symptoms		
	NPI	128
Frontal lobe function	Executive Interview	102
	Frontal Behavioural Inventory	93
Neuropsychiatric features of dementia:		
General measures	NPI	128
	BEHAVE-AD	125
	CUSPAD	130
	MOUSEPAD	133
	CERAD	138

Clinical or research issue	Suggested scales	Page No.
Specific features:		
Personality change	Brooks and McKinlay scale	124
Agitation	CMAI	159
	BARS	158
Aggression	RAGE	142
	Overt Aggression Scale	144
	Ryden Aggression Scale	154
Behavioural disturbances in dementia	NRS	146
	COBRA	148
	PGDRS	243
	NOSGER	288
	DBRS	152
Global ratings of dementia severity	Dementia Behavior Disturbance Scale	162
Activities of Daily Living:		
Specific for dementia	IADL	186
	IDDD	188
	FAQ	192
	DAFS	197
	CSADL	200
	DAD	219
	ADFACS	220
Generic scales	ADL index	199
	FDS	209
	Rapid Disability Rating Scale – 2 (RDRS-2)	207
Mild cognitive impairment	All neuropsychiatric scales	123
Other disorders		
Global measures of psychiatric symptomatology	BPRS	272
	RAGS	274
	GAPS	276
	Psychogeriatric Assessment Scales	278
	GMSS	279
	SPAS	281
Parkinsonian signs/side-effects of drugs	Webster Scale	302
	TDRS	304
Caregiver burden	Revised Memory and Behavior Problems Checklist	332
	Problem Checklist and Strain Scale	322
	SCB	326
	CAS	333
Caregiver stress	BDI	7
	Problem Checklist and Strain Scale	322
	Ways of Coping Checklist	324
	Caregiving Hassles Scale	328
	GHQ	334

Clinical or research issue	Suggested scales	Page No.
	Zung Self-Rating Depression Scale	339
Quality of life measures	QOL-AD	232
Memory complaints	CFQ	346
Delirium	CAM	315
	DSI	314
	DRS	317
	DI	319
Scales to consider when starting a memory clinic	MMSE	36
	Blessed	46
	ADAS-Cog	48
	ADAS	48
	BEHAVE-AD	125
	NPI	128
	DAD	219
	Bristol ADL	195
	CFQ	346
	Ischaemic Score	365
	Neuropsychological Tests	104–122

Alphabetic list of scales

A Cognitive Screening Battery for Dementia in the Elderly	90	Canberra Interview for the Elderly (CIE)	280
A Collateral Source Version of the Geriatric Depression Rating Scale	5	Caregiver Activity Survey (CAS)	333
		Caregiver Time Use	343
Activities of Daily Living (ADL) Index	199	Caregiving Hassles Scale	328
ADAS/ADAS-Cog; ADAS-Non-Cog	48	Carenap D	258
Agitated Behaviour Mapping Instrument (ABMI)	157	Caretaker Obstreperous Behaviour Rating Assessment (COBRA) scale	148
Agitated Behavior in Dementia Scale	182	Carroll Rating Scale (CRS)	16
Alzheimer's Disease Functional Assessment and Change Scale (ADFACS)	220	Center for Epidemiological Studies – Depression Scale (CES-D)	13
An Instrument for Assessing Health-Related QoL in Persons with AD (ADRQL)	265	CERAD Behavioural Rating Scale	138
		Challenging Behaviour Scale (CBS)	177
Apathy Scale for Parkinson's Disease	168	Checklist Differentiating Pseudodementia from Dementia	21
AUDIT	370	Cleveland Scale for ADL (CASADL)	200
Barnes Akathisia Rating Scale (BAS, BARS)	311	Clifton Assessment Procedures for the Elderly (CAPE)	56
Bayer ADL Scale	218		
BEAM-D	169	Clinical Dementia Rating (CDR)	238
Beck Depression Inventory (BDI)	7	Clinical Rating Scale for Symptoms of Psychosis in AD (SPAD)	171
Bedford Alzheimer Nursing Severity Scale for the Severely Demented	267	Clinicians Global Impression of Change	240
BEHAVE-AD	125	Clock Drawing Test	51
Behavior Rating Scale for Dementia (BRSD)	179	Cognitive Abilities Screening Instrument (CASI)	70
Behavioural Activities in Demented Geriatric Patients	178	Cognitive Capacity Screening Examination	76
Behavioural and Mood Disturbance Scale (BDMS)	340	Cognitive Drug Research Assessment System (COGDRAS)	71
Blessed Dementia Scale	46	Cognitive Failures Questionnaire (CFQ)	346
Boston Naming Test	116	Cognitive Performance Test	201
Brief Agitation Rating Scale (BARS)	158	Cognitively Impaired Life Quality Scale (CILQ)	262
Brief Assessment Scale for Depression	29	Cohen-Mansfield Agitation Inventory (CMAI) – Long Form	159
Brief Assessment Schedule Depression Cards (BASDEC)	10	Columbia University Scale for Psychopathology in AD (CUSPAD)	130
Brief Cognitive Rating Scale (BCRS)	61		
Brief Psychiatric Rating Scale (BPRS)	272	Community Screening Instrument for Dementia (CSI-D)	269
Bristol Activities of Daily Living Scale	195		
Burden Interview	327	Comprehensive Assessment and Referral Evaluation (CARE)	290
Buschke Selective Reminding Test	106	Comprehensive Psychopathological Rating Scale (CPRS)	255
CAGE Questionnaire	368		
Camberwell Assessment of Need for the Elderly (CANE)	294	Computerized Cognitive Examination of the Elderly (ECO)	97
Cambridge Mental Disorders of the Elderly Examination (CAMDEX)	286	Confusion Assessment Method (CAM)	318
Cambridge Neurological Inventory	301	Core Assessment and Outcomes Package for Older People	277
Cambridge Neuropsychological Test Automated Battery (CANTAB)	63		

Cornell Scale for Depression in Dementia	9
Cornell-Brown Scale for QoL in Dementia	266
Crichton Royal Behavioural Rating Scale (CRBRS)	241
Cumulative Illness Rating Scale (CIRS)	359
Daily Activities Questionnaire (DAQ)	194
Delirium Rating Scale (DRS)	317
Delirium Symptom Interview (DSI)	314
Dementia Behavior Disturbance Scale	162
Dementia Quality of Life Instrument	264
Dementia Rating Scale	245
Dependence Scale	222
Depressive Signs Scale (DSS)	15
Détérioration de Cognition Observée (DECO)	83
Direct Assessment of ADL in AD	215
Direct Assessment of Functional Status (DAFS)	197
Disability Assessment for Dementia (DAD)	219
Disruptive Behaviour Rating Scales (DBRS)	152
Dressing Performance Scale	205
Dysfunctional Behaviour Rating Instrument (DBRI)	165
Early Signs of Dementia Checklist	89
Easycare: Elderly Assessment System	295
Echelle Comportement et Adaptation (ECA) Scale	257
Emotionalism and Mood Disorders after Stroke	26
EURO-D scale	28
EuroQol	228
Functional Assessment Staging (FAST)	235
Functional Dementia Scale	209
GBS Scale	246
General Health Questionnaire GHQ)	334
General Medical Health Rating (GMHR)	309
Georagsobber Vatieschaal voor de Intramurale Psycogeriatrie (GIP)	173
Geriatric Depression Scale (GDS)	2
Geriatric Depression Scale (Residential)	4
Geriatric Evaluation by Relative's Rating Instrument (GERRI)	337
Geriatric Mental State Schedule (GMSS)	279
Geriatric Rating Scale (GRS)	247
Global Assessment of Psychiatric Symptoms (GAPS)	276
Global Deterioration Scale (GDS)	236
Hamilton Depression Rating Scale	6
Harmful Behaviours Scale	176
Hierarchic Dementia Scale	251
HoNOS 65+	297
INSIGHT	366
IQCODE	348
Irritability, Aggression and Apathy Scale	166
Ischaemic Score	365
Kew Cognitive Test	73
Lancashire QoL Profile (Residential)	230
Lay Person-Based Screening for Early Detection of AD	85
London Handicap Scale	307
Manchester and Oxford Universities Scales for the Psychopathological Assessment of Dementia (MOUSEPAD)	133
Mania Rating Scale	19
Marital Intimacy Scale	330
Mattis Dementia Rating Scale (DRS)	50
MAST-G	369
Measurement of Morale in the Elderly	360
Memory Functioning Questionnaire (MFQ)	351
Memory Impairment Screen	80
Mental Status Questionnaire (MSQ)/Face–Hand test (FHT)	75
Mental Test Score (MTS)/Abbreviated Mental Test Score (AMTS)	44
Metamemory in Adulthood (MIA) Questionnaire	350
Middlesex Elderly Assessment of Mental State	101
Milan Overall Dementia Assessment	260
Mini Nutritional Assessment	371
Mini-Mental State Examination (MMSE)	36
Montgomery and Asberg Depression Rating Scale (MADRS)	8
Mood Scales – Elderly (MS–E)	18
Multidimensional Caregiver Burden Inventory	344
Multidimensional Observation Scale for Elderly Subjects (MOSES)	284
Multiphasic Environmental Assessment Procedure (MEAP)	356
National Adult Reading Test (NART)	113
Neurobehavioural Rating Scale (NRS)	146
Neurological Evaluation Scale (NES)	305
Neuropsychiatric Inventory (NPI)	128
Neuropsychiatric Inventory with Caregiver Distress Scale	129
NIMH Dementia Mood Assessment Scale (DMAS)	23
Nurses' Observation Scale for Geriatric Patients (NOSGER)	288
Nurses' Observation Scale for Inpatient Evaluation (NOSIE)	150
Nursing Home Behavior Problem Scale (NHBPS)	174
OARS Depressive Scale (ODS)	14
Objective Assessment of Praxis	84
Observation List for Early Signs of Dementia (OLD)	88
Observed Agitation in Patients with DAT (SOAPD)	160
Overt Aggression Scale (OAS)	144
PAMIE Scale	248
Performance Test of ADL	210
Personality Inventory	124
Philadelphia Geriatric Center Morale Scale	357
Physical Self-Maintenance Scale and Instrumental Activities of Daily Living (IADL)	221
Pittsburgh Agitation Scale (PAS)	163
Present Behavioural Examination (PBE)	137
Present Functioning Questionnaire and Functional Rating Scale	202

PRIME-MD	293	Structured Assessment of Independent Living Skills (SALES)	212
Problem Checklist and Strain Scale	322	Structured Telephone Interview for Dementia (STIDA)	81
Progressive Deterioration Scale (PDS)	191		
Psychogeriatric Assessment Scales (PAS)	278	Survey Psychiatric Assessment Schedule (SPAS)	281
Psychogeriatric Dependency Rating Scales (PGDRS)	243	Syndrom Kurztest (SKT)	69
QoL in AD: Patient and Caregiver Report (QOL-AD)	232	Tardive Dyskinesia Rating Scale (TDRS)	304
		Test Battery for the Diagnosis of Dementia in Individuals with Intellectual Disability	91
Quality of Interactions Schedule (QUIS)	365	Texas Functional Living Scale	227
Quality of Life Assessment Schedule	263	The Alzheimer's Disease ADL International Scale	223
Quality of Life in Dementia	229	The Alzheimer's Disease Knowledge Test	373
Quality of Well-Being Scale	268	The California Dementia Behavior Questionnaire	175
Quantification of Physical Illness in Psychiatric Research in the Elderly	306	The Delirium Index (DI)	319
Rapid Disability Rating Scale – 2	207	The Even Briefer Assessment Scale for Depression (EBAS-DEP)	31
Rating Anxiety in Dementia (RAID)	183	The Executive Interview	102
Rating Scale for Aggressive Behaviour in the Elderly (RAGE)	142	The Frontal Behavioural Inventory	93
		The FSAB Battery	259
Refined ADL Assessment Scale (RADL)	216	The General Practitioner Assessment of Cognition (GPCOG)	95
Relative's Assessment of Global Symptomatology (RAGS)	274	The Knowledge of Memory Aging Questionnaire	352
Resistiveness to Care Scale (RTC-DAT)	181	The Mini-Cog	60
Retrospective Postmortem Dementia Assessment (RCD-1)	364	The Modified MMSE (3MS) Examination	42
		The MOS 36-Item Short Form Health Survey (SF-36)	296
Revised Hasegawa's Dementia Scale (HDS-R)	78		
Revised Memory and Behavior Problems Checklist	332	The Neuropsychological Impairment Scale – Snr	98
Rey Auditory Verbal Learning Test	107	The Philadelphia Geriatric Center Multilevel Assessment Instrument	292
Rey Osterrieth Complex Figure	108		
Ryden Aggression Scale	154	The Pleasant Events Schedule – AD	341
Sandoz Clinical Assessment – Geriatric (SCAG)	253	The Resource Utilization in Dementia (RUD) Instrument	372
Screen for Caregiver Burden (SCB)	326		
SELFCARE (D)	11	The Severe MMSE	38
SET Test	66	The Telephone Interview for Cognitive Status	86
Seven-Minute Neurocognitive Screening Battery	77	The Ten-Point Clock Test	55
Severe Impairment Battery (SIB)	74	The Test for Severe Impairment (TSI)	92
Short and Sweet Screening Instrument (SAS-SI)	100	The Time and Change Test	79
Short Anxiety Screening Test	32	Trail Making Test	109
Short Cognitive/Neuropsychological Test Battery for First-Tier Fitness-to-Drive Assessment of Older Adults	103	TRIMS Behavioral Problem Checklist (BPC)	336
		Validity and Reliability of the Alzheimer's Disease Co-operative Study (ADCS-CGIC)	256
Short Mental Status Questionnaire	67	Verbal Fluency: Fast Test/Category Fluency	114
Short Orientation–Memory–Concentration Test	68	Ways of Coping Checklist: Revision and Psychometric Properties	324
Short Portable Mental Status Questionnaire (SPMSQ)	64		
		Webster Scale	302
SIDAM	275	Wechsler Adult Intelligence Scale (WAIS-III)	110
Simpson-Angus Scale (SAS)	310	Wechslet Memory Scale (WMS-III)	111
Standardized MMSE (SMMSE)	40	Wisconsin Card Sorting Test (WCST)	112
Stepwise Comparative Status Analysis (STEP)	117	Zung Self-Rating Depression Scale	339
Stockton Geriatric Rating Scale	250		
Stroop Colour–Word Test	115		